Exercise Physiology

Exercise Physiology

Edited by
Jorge Green

Larsen & Keller
www.larsen-keller.com

Exercise Physiology
Edited by Jorge Green
ISBN: 978-1-63549-117-3 (Hardback)

Larsen & Keller
Published by Larsen and Keller Education,
5 Penn Plaza,
19th Floor,
New York, NY 10001, USA

Cataloging-in-Publication Data

Exercise physiology / edited by Jorge Green.
p. cm.
Includes bibliographical references and index.
ISBN 978-1-63549-117-3
1. Exercise--Physiological aspects. 2. Exercise. 3. Physical fitness--Physiological aspects. 4. Human mechanics.
I. Green, Jorge.
QP301 .E84 2017
612.044--dc23

Printed and bound in China.

For more information regarding Larsen and Keller Education and its products, please visit the publisher's website www.larsen-keller.com

Table of Contents

Preface

This book is a compilation of chapters that discuss the most vital concepts in the field of exercise physiology. It provides deep insights about the fundamental theory and practice related to this area. Exercise physiology refers to the study of the effects and results of different exercises. It examines the effect exercise has on the body like the various metabolic changes occurring in the muscular and circulatory systems as well as fatigue and its effects on the brain. This textbook unfolds the innovative aspects of exercise physiology that will be crucial for the holistic understanding of the subject matter. Coherent flow of topics, student-friendly language and extensive use of examples make this text an invaluable source of knowledge.

To facilitate a deeper understanding of the contents of this book a short introduction of every chapter is written below:

Chapter 1- Physical fitness is the well-being and the ability to perform physical activities and it is achieved by eating healthy and exercising properly. Physical fitness may change drastically with the increase in a person's age. This chapter is an overview of the subject matter incorporating all the major aspects of exercise physiology.

Chapter 2- Physical exercise can be classified into aerobic exercise, strength training, stretching and anaerobic exercise. Common aerobic exercises which are explained in this chapter are cycling, burpee, skipping rope and jogging. Exercising enhances the immune system and helps in the prevention of diseases such as diabetes and obesity.

Chapter 3- Exercise has many benefits, but it also has effects. Excess of exercise can cause exercise induced nausea, exercise hypertension, exercise intolerance and muscle fatigue. Exercise should be properly done, initially under the assistance of an instructor to avoid any injury. Excess of exercise can never be good; overtraining can cause suppressed immune function.

Chapter 4- To maintain a physically fit body with a fit mind, it is very important to exercise. The benefits of exercising include physical strength, fighting depression, obesity and diabetes. The aspects elucidated in this chapter are of vital importance, and provide a better understanding of exercise. The topics discussed in the chapter are of great importance to broaden the existing knowledge on exercise physiology.

Chapter 5- To understand the effect that physical activity has at the cellular level and on the body as a whole is the main concern of sports science. Kinesiology on the other hand concentrates on the biomechanics and orthopedics of a body in motion. This chapter also discusses movement assessment and kinathropometry. Exercise physiology is an emerging field of study; the following chapter will not only provide an overview, it will also delve deep into the variegated topics related to it.

Chapter 6- The sum total of all the chemical processes that occur in the body and help sustain life is referred to as metabolism. Some of the mechanisms explained in this chapter are metabolic equivalent, basal metabolic rate and metabolic age. The aspects elucidated in this chapter are of vital importance, and provide a better understanding of exercise physiology.

Chapter 7- Exercise intensity is the amount of energy spent while exercising, and every individual has a different exercise intensity. A typical measure of exercise intensity is the heart rate. Muscle contraction determines the flow of blood inside the body. All the aspects of exercise physiology have been carefully analyzed in this chapter.

I would like to share the credit of this book with my editorial team who worked tirelessly on this book. I owe the completion of this book to the never-ending support of my family, who supported me throughout the project.

Editor

Introduction to Exercise Physiology

Physical fitness is the well-being and the ability to perform physical activities and it is achieved by eating healthy and exercising properly. Physical fitness may change drastically with the increase in a person's age. This chapter is an overview of the subject matter incorporating all the major aspects of exercise physiology.

Exercise Physiology

Exercise physiology is the physiology of physical exercise. It is the study of the acute responses and chronic adaptations to a wide range of exercise conditions.

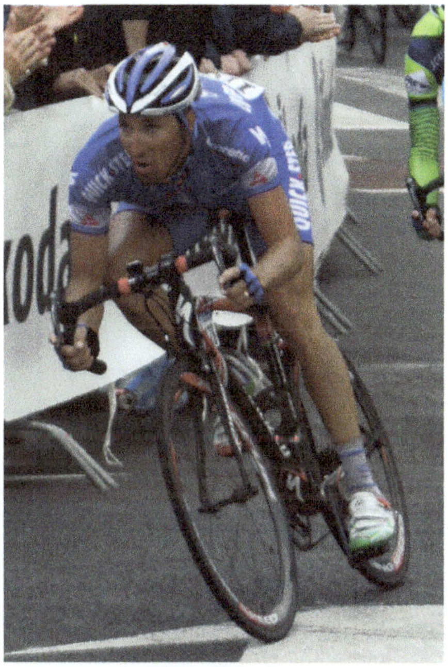

Cyclists are known for using knowledge in exercise physiology in order to optimize training to reach the maximal level of performance.

Exercise physiologists study the effect of exercise on pathology, and the mechanisms by which exercise can reduce or reverse disease progression.

Energy Expenditure

Humans have a high capacity to expend energy for many hours during sustained exertion. For example, one individual cycling at a speed of 26.4 km/h (16.4 mph) through 8,204 km (5,098 mi) over 50 consecutive days expended a total of 1,145 MJ (273,850 kcal; 273,850 dieter calories) with an average power output of 182.5 W.

Skeletal muscle burns 90 mg (0.5 mmol) of glucose each minute during continuous activity (such as when repetitively extending the human knee), generating ≈24 W of mechanical energy, and since muscle energy conversion is only 22–26% efficient, ≈76 W of heat energy. Resting skeletal muscle has a basal metabolic rate (resting energy consumption) of 0.63 W/kg making a 160 fold difference between the energy consumption of inactive and active muscles. For short duration muscular exertion, energy expenditure can be far greater: an adult human male when jumping up from a squat can mechanically generate 314 W/kg. Such rapid movement can generate twice this amount in nonhuman animals such as bonobos, and in some small lizards.

This energy expenditure is very large compared to the basal resting metabolic rate of the adult human body. This rate varies somewhat with size, gender and age but is typically between 45 W and 85 W. Total energy expenditure (TEE) due to muscular expended energy is much higher and depends upon the average level of physical work and exercise done during a day. Thus exercise, particularly if sustained for very long periods, dominates the energy metabolism of the body. Physical activity energy expenditure correlates strongly with the gender, age, weight, heart rate, and VO_2 max of an individual, during physical activity.

Metabolic Changes

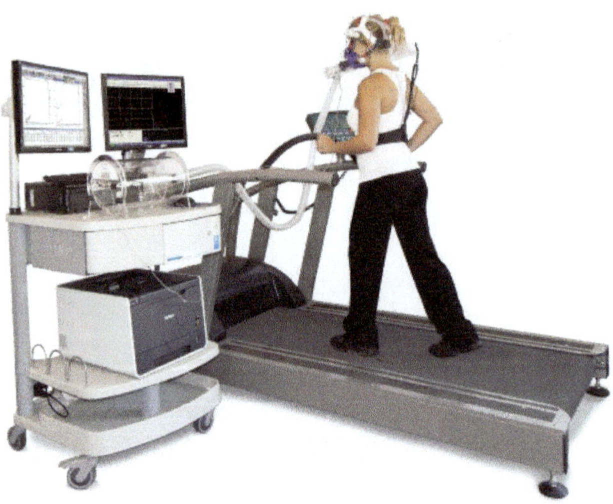

Ergospirometry laboratory for the measurement of metabolic changes during a graded exercise test on a treadmill

Rapid Energy Sources

Energy needed to perform short lasting, high intensity bursts of activity is derived from anaerobic metabolism within the cytosol of muscle cells, as opposed to aerobic respiration which utilizes oxygen, is sustainable, and occurs in the mitochondria. The quick energy sources consist of the phosphocreatine (PCr) system, fast glycolysis, and adenylate kinase. All of these systems re-synthesize adenosine triphosphate (ATP), which is the universal energy source in all cells. The most rapid source, but the most readily depleted of the above sources is the PCr system which utilizes the enzyme creatine kinase. This enzyme catalyzes a reaction that combines phosphocreatine and adenosine diphosphate (ADP) into ATP and creatine. This resource is short lasting because oxygen is required for the resynthesis of phosphocreatine via mitochondrial creatine kinase. Therefore, under anaerobic conditions, this substrate is finite and only lasts between approximately 10 to 30 seconds of high intensity work. Fast glycolysis, however, can function for approximately 2 minutes prior to fatigue, and predominately uses intracellular glycogen as a substrate. Glycogen is broken down rapidly via glycogen phosphorylase into individual glucose units during intense exercise. Glucose is then oxidized to pyruvate and under anaerobic condition is reduced to lactic acid. This reaction oxidizes NADH to NAD, thereby releasing a hydrogen ion, promoting acidosis. For this reason, fast glycolysis can not be sustained for long periods of time. Lastly, adenylate kinase catalyzes a reaction by which 2 ADP are combined to form ATP and adenosine monophosphate (AMP). This reaction takes place during low energy situations such as extreme exercise or conditions of hypoxia, but is not a significant source of energy. The creation of AMP resulting from this reaction stimulates AMP-activated protein kinase (AMP kinase) which is the energy sensor of the cell. After sensing low energy conditions, AMP kinase stimulates various other intracellular enzymes geared towards increasing energy supply and decreasing all anabolic, or energy requiring, cell functions.

Plasma Glucose

Plasma glucose is said to be maintained when there is an equal rate of glucose appearance (entry into the blood) and glucose disposal (removal from the blood). In the healthy individual, the rates of appearance and disposal are essentially equal during exercise of moderate intensity and duration; however, prolonged exercise or sufficiently intense exercise can result in an imbalance leaning towards a higher rate of disposal than appearance, at which point glucose levels fall producing the onset of fatigue. Rate of glucose appearance is dictated by the amount of glucose being absorbed at the gut as well as liver (hepatic) glucose output. Although glucose absorption from the gut is not typically a source of glucose appearance during exercise, the liver is capable of catabolizing stored glycogen (glycogenolysis) as well as synthesizing new glucose from specific reduced carbon molecules (glycerol, pyruvate, and lactate) in a process called gluconeogenesis. The ability of the liver to release glucose into the blood from glycogenolysis is unique, since skeletal muscle, the other major glycogen reservoir, is incapable of doing so. Unlike skeletal muscle, liver cells contain the enzyme glycogen phosphatase, which removes a phosphate group from glucose-6-P to release free glucose. In order for glucose to exit a cell membrane, the removal of this phosphate group is essential. Although gluconeogenesis is an important component of hepatic glucose output, it alone can not sustain exercise. For this reason, when glycogen stores are depleted during exercise, glucose levels fall and fatigue sets in. Glucose disposal, the other side of the equation, is controlled by uptake of glucose at the working skeletal muscles. During exercise, despite decreased insulin concentrations, muscle increases GLUT4 translocation of and glucose uptake. The mechanism for increased GLUT4 translocation is an area of ongoing research.

glucose control: As mentioned above, insulin secretion is reduced during exercise, and does not play a major role in maintaining normal blood glucose concentration during exercise, but its counter-regulatory hormones appear in increasing concentrations. Principle among these are glucagon, epinephrine, and growth hormone. All of these hormones stimulate liver (hepatic) glucose output, among other functions. For instance, both epinephrine and growth hormone also stimulate adipocyte lipase, which increases non-esterified fatty acid (NEFA) release. By oxidizing fatty acids, this spares glucose utilization and helps to maintain blood sugar level during exercise.

Exercise for diabetes: Exercise is a particularly potent tool for glucose control in those who have diabetes mellitus. In a situation of elevated blood glucose (hyperglycemia), moderate exercise can induce greater glucose disposal than appearance, thereby decreasing total plasma glucose concentrations. As stated above, the mechanism for this glucose disposal is independent of insulin, which makes it particularly well-suited for people with diabetes. In addition, there appears to be an increase in sensitivity to insulin for approximately 12–24 hours post-exercise. This is particularly useful for those who have type II diabetes and are producing sufficient insulin but demonstrate peripheral resistance to insulin signaling. However, during extreme hyperglycemic episodes, people with diabetes should avoid exercise due to potential complications associated with ketoacidosis. Exercise could exacerbate ketoacidosis by increasing ketone synthesis in response to increased circulating NEFA's.

Type II diabetes is also intricately linked to obesity, and there may be a connection between type II diabetes and how fat is stored within pancreatic, muscle, and liver cells. Likely due to this connection, weight loss from both exercise and diet tends to increase insulin sensitivity in the majority of people. In some people, this effect can be particularly potent and can result in normal glucose control. Although nobody is technically cured of diabetes, individuals can live normal lives without the fear of diabetic complications; however, regain of weight would assuredly result in diabetes signs and symptoms.

Oxygen

Vigorous physical activity (such as exercise or hard labor) increases the body's demand for oxygen. The first-line physiologic response to this demand is an increase in heart rate, breathing rate, and depth of breathing.

Oxygen consumption (VO_2) during exercise is best described by the Fick Equation: $VO_2=Q \times (a\text{-}vO_2diff)$, which states that the amount of oxygen consumed is equal to cardiac output (Q) multiplied by the difference between arterial and venous oxygen concentrations. More simply put, oxygen consumption is dictated by the quantity of blood distributed by the heart as well as the working muscle's ability to take up the oxygen within that blood; however, this is a bit of an oversimplification. Although cardiac output is thought to be the limiting factor of this relationship in healthy individuals, it is not the only determinant of VO2 max. That is, factors such as the ability of the lung to oxygenate the blood must also be considered. Various pathologies and anomalies cause conditions such as diffusion limitation, ventilation/perfusion mismatch, and pulmonary shunts that can limit oxygenation of the blood and therefore oxygen distribution. In addition, the oxygen carrying capacity of the blood is also an important determinant of the equation. Oxygen carrying capacity is often the target of exercise (ergogenic aids) aids used in endurance sports to increase the volume percentage of red blood cells (hematocrit), such as through blood doping or the use of erythropoietin (EPO). Furthermore, peripheral oxygen uptake is reliant on a rerouting of blood flow from relatively inactive viscera to the working skeletal muscles, and within the skeletal muscle, capillary to muscle fiber ratio influences oxygen extraction.

Dehydration

Dehydration refers both to hypohydration (dehydration induced prior to exercise) and to exercise-induced dehydration (dehydration that develops during exercise). The latter reduces aerobic endurance performance and results in increased body temperature, heart rate, perceived exertion, and possibly increased reliance on carbohydrate as a fuel source. Although the negative effects of exercise-induced dehydration on exercise performance were clearly demonstrated in the 1940s, athletes continued to believe for years thereafter that fluid intake was not beneficial. More recently, negative effects on performance have been demonstrated with modest (<2%) dehydration, and these effects are exacerbated when the exercise is performed in a hot environment. The effects of hypohydration may vary, depending on whether it is induced through diuretics or sauna exposure, which substantially reduce plasma volume, or prior exercise, which has much less impact on plasma volume. Hypohydration reduces aerobic endurance, but its effects on muscle strength and endurance are not consistent and require further study. Intense prolonged exercise produces metabolic waste heat, and this is removed by sweat-based thermoregulation. A male marathon runner loses each hour around 0.83 L in cool weather and 1.2 L in warm (losses in females are about 68 to 73% lower). People doing heavy exercise may lose two and half times as much fluid in sweat as urine. This can have profound physiological effects. Cycling for 2 hours in the heat (35 °C) with minimal fluid intake causes body mass decline by 3 to 5%, blood volume likewise by 3 to 6%, body temperature to rise constantly, and in comparison with proper fluid intake, higher heart rates, lower stroke volumes and cardiac outputs, reduced skin blood flow, and higher systemic vascular resistance. These effects are largely eliminated by replacing 50 to 80% of the fluid lost in sweat.

Other

- Plasma catecholamine concentrations increase 10-fold in whole body exercise.
- Ammonia is produced by exercised skeletal muscles from ADP (the precursor of ATP) by purine nucleotide deamination and amino acid catabolism of myofibrils.
- interleukin-6 (IL-6) increases in blood circulation due to its release from working skeletal muscles. This release is reduced if glucose is taken, suggesting it is related to energy depletion stresses.
- Sodium absorption is affected by the release of interleukin-6 as this can cause the secretion of arginine vasopressin which, in turn, can lead to exercise-associated dangerously low sodium levels (hyponatremia). This loss of sodium in blood plasma can result in swelling of the brain. This can be prevented by awareness of the risk of drinking excessive amounts of fluids during prolonged exercise.

Brain

At rest, the human brain receives 15% of total cardiac output, and uses 20% of the body's energy consumption. The brain is normally dependent for its high energy expenditure upon aerobic metabolism. The brain as a result is highly sensitive to failure of its oxygen supply with loss of consciousness occurring within six to seven seconds, with its EEG going flat in 23 seconds. If it affected the oxygen and glucose supply to the brain, the metabolic demands of exercise could therefore quickly disrupt its functioning.

Protecting the brain from even minor disruption is important since exercise depends upon motor control, and particularly, because humans are bipeds, the motor control needed for keeping balance. Indeed, for this reason, brain energy consumption is increased during intense physical exercise due to the demands in the motor cognition needed to control the body.

Cerebral Oxygen

Cerebral autoregulation usually ensures the brain has priority to cardiac output, though this is impaired slightly by exhaustive exercise. During submaximal exercise, cardiac output increases and cerebral blood flow increases beyond the brain's oxygen needs. However, this is not the case for continuous maximal exertion: "Maximal exercise is, despite the increase in capillary oxygenation [in the brain], associated with a reduced mitochondrial O_2 content during whole body exercise" The autoregulation of the brain's blood supply is impaired particularly in warm environments

Glucose

In adults, exercise depletes the plasma glucose available to the brain: short intense exercise (35 min ergometer cycling) can reduce brain glucose uptake by 32%.

At rest, energy for the adult brain is normally provided by glucose but the brain has a compensatory capacity to replace some of this with lactate. Research suggests that this can be raised, when a person rests in a brain scanner, to about 17%, with a higher percentage of 25% occurring during hypoglycemia. During intense exercise, lactate has been estimated to provide a third of the brain's energy needs. There is evidence that the brain might, however, in spite of these alternative sources of energy, still suffer an energy crisis since IL-6 (a sign of metabolic stress) is released during exercise from the brain.

Hyperthermia

Humans use sweat thermoregulation for body heat removal, particularly to remove the heat produced during exercise. Moderate dehydration as a consequence of exercise and heat is reported to impair cognition. These impairments can start after body mass lost that is greater than 1%. Cognitive impairment, particularly due to heat and exercise is likely to be due to loss of integrity to the blood brain barrier. Hyperthermia also can lower cerebral blood flow, and raise brain temperature.

Fatigue

Intense Activity

Researchers once attributed fatigue to a build-up of lactic acid in muscles. However, this is no longer believed. Rather, lactate may stop muscle fatigue by keeping muscles fully responding to nerve signals. The available oxygen and energy supply, and disturbances of muscle ion homeostasis are the main factor determining exercise performance, at least during brief very intense exercise.

Each muscle contraction involves an action potential that activates voltage sensors, and so releases Ca^{2+} ions from the muscle fibre's sarcoplasmic reticulum. The action potentials that cause this require also ion changes: Na influxes during the depolarization phase and K effluxes for the repolarization phase. Cl^- ions also diffuse into the sarcoplasm to aid the repolarization phase. During intense muscle contraction, the ion pumps that maintain homeostasis of these ions are inactivated and this (with other ion related disruption) causes ionic disturbances. This causes cellular membrane depolarization, inexcitability, and so muscle weakness. Ca^{2+} leakage from type 1 ryanodine receptor) channels has also been identified with fatigue.

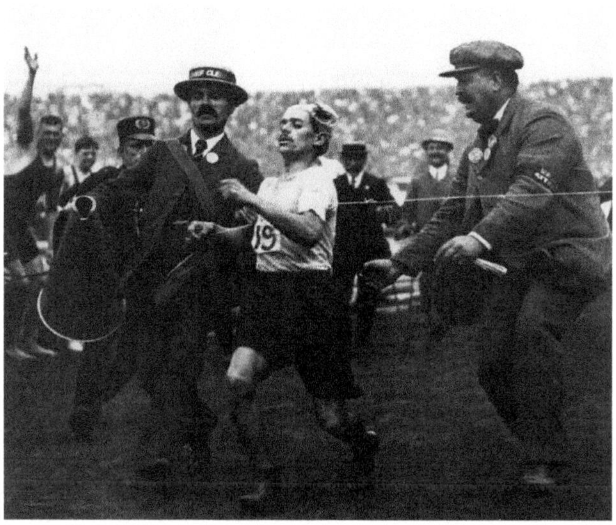

Dorando Pietri about to collapse at the Marathon finish at the 1908 London Olympic Games

Endurance Failure

After intense prolonged exercise, there can be a collapse in body homeostasis. Some famous examples include:

- Dorando Pietri in the 1908 Summer Olympic men's marathon ran the wrong way and collapsed several times.
- Jim Peters in the marathon of the 1954 Commonwealth Games staggered and collapsed several times, and though he had a five-kilometre (three-mile) lead, failed to finish. Though it was formerly believed that this was due to severe dehydration, more recent research suggests it was the combined effects upon the brain of hyperthermia, hypertonic hypernatraemia associated with dehydration, and possibly hypoglycaemia.
- Gabriela Andersen-Schiess in the woman's marathon at the Los Angeles 1984 Summer Olympics in the race's final 400 meters, stopping occasionally and shown signs of heat exhaustion. Though she fell across the finish line, she was released from medical care only two hours later.

Central Governor

Tim Noakes, based on an earlier idea by the 1922 Nobel Prize in Physiology or Medicine winner Archibald Hill has proposed the existence of a central governor. In this, the brain continuously adjusts the power output by muscles during exercise in regard to a safe level of exertion. These neural calculations factor in prior length of strenuous exercise, the planned duration of further exertion, and the present metabolic state of the body. This adjusts the number of activated skeletal muscle motor units, and is subjectively experienced as fatigue and exhaustion. The idea of a central governor rejects the earlier idea that fatigue is only caused by mechanical failure of the exercising muscles (“peripheral fatigue”). Instead, the brain models the metabolic limits of the body to ensure that whole body homeostasis is protected, in particular that the heart is guarded from hypoxia, and an emergency reserve is always maintained. The idea of the central governor has been questioned since ‘physiological catastrophes’ can and do occur suggesting athletes (such as Dorando Pietri, Jim Peters and Gabriela Andersen-Schiess) can over-ride the “central governor’.

Other Factors

The exercise fatigue has also been suggested to be effected by:

- brain hyperthermia
- glycogen depletion in brain cells
- reactive oxygen species impairing skeletal muscle function
- reduced level of glutamate secondary to uptake of ammonia in the brain
- Fatigue in diaphragm and abdominal respiratory muscles limiting breathing
- Impaired oxygen supply to muscles
- Ammonia effects upon the brain
- Serotonin pathways in the brain

Cardiac Biomarkers

Prolonged exercise such as marathons can increase cardiac biomarkers such as troponin, B-type natriuretic peptide (BNP), and ischemia-modified (aka MI) albumin. This can be misinterpreted by medical personnel as signs of myocardial infarction, or cardiac dysfunction. In these clinical conditions, such cardiac biomarkers are produced by irreversible injury of muscles. In contrast, the processes that create them after strenuous exertion in endurance sports are reversible, with their levels returning to normal within 24-hours (further research, however, is still needed).

Human Adaptations

Humans are specifically adapted to engage in prolonged strenuous muscular activity (such as efficient long distance bipedal running). This capacity for endurance running evolved to allow the running down of game animals by persistent slow but constant chase over many hours.

Central to the success of this is the ability of the human body, unlike that of the animals they hunt, to effectively remove muscle heat waste. In most animals, this is stored by allowing a temporary increase in body temperature. This allows them to escape from animals that quickly speed after them for a short duration (the way nearly all predators catch their prey). Humans, unlike other animals that catch prey, remove heat with a specialized thermoregulation based on sweat evaporation. One gram of sweat can remove 2,598 J of heat energy. Another mechanism is increased skin blood flow during exercise that allows for greater convective heat loss that is aided by our upright posture. This skin based cooling has resulted in humans acquiring an increased number of sweat glands, combined with a lack of body fur that would otherwise stop air circulation and efficient evaporation. Because humans can remove exercise heat, they can avoid the fatigue from heat exhaustion that affects animals chased in a persistent manner, and so eventually catch them.

Selective Breeding Experiments With Rodents

Rodents have been specifically bred for exercise behavior or performance in several different studies. For example, laboratory rats have been bred for high or low performance on a motorized treadmill with electrical stimulation as motivation. The high-performance line of rats also exhibits increased voluntary wheel-running behavior as compared with the low-capacity line. In an experimental evolution approach, four replicate lines of laboratory mice have been bred for high levels of voluntary exercise on wheels, while four additional control lines are maintained by breeding without regard to the amount of wheel running. These selected lines of mice also show increased endurance capacity in tests of forced endurance capacity on a motorized treadmill. However, in neither selection experiment have the precise causes of fatigue during either forced or voluntary exercise been determined.

Exercise-induced Muscle Pain

Physical exercise may cause pain both as an immediate effect that may result from stimulation of free nerve endings by low pH, as well as a delayed onset muscle soreness. The delayed soreness is fundamentally the result of ruptures within the muscle, although apparently not involving the rupture of whole muscle fibers.

Muscle pain can range from a mild soreness to a debilitating injury depending on intensity of exercise, level of training, and other factors.

Education in Exercise Physiology

Accreditation programs exist with professional bodies in most developed countries, ensuring the quality and consistency of education. In Canada, one may obtain the professional certification title – Certified Exercise Physiologist for those working with clients (both clinical and non clinical) in the health and fitness industry. An exercise physiologist's area of study may include but is not limited to biochemistry, bioenergetics, cardiopulmonary function, hematology, biomechanics, skeletal muscle physiology, neuroendocrine function, and central and peripheral nervous system function. Furthermore, exercise physiologists range from basic scientists, to clinical researchers, to clinicians, to sports trainers.

Colleges and universities offer exercise physiology as a program of study on various different levels, including undergraduate, graduate, and doctoral programs. The basis of Exercise Physiology as a major is to prepare students for a career in field of health sciences. A program that focuses on the scientific study of the physiological processes involved in physical or motor activity, including sensorimotor interactions, response mechanisms, and the effects of injury, disease, and disability. Includes instruction in muscular and skeletal anatomy; molecular and cellular basis of muscle contraction; fuel utilization; neurophysiology of motor mechanics; systemic physiological responses (respiration, blood flow, endocrine secretions, and others); fatigue and exhaustion; muscle and body training; physiology of specific exercises and activities; physiology of injury; and the effects of disabilities and disease. Careers available with a degree in Exercise Physiology can include: non-clinical, client-based work; strength and conditioning specialists; cardiopulmonary treatment; and clinical-based research.

In order to gauge the multiple areas of study, students are taught processes in which to follow on a client-based level. Practical and lecture teachings are instructed in the classroom and in a laboratory setting. These include:

- Health and risk assessment: In order to safely work with a client on the job, you must first be able to know the benefits and risks associated with physical activity. Examples of this include knowing specific injuries the body can experience during exercise, how to properly screen a client before their training begins, and what factors to look for that may inhibit their performance.
- Exercise testing: Coordinating exercise tests in order to measure body compositions, cardiorespiratory fitness, muscular strength/endurance, and flexibility. Functional tests are also used in order to gain understanding on a more specific part of the body. Once the information is gathered about a client, exercise physiologists must also be able to interpret the test data and decide what health-related outcomes have been discovered.
- Exercise prescription: Forming training programs that best meet an individuals health and fitness goals. Must be able to take into account different types of exercises, the reasons/ goal for a clients workout, and pre-screened assessments. Knowing how to prescribe exercises for special considerations and populations is also required. These may include age differences, pregnancy, joint diseases, obesity, pulmonary disease, etc.

Curriculum

The curriculum for exercise physiology includes biology, chemistry, and applied sciences. The purpose of the classes selected for this major is to have a proficient understanding of human anatomy, human physiology, and exercise physiology. Includes instruction in muscular and skeletal anatomy; molecular and cellular basis of muscle contraction; fuel utilization; neurophysiology of motor mechanics; systemic physiological responses (respiration, blood flow, endocrine secretions, and others); fatigue and exhaustion; muscle and body training; physiology of specific exercises and activities; physiology of injury; and the effects of disabilities and disease. Not only is a full class schedule needed to complete a degree in Exercise Physiology, but a minimum amount of practicum experience is required and internships are recommended.

Physical Fitness

Physical fitness is a general state of health and well-being and, more specifically, the ability to perform aspects of sports, occupations and daily activities. Physical fitness is generally achieved through proper nutrition, moderate-vigorous physical exercise, and sufficient rest.

Before the industrial revolution, *fitness* was defined as the capacity to carry out the day's activities without undue fatigue. However, with automation and changes in lifestyles *physical fitness* is now considered a measure of the body's ability to function efficiently and effectively in work and leisure activities, to be healthy, to resist hypokinetic diseases, and to meet emergency situations.

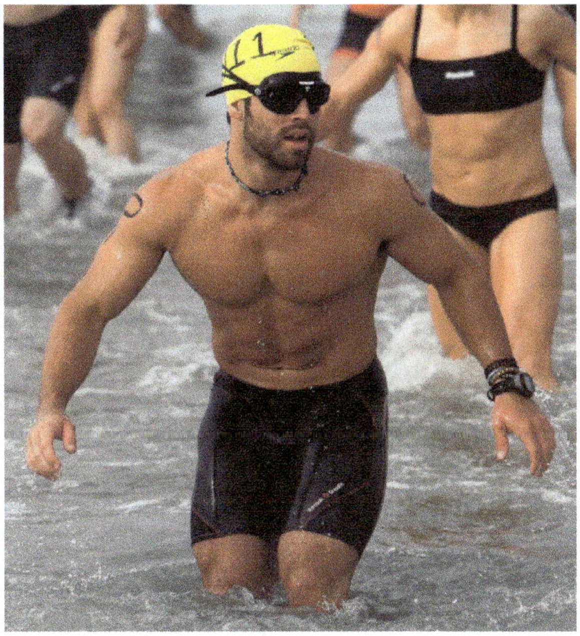

Physical fitness can be achieved through exercise. Photo shows Rich Froning Jr. – four-time winner of "Fittest Man on Earth" title.

Fitness

Fitness is defined as the quality or state of being fit. Around 1950, perhaps consistent with the Industrial Revolution and the treatise of World War II, the term "fitness" increased in western vernacular by a factor of ten. Modern definition of fitness describe either a person or machine's ability to perform a specific function or a holistic definition of human adaptability to cope with various situations. This has led to an interrelation of human fitness and attractiveness which has mobilized global fitness and fitness equipment industries. Regarding specific function, fitness is attributed to personnel who possess significant aerobic or anaerobic ability, i.e. strength or endurance. A holistic definition of fitness is described by Greg Glassman in the CrossFit journal as an increased work capacity across broad times and modal domains; mastery of several attributes of fitness including strength, endurance, power, speed, balance and coordination and being able to improve the amount of work done in a given time with any of these domains. A well rounded fitness program will improve a person in all aspects of fitness, rather than one, such as only cardio/respiratory endurance or only weight training.

A comprehensive fitness program tailored to an individual typically focuses on one or more specific skills, and on age- or health-related needs such as bone health. Many sources also cite mental, social and emotional health as an important part of overall fitness. This is often presented in textbooks as a triangle made up of three points, which represent physical, emotional, and mental fitness. Physical fitness can also prevent or treat many chronic health conditions brought on by unhealthy lifestyle or aging. Working out can also help some people sleep better and possibly alleviate some mood disorders in certain individuals.

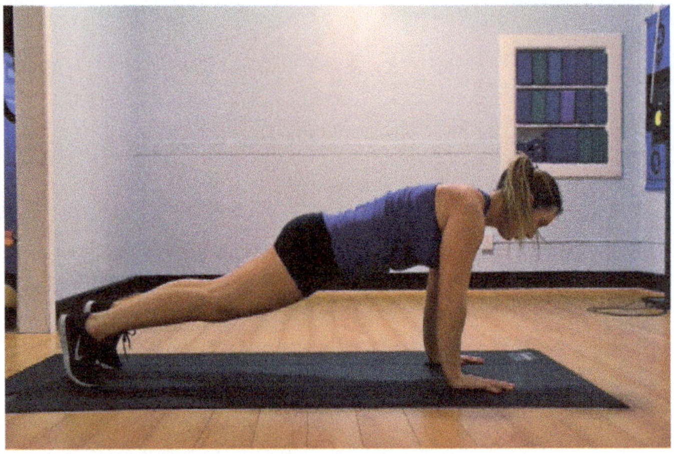

A woman performs plank exercise for strengthening of muscles

Developing research has demonstrated that many of the benefits of exercise are mediated through the role of skeletal muscle as an endocrine organ. That is, contracting muscles release multiple substances known as myokines which promote the growth of new tissue, tissue repair, and various anti-inflammatory functions, which in turn reduce the risk of developing various inflammatory diseases.

Activity Guidelines

The Physical Activity Guidelines for Americans was created by the Office of Disease Prevention and Health Promotion. This publication suggests that all adults should avoid inactivity to promote good health mentally and physically. For substantial health benefits, adults should participate in at least 150 minutes (two hours and 30 minutes) a week of moderate-intensity, or 75 minutes (1 hour and 15 minutes) a week of vigorous-intensity aerobic physical activity, or an equivalent combination of moderate- and vigorous-intensity aerobic activity. Aerobic activity should be performed in episodes of at least 10 minutes, and preferably, it should be spread throughout the week. For additional and more extensive health benefits, adults should increase their aerobic physical activity to 300 minutes (5 hours) a week of moderate-intensity, or 150 minutes a week of vigorous-intensity aerobic physical activity, or an equivalent combination of moderate- and vigorous-intensity activity. Additional health benefits are gained by engaging in physical activity beyond this amount. Adults should also do muscle-strengthening activities that are moderate or high intensity and involve all major muscle groups on 2 or more days a week, as these activities provide additional health benefits.

Training

Specific or task-oriented fitness is a person's ability to perform in a specific activity with a reasonable efficiency: for example, sports or military service. Specific training prepares athletes to perform well in their sports.

Examples are:

- 100 m sprint: in a sprint the athlete must be trained to work anaerobically throughout the race, an example of how to do this would be interval training.

- Middle distance running: athletes require both speed and endurance to gain benefit out of this training. The hard working muscles are at their peak for a longer period of time as they are being used at that level for longer period of time.
- Marathon: in this case the athlete must be trained to work aerobically and their endurance must be built-up to a maximum.
- Many fire fighters and police officers undergo regular fitness testing to determine if they are capable of the physically demanding tasks required of the job.
- Members of armed forces will often be required to pass a formal fitness test – for example soldiers of the US Army must be able to pass the Army Physical Fitness Test (APFT).
- Hill sprints: requires a level of fitness to begin with, the exercise is particularly good for the leg muscles. The army often trains doing mountain climbing and races.
- Plyometric and Isometric Exercises: An excellent way to build strength and increase muscular endurance.
- Sand running creates less strain on leg muscles than running on grass or concrete. This is because sand collapses beneath the foot softening the landing. Sand training is an effective way to lose weight and become fit as its proven you need more effort (one and a half times more) to run on the soft sand than on a hard surface.
- Aquajogging is a form of exercise that decreases strain on joints and bones. The water supplies minimal impact to muscles and bones which is good for those recovering from injury. Furthermore, the resistance of the water as one jogs through it provides an enhanced effect of exercise (the deeper you are the greater the force needed to pull your leg through).

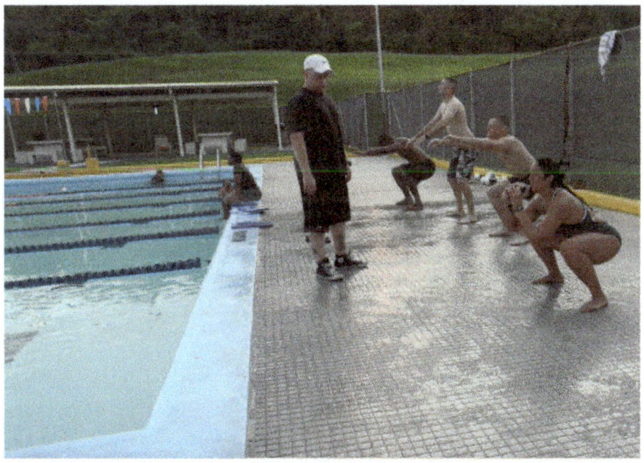

Swimmers perform squats prior to entering the pool in a U.S. military base, 2011

- Swimming: Squatting exercise helps in enhancing a swimmer's start.

In order for physical fitness to benefit the health of an individual, an unknown response in the person called a stimulus will be triggered by the exertion. When exercise is performed with the correct amount of intensity, duration and frequency, a significant amount of improvement can occur. The person may overall feel better but the physical effects on the human body take weeks or months to notice and possibly years for full development. For training purposes, exercise must provide a stress or demand on either a function or tissue. To continue improvements, this demand must eventually increase little over an extended period of time. This sort of exercise training has three basic principles: overload, specificity, and progression. These principles are related to health but also enhancement of physical working capacity.

High Intensity Interval Training (HIIT)

High Intensity Interval Training consists of repeated, short bursts of exercise, completed at a high level of intensity. These sets of intense activity are followed by a predetermined time of rest or low intensity activity. Studies have shown that exercising at a higher intensity has increased cardiac benefits for humans, compared to when exercising at a low or moderate level. When your workout consists of an HIIT session, your body has to work harder to replace the oxygen it lost. Research into the benefits of HIIT have revealed that it can be very successful for reducing fat, especially around the abdominal region. Furthermore, when compared to continuous moderate exercise, HIIT proves to burn more calories and increase the amount of fat burned post- HIIT session. Lack of time is one of the main reasons stated for not exercising; HIIT is a great alternative for those people because the duration of an HIIT session can be as short as 10 minutes, making it much quicker than conventional workouts.

Aerobic Exercise

Cardiorespiratory fitness can be measured using VO2 max, a measure of the amount of oxygen the body can uptake and utilize. Aerobic exercise, which improves cardiorespiratory fitness, involves movement that increases the heart rate to improve the body's oxygen consumption. This form of exercise is an important part of all training regiments ranging from professional athletes to the everyday person. Also, it helps increase stamina.

Examples are:

- Jogging – Running at a steady and gentle pace. This form of exercise is great for maintaining weight.
- Elliptical Training – This is a stationary exercise machine used to perform walking, or running without causing excessive stress on the joints. This form of exercise is perfect for people with achy hips, knees and ankles.
- Walking – Moving at a fairly regular pace for a short, medium or long distance.
- Treadmill training – Many treadmills have programs set up that offers a numerous amount of different workout plans. One effective cardiovascular activity would be to switch between running and walking. Typically warm up first by walking and then switch off between walking for three minutes and running for three minutes.
- Swimming – Using the arms and legs to keep oneself afloat and moving either forwards or backwards. This is a good full body exercise for those who are looking to strengthen their core while improving cardiovascular endurance.
- Cycling – Riding a bicycle typically involves longer distances than walking or jogging. This is another low stress exercise on the joints and is great for improving leg strength.

Effects

Controlling Blood Pressure

Physical fitness has proven to result in positive effects on the body's blood pressure because staying active and exercising regularly builds up a stronger heart. The heart is the main organ in charge of systolic blood pressure and diastolic blood pressure. Engaging in a physical activity will create a rise in blood pressure, once the activity is stopped, however, the individual's blood pressure will return to normal. The more physical activity that one engages in, the easier this process becomes, resulting in a more 'fit' individual. Through regular physical fitness, the heart does not have to work as hard to create a rise in blood pressure, which lowers the force on the arteries, and lowers the over all blood pressure.

Cancer Prevention

Centers for disease control and prevention provide lifestyle guidelines of maintaining a balanced diet and engaging in physical activity to reduce the risk of disease. The WCRF/ American Institute for Cancer Research (AICR) published a list of recommendations that reflect the evidence they have found through consistency in fitness and dietary factors that directly relate to Cancer prevention.

The WCRF/AICR recommendations include the following:

- "Be as lean as possible without becoming underweight
- Each week, adults should engage in at least 150 minutes of moderate intensity physical activity or 75 minutes of vigorous intensity physical activity
- Children should engage in at least one hour of moderate or vigorous physical activity each week
- Be physically active for at least thirty minutes every day
- Avoid sugar, limit the consumption of energy packed foods
- Balance your diet with a variety of vegetables, grains, fruits, legumes, etc.
- Limit sodium intake, the consumption of red meats and the consumption of processed meats
- Limit alcoholic drinks to two for men and one for women a day"

These recommendations are also widely supported by the American Cancer Society. The guidelines have been evaluated and individuals that have higher guideline adherence scores substantially reduce cancer risk as well as help towards control with a multitude of chronic health problems. Regular physical activity is a factor that helps reduce an individual's blood pressure and improves cholesterol levels, two key components that correlate with heart disease and Type 2 Diabetes. The American Cancer Society encourages the public to "adopt a physically active lifestyle" by meeting the criteria in a variety of physical activities such as hiking, swimming, circuit training, resistance raining, lifting, etc. It is understood that cancer is not a disease that can be cured by physical fitness alone, however because it is a multifactorial disease, physical fitness is a controllable prevention. The large associations tied with being physically fit and reduced cancer risk are enough to provide a strategy to reduce cancer risk. The American Cancer Society assorts different levels of activity ranging from moderate to vigorous to clarify the recommended time spent on a physical activity. These classifications of physical activity consider the intentional exercise and basic activities done on a daily basis and give the public a greater understanding by what fitness levels suffice as future disease prevention.

Inflammation

Studies have shown an association between increased physical activity and reduced inflammation. It produces both a short-term inflammatory response and a long-term anti-inflammatory effect. Physical activity reduces inflammation in conjunction with or independent of changes in body weight. However, the mechanisms linking physical activity to inflammation are unknown.

Immune System

Physical activity boosts the immune system. This is dependent on the concentration of endogenous factors (such as sex hormones, metabolic hormones and growth hormones), body temperature, blood flow, hydration status and body position. Physical activity has shown to increase the levels of natural killer (NK) cells, NK T cells, macrophages, neutrophils and eosinophils, complements, cytokines, antibodies and T cytotoxic cells. However, the mechanism linking physical activity to immune system is not fully understood.

Cardiovascular Disease Prevention

Physical activity affects one's blood pressure, cholesterol levels, blood lipid levels, blood clotting factors and the strength of blood vessels. All factors that directly correlate to cardiovascular disease. It also improves the body's use of insulin. People who are at risk for diabetes, Type 2 (insulin resistant) especially, benefit greatly from physical activity because it activates a better usage of insulin and protects the heart. Those who develop diabetes have an increased risk of developing cardiovascular disease. In a study where a sample of around ten thousand adults from the Third National Health and Nutrition Examination Survey, physical activity and metabolic risk factors such as insulin resistance, inflammation, dyslipidemia were assessed. The study adjusted basic confounders with moderate/vigorous physical activity and the relation with CVD mortality. The results displayed physical activity being associated with a lower risk of CVD mortality that was independent of traditional metabolic risk factors.

The American Heart Association recommendations include the same findings as provided in the WCRF/ AICR recommendations list for people who are healthy. In regards to people with lower blood pressure or cholesterol, the association recommends that these individuals aim for around forty minutes of moderate to vigorous physical activity around three or four times a week.

Weight Control

Achieving resilience through physical fitness promotes a vast and complex range of health related benefits. Individuals who keep up physical fitness levels generally regulate their distribution of body fat and stay away from obesity. Abdominal fat, specifically visceral fat, is most directly affected by engaging in aerobic exercise. Strength training has been known to increase the amount of muscle in the body, however it can also reduce body fat. Sex steroid hormones, insulin, and an appropriate immune response are factors that mediate metabolism in relation to the abdominal fat. Therefore, physical fitness provides weight control through regulation of these bodily functions.

Menopause and Physical Fitness

Menopause is the term that is used to refer to the stretch of both before and after a woman's last menstrual cycle. There are an instrumental amount of symptoms connected to menopause, most of which can affect the quality of life of the women involved in this stage of her life. One way to reduce the severity of the symptoms is exercise and keeping a healthy level of fitness. Prior to and during menopause as the female body changes there can be physical, physiological or internal changes to the body. These changes can be prevented or even reduced with the use of regular exercise. These changes include;

- Prevention of weight gain: around menopause women tend to experience r a reduction in muscle mass and an increase in fat levels. Slight increases in physical exercise can help to prevent these changes.
- Reduce the risk of breast cancer: due to the weight loss from regular exercise may offer protection from breast cancer.
- Strengthen the bones: Physical activity can slow the bone loss associated with menopause, reducing the chance of bone fractures and osteoporosis.
- Reduce the risk of disease: Excess weight can increase the risk of heart disease and type 2 diabetes, and the regular physical activity can counter these effects.
- Boost the mood: By being involved in regular activities it can improve the psychological health, this can be the case at any age and not only for times during or after menopause.

The Melbourne Women's Midlife Health Project provided evidence that showed over an eight-year time period 438 were followed. Even though the physical activity was not associated with VMS in this cohort at the beginning. Women who reported they were physically active everyday at the beginning were 49% less likely to have reported bothersome hot flushes. This is in contrast to women whose level of activity decreased and were more likely to experience bothersome hot flushes.

References

- Elia, M. (1992) "Energy expenditure in the whole body". Energy metabolism. Tissue determinants and cellular corollaries. 61–79 Raven Press New York. ISBN 978-0-88167-871-0
- Nosaka, Ken (2008). "Muscle Soreness and Damage and the Repeated-Bout Effect". In Tiidus, Peter M. Skeletal muscle damage and repair. Human Kinetics. pp. 59–76. ISBN 978-0-7360-5867-4.
- American College of Sports Medicine (2010). ACSM's guidelines for exercise testing and prescription (8th ed.). Philadelphia: Lippincott Williams & Wilkins. ISBN 978-0-7817-6903-7.

- Eschbach, Chris (January 12, 2012). "Exercise Recommendations for Menopause-Aged Women". American College of Sports Medicine. American College of Sports Medicine. Retrieved 12 April 2015.
- Keytel, L.R. (March 2005). "Prediction of energy expenditure from heart rate monitoring during submaximal exercise." (PDF). Journal of Sports Sciences: 10. Retrieved 16 April 2015.
- "How much physical activity do adults need?". Centers for Disease Control and Prevention. 1 December 2011. Retrieved 29 April 2013.

2

Physical Exercise and its Classification

Physical exercise can be classified into aerobic exercise, strength training, stretching and anaerobic exercise. Common aerobic exercises which are explained in this chapter are cycling, burpee, skipping rope and jogging. Exercising enhances the immune system and helps in the prevention of diseases such as diabetes and obesity.

Physical Exercise

Physical exercise is any bodily activity that enhances or maintains physical fitness and overall health and wellness. It is performed for various reasons, including increasing growth and development, preventing aging, strengthening muscles and the cardiovascular system, honing athletic skills, weight loss or maintenance, and merely enjoyment. Frequent and regular physical exercise boosts the immune system and helps prevent "diseases of affluence" such as cardiovascular disease, type 2 diabetes, and obesity. It may also help prevent stress and depression, increase quality of sleep and act as a non-pharmaceutical sleep aid to treat diseases such as insomnia, help promote or maintain positive self-esteem, improve mental health, maintain steady digestion and treat constipation and gas, regulate fertility health, and augment an individual's sex appeal or body image, which has been found to be linked with higher levels of self-esteem. Childhood obesity is a growing global concern, and physical exercise may help decrease some of the effects of childhood and adult obesity. Some care providers call exercise the "miracle" or "wonder" drug—alluding to the wide variety of benefits that it can provide for many individuals.

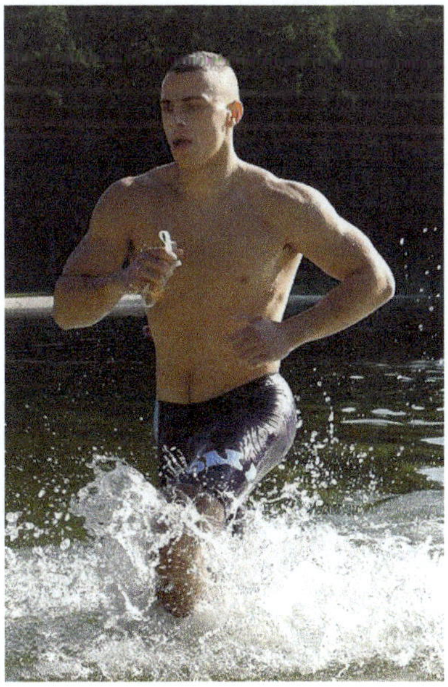

Running in water

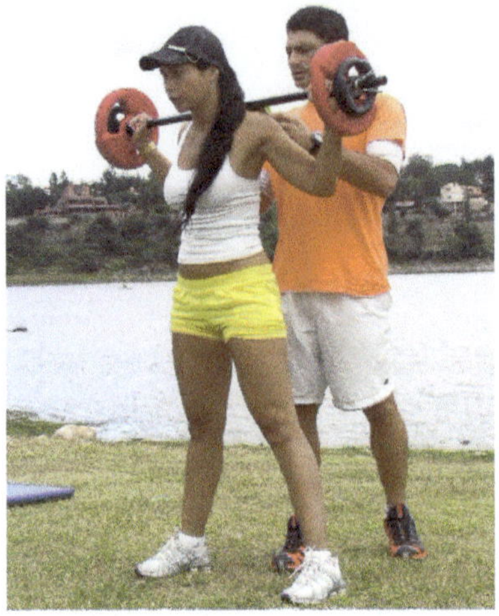

In the United Kingdom two to four hours of light activity are recommended during working hours. This includes walking and standing. In the United States, the CDC/ACSM consensus statement and the Surgeon General's report states that every adult should participate in moderate exercise, such as walking, swimming, and household tasks, for a minimum of 30 minutes daily.

Classification

Physical exercises are generally grouped into three types, depending on the overall effect they have on the human body:

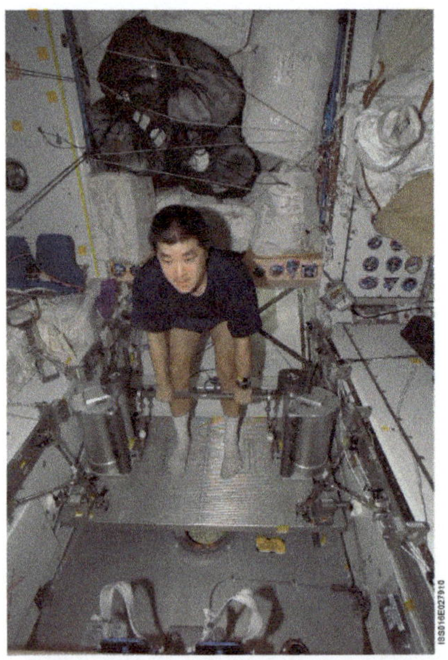

Exercise in space: Astronaut Daniel Tani, Expedition 16 flight engineer, works out at the Unity node of the International Space Station using the short bar of the Interim Resistive Exercise Device (IRED) to perform pull-ups to increase his upper body strength while in a microgravity environment

- Aerobic exercise is any physical activity that uses large muscle groups and causes the body to use more oxygen than it would while resting. The goal of aerobic exercise is to increase cardiovascular endurance. Examples of aerobic exercise include cycling, swimming, brisk walking, skipping rope, rowing, hiking, playing tennis, continuous training, and long slow distance training.

- Anaerobic exercise, which includes strength and resistance training, can firm, strengthen, and tone muscles, as well as improve bone strength, balance, and coordination. Examples of strength moves are push-ups, pull-ups, lunges, and bicep curls using dumbbells. Anaerobic exercise also include weight training, functional training, eccentric training, Interval training, sprinting, and high-intensity interval training increase short-term muscle strength.
- Flexibility exercises stretch and lengthen muscles. Activities such as stretching help to improve joint flexibility and keep muscles limber. The goal is to improve the range of motion which can reduce the chance of injury.

Physical exercise can also include training that focuses on accuracy, agility, power, and speed.

Sometimes the terms 'dynamic' and 'static' are used. 'Dynamic' exercises such as steady running, tend to produce a lowering of the diastolic blood pressure during exercise, due to the improved blood flow. Conversely, static exercise (such as weight-lifting) can cause the systolic pressure to rise significantly (during the exercise).

Health Effects

A review of correlational studies suggest that physical exercise is important for maintaining physical fitness and can contribute positively to maintaining a healthy weight, regulating digestive health, building and maintaining healthy bone density, muscle strength, and joint mobility, promoting physiological well-being, reducing surgical risks, and strengthening the immune system. Some studies indicate that exercise may increase life expectancy and quality of life. Moderate levels of exercise have been correlated with preventing aging and improving quality of life by reducing inflammatory potential. People who participate in moderate to high levels of physical exercise have a lower mortality rate compared to individuals who are not physically active.

According to the World Health Organization, lack of physical activity contributes to approximately 17% of heart disease and diabetes, 12% of falls in the elderly, and 10% of breast cancer and colon cancer.

Not everyone benefits equally from exercise. There is tremendous variation in individual response to training; where most people will see a moderate increase in endurance from aerobic exercise, some individuals will as much as double their oxygen uptake, while others can never augment endurance. However, muscle hypertrophy from resistance training is primarily determined by diet and testosterone. This genetic variation in improvement from training is one of the key physiological differences between elite athletes and the larger population. Studies have shown that exercising in middle age leads to better physical ability later in life.

Cardiovascular System

The beneficial effect of exercise on the cardiovascular system is well documented. There is a direct correlation between physical inactivity and cardiovascular mortality, and physical inactivity is an independent risk factor for the development of coronary artery disease. Low levels of physical exercise increase the risk of cardiovascular diseases mortality.

Children who participate in physical exercise experience greater loss of body fat and increased cardiovascular fitness. Studies have shown that academic stress in youth increases the risk of cardiovascular disease in later years; however, these risks can be greatly decreased with regular physical exercise. There is a dose-response relation between the amount of exercise performed from approximately 700 to 2000 kcal of energy expenditure per week and all-cause mortality and cardiovascular disease mortality in middle-aged and elderly populations. The greatest potential for reduced mortality is in the sedentary who become moderately active. Studies have shown that since heart disease is the leading cause of death in women, regular exercise in aging women leads to healthier cardiovascular profiles. Most beneficial effects of physical activity on cardiovascular disease mortality can be attained through moderate-intensity activity (40% to 60% of maximal oxygen uptake, depending on age). Persons who modify their behavior after myocardial infarction to include regular exercise have improved rates of survival. Persons who remain sedentary have the highest risk for all-cause and cardiovascular disease mortality. According to the American Heart Association, exercise reduces blood pressure, LDL and total cholesterol, and body weight. It increases HDL cholesterol, insulin sensitivity, and exercise tolerance.

Immune System

Although there have been hundreds of studies on exercise and the immune system, there is little direct evidence on its connection to illness. Epidemiological evidence suggests that moderate exercise has a beneficial effect on the human immune system; an effect which is modeled in a J curve. Moderate exercise has been associated with a 29% decreased incidence of upper respiratory tract infections (URTI), but studies of marathon runners found that their prolonged high-intensity exercise was associated with an increased risk of infection occurrence. However, another study did not find the effect. Immune cell functions are impaired following acute sessions of prolonged, high-intensity exercise, and some studies have found that athletes are at a higher risk for infections. Studies have shown that strenuous stress for long durations, such as training for a marathon, can suppress the immune system by decreasing the concentration of lymphocytes. The immune systems of athletes and nonathletes are generally similar. Athletes may have slightly elevated natural killer cell count and cytolytic action, but these are unlikely to be clinically significant.

Vitamin C supplementation has been associated with lower incidence of URTIs in marathon runners.

Biomarkers of inflammation such as C-reactive protein, which are associated with chronic diseases, are reduced in active individuals relative to sedentary individuals, and the positive effects of exercise may be due to its anti-inflammatory effects. In individuals with heart disease, exercise interventions lower blood levels of fibrinogen and C-reactive protein, an important cardiovascular risk marker. The depression in the immune system following acute bouts of exercise may be one of the mechanisms for this anti-inflammatory effect.

Cancer

A systematic review evaluated 45 studies that examined the relationship between physical activity and cancer survivorship. According to the study results "There was consistent evidence from 27 observational studies that physical activity is associated with reduced all-cause, breast cancer–specific, and colon cancer–specific mortality".

Epigenetic Effects

Physical exercise was correlated with a lower methylation frequency of two tumor suppressor genes, CACNA2D3 and L3MBTL. Hypermethylation of CACNA2D3 is associated with gastric cancer, while hypermethylation of L3MBTL is associated with breast cancer, brain tumors and hematological malignancies. A recent study indicates that exercise results in reduced DNA methylation at CpG sites on genes associated with breast cancer.

Cancer Cachexia

Physical exercise is becoming a widely accepted non-pharmacological intervention for the prevention and attenuation of cancer cachexia. "Cachexia is a multiorganic syndrome associated with cancer, characterized by inflammation, body weight loss (at least 5%) and muscle and adipose tissue wasting". Exercise triggers the activation of the transcriptional coactivator peroxisome proliferator-activated receptor gamma coactivator-1α (PGC-1α), which suppresses FoxO- and NF-κB-dependent gene transcription during muscle atrophy that is induced by fasting or denervation; thus, PGC-1α may be a key intermediate responsible for the beneficial antiatrophic effects of physical exercise on cancer cachexia. The exercise-induced isoform PGC-1α4, which can repress myostatin and induce IGF1 and hypertrophy, is a potential drug target for treatment of cancer cachexia. Other factors, such as JUNB and SIRT1, that maintain skeletal muscle mass and promote hypertrophy are also induced with regular physical exercise.

Neurobiological

The neurobiological effects of physical exercise are numerous and involve a wide range of interrelated effects on brain structure, brain function, and cognition. A large body of research in humans has demonstrated that consistent aerobic exercise (e.g., 30 minutes every day) induces persistent improvements in certain cognitive functions, healthy alterations in gene expression in the brain, and beneficial forms of neuroplasticity and behavioral plasticity; some of these long-term effects include: increased neuron growth, increased neurological activity (e.g., c-Fos and BDNF signaling), improved stress coping, enhanced cognitive control of behavior, improved declarative, spatial, and working memory, and structural and functional improvements in brain structures and pathways associated with cognitive control and memory. The effects of exercise on cognition have important implications for improving academic performance in children and college students, improving adult productivity, preserving cognitive function in old age, preventing or treating certain neurological disorders, and improving overall quality of life.

People who regularly perform aerobic exercise (e.g., running, jogging, brisk walking, swimming, and cycling) have greater scores on neuropsychological function and performance tests that measure certain cognitive functions, such as attentional control, inhibitory control, cognitive flexibility, working memory updating and capacity, declarative memory, spatial memory, and information processing speed. Aerobic exercise is also a potent antidepressant and euphoriant; as a result, consistent exercise produces general improvements in mood and self-esteem.

Regular aerobic exercise improves symptoms associated with a variety of central nervous system disorders and may be used as an adjunct therapy for these disorders. There is clear evidence of exercise treatment efficacy for major depressive disorder and attention deficit hyperactivity disorder. A large body of preclinical evidence and emerging clinical evidence supports the use of exercise therapy for treating and preventing the development of drug addictions. Reviews of clinical evidence also support the use of exercise as an adjunct therapy for certain neurodegenerative disorders, particularly Alzheimer's disease and Parkinson's disease. Regular exercise is also associated with a lower risk of developing neurodegenerative disorders. Regular exercise has also been proposed as an adjunct therapy for brain cancers.

Depression

Physical exercise has established efficacy as an antidepressant in individuals with depression and current medical evidence supports the use of exercise as both a preventive measure against and an adjunct therapy with antidepressant medication for depressive disorders. A July 2016 meta-analysis concluded that physical exercise improves overall quality of life in individuals with depression relative to controls. One systematic review noted that yoga may be effective in alleviating symptoms of prenatal depression. The biomolecular basis for exercise-induced antidepressant effects is believed to be a result of increased neurotrophic factor signaling, particularly brain-derived neurotrophic factor.

Continuous aerobic exercise can induce a transient state of euphoria, colloquially known as a "runner's high" in distance running or a "rower's high" in crew, through the increased biosynthesis of at least three euphoriant neurochemicals: anandamide (an endocannabinoid), β-endorphin (an endogenous opioid), and phenethylamine (a trace amine and amphetamine analog).

A systematic review noted that, although limited, some evidence suggests that the duration of engagement in a sedentary lifestyle is positively correlated with a risk of developing an anxiety disorder or experiencing anxiety symptoms. It noted that additional research is needed in order to confirm these findings.

Sleep

A 2010 review of published scientific research suggested that exercise generally improves sleep for most people, and helps sleep disorders such as insomnia. The optimum time to exercise *may* be 4 to 8 hours before bedtime, though exercise at any time of day is beneficial, with the possible exception of heavy exercise taken shortly before bedtime, which may disturb sleep. There is, in any case, insufficient evidence to draw detailed conclusions about the relationship between exercise and sleep.

According to a 2005 study, exercise is the most recommended alternative to sleeping pills for resolving insomnia. Sleeping pills are more costly than to make time for a daily routine of staying fit, and may have dangerous side effects in the long run. Exercise can be a healthy, safe and inexpensive way to achieve more and better sleep.

Excessive Exercise

Too much exercise can be harmful. Without proper rest, the chance of stroke or other circulation problems increases, and muscle tissue may develop slowly. Extremely intense, long-term cardiovascular exercise, as can be seen in athletes who train for multiple marathons, has been associated with scarring of the heart and heart rhythm abnormalities. Specifically, high cardiac output has been shown to cause enlargement of the left and right ventricle volumes, increased ventricle wall thickness, and greater cardiac mass. These changes further result in myocardial cell damage in the lining of the heart, leading to scar tissue and thickened walls. During these processes, the protein troponin increases in the bloodstream, indicating cardiac muscle cell death and increased stress on the heart itself.

Inappropriate exercise can do more harm than good, with the definition of "inappropriate" varying according to the individual. For many activities, especially running and cycling, there are significant injuries that occur with poorly regimented exercise schedules. Injuries from accidents also remain a major concern, whereas the effects of increased exposure to air pollution seem only a minor concern.

In extreme instances, over-exercising induces serious performance loss. Unaccustomed overexertion of muscles leads to rhabdomyolysis (damage to muscle) most often seen in new army recruits. Another danger is overtraining, in which the intensity or volume of training exceeds the body's capacity to recover between bouts. One sign of Overtraining Syndrome (OTS) is suppressed immune function, with an increased incidence of upper respiratory tract infection (URTI). An increased incidence of URTIs is also associated with high volume/intensity training, as well as with excessive exercise (EE), such as in a marathon.

Stopping excessive exercise suddenly may create a change in mood. Exercise should be controlled by each body's inherent limitations. While one set of joints and muscles may have the tolerance to withstand multiple marathons, another body may be damaged by 20 minutes of light jogging. This must be determined for each individual.

Too much exercise may cause a woman to miss her periods, a symptom known as amenorrhea. This is a very serious condition which indicates a woman is pushing her body beyond its natural boundaries.

Mechanism of Effects

Skeletal Muscle

Resistance training and subsequent consumption of a protein-rich meal promotes muscle hypertrophy and gains in muscle strength by stimulating myofibrillar muscle protein synthesis (MPS) and inhibiting muscle protein breakdown (MPB). The stimulation of muscle protein synthesis by resistance training occurs via phosphorylation of the mechanistic target of rapamycin (mTOR) and subsequent activation of mTORC1, which leads to protein biosynthesis in the ribosome via phosphorylation of mTORC1's immediate targets (the p70S6 kinase and the translation initiation factor 4EBP1). The suppression of muscle protein breakdown following food consumption occurs primarily via increases in plasma insulin; however, a suppression of MPB of comparable magnitude has also been shown to occur in humans from a sufficient elevation of plasma β-hydroxy β-methylbutyric acid.

Aerobic exercise induces mitochondrial biogenesis and an increased capacity for oxidative phosphorylation in the mitochondria of skeletal muscle, which is one mechanism by which aerobic exercise enhances submaximal endurance performance. These effects occur via an exercise-induced increase in the intracellular AMP:ATP ratio, thereby triggering the activation of AMP-activated protein kinase (AMPK) which subsequently phosphorylates peroxisome proliferator-activated receptor gamma coactivator-1α (PGC-1α), the master regulator of mitochondrial biogenesis.

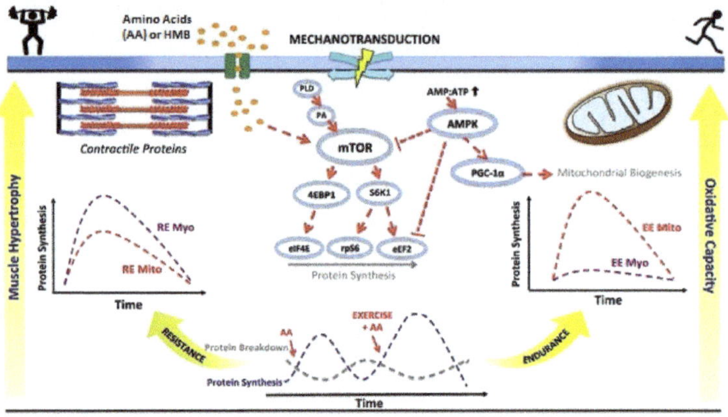

Diagram of the molecular signaling cascades that are involved in myofibrillar muscle protein synthesis and mitochondrial biogenesis in response to physical exercise and specific amino acids or their derivatives (primarily leucine and HMB).

Abbreviations and Representations:

• PLD: phospholipase D • PA: phosphatidic acid • mTOR: mechanistic target of rapamycin • AMP: adenosine monophosphate • ATP: adenosine triphosphate • AMPK: AMP-activated protein kinase • PGC-1α: peroxisome proliferator-activated receptor gamma coactivator-1α • 4EBP1: eukaryotic translation initiation factor 4E-binding protein 1 • S6K1: p70S6 kinase • eIF4E: eukaryotic translation initiation factor 4E • RPS6: ribosomal protein S6 • eEF2: eukaryotic elongation factor 2 • RE: resistance exercise; EE: endurance exercise • Myo: myofibrillar; Mito: mitochondrial • AA: amino acids • ↑ represents activation • T represents inhibition

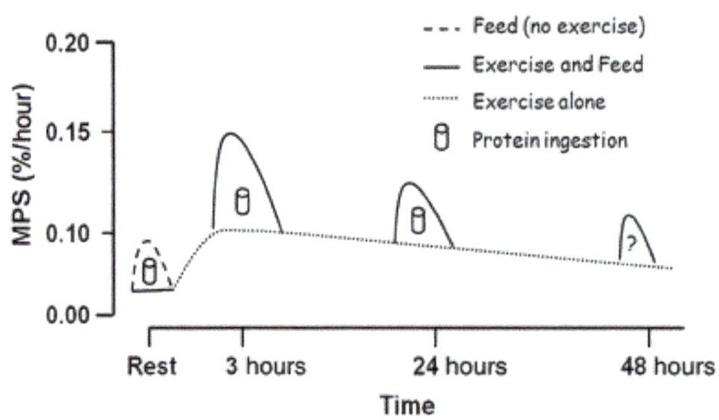

Resistance training stimulates myofibrillar muscle protein synthesis for a period of up to 48 hours following exercise (shown by dotted line). Ingestion of a protein-rich meal at any point during this period will augment the exercise-induced increase in muscle protein synthesis (shown by solid lines).

Other Peripheral Organs

Developing research has demonstrated that many of the benefits of exercise are mediated through the role of skeletal muscle as an endocrine organ. That is, contracting muscles release multiple substances known as myokines which promote the growth of new tissue, tissue repair, and multiple anti-inflammatory functions, which in turn reduce the risk of developing various inflammatory diseases. Exercise reduces levels of cortisol, which causes many health problems, both physical and mental. Endurance exercise before meals lowers blood glucose more than the same exercise after meals. There is evidence that vigorous exercise (90–95% of VO_2 max) induces a greater degree of physiological cardiac hypertrophy than moderate exercise (40 to 70% of VO_2 max), but it is unknown whether this has any effects on overall morbidity and/or mortality. Both aerobic and anaerobic exercise work to increase the mechanical efficiency of the heart by increasing cardiac volume (aerobic exercise), or myocardial thickness (strength training). Ventricular hypertrophy, the thickening of the ventricular walls, is generally beneficial and healthy if it occurs in response to exercise.

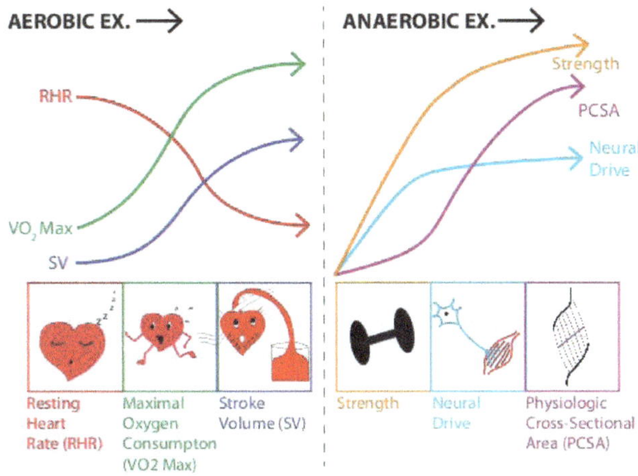

Summary of long-term adaptations to regular aerobic and anaerobic exercise. Aerobic exercise can cause several central cardiovascular adaptations, including an increase in stroke volume (SV) and maximal aerobic capacity (VO_2 max), as well as a decrease in resting heart rate (RHR). Long-term adaptations to resistance training, the most common form of anaerobic exercise, include muscular hypertrophy, an increase in the physiological cross-sectional area (PCSA) of muscle(s), and an increase in neural drive, both of which lead to increased muscular strength. Neural adaptations begin more quickly and plateau prior to the hypertrophic response.

Central Nervous System

The persistent long-term neurobiological effects of regular physical exercise are believed to be mediated by transient exercise-induced increases in the concentration of neurotrophic factors (e.g., BDNF, IGF-1, VEGF, and GDNF) and other biomolecules in peripheral blood plasma, which subsequently cross the blood–brain barrier and blood–cerebrospinal fluid barrier and bind to their associated receptors in the brain. Upon binding to their receptors in cerebral vasculature and brain cells (i.e., neurons and glial cells), these biomolecules trigger intracellular signaling cascades that lead to neuroplastic biological responses – such as neurogenesis, synaptogenesis, oligodendrogenesis, and angiogenesis, among others – which ultimately mediate the exercise-induced improvements in cognitive function.

Public Health Measures

Multiple component community-wide campaigns are frequently used in an attempt to increase a population's level of physical activity. A 2015 Cochrane review, however, did not find evidence supporting a benefit. The quality of the underlying evidence was also poor. Survery of brief interventions promoting physical activity found that they are cost-effective, although there are variations between studies.

Environmental approaches appear promising: signs that encourage the use of stairs, as well as community campaigns, may increase exercise levels. The city of Bogotá, Colombia, for example, blocks off 113 kilometers (70 mi) of roads on Sundays and holidays to make it easier for its citizens to get exercise. These pedestrian zones are part of an effort to combat chronic diseases, including obesity.

To identify which public health strategies are effective, a Cochrane overview of reviews is in preparation.

Physical exercise was said to decrease healthcare costs, increase the rate of job attendance, as well as increase the amount of effort women put into their jobs.

Children will mimic the behavior of their parents in relation to physical exercise. Parents can thus promote physical activity and limit the amount of time children spend in front of screens which may decrease the risk of childhood obesity.

Overweight children who participate in physical exercise experience greater loss of body fat and increased cardiovascular fitness. According to the Centers for Disease Control and Prevention in the United States, both children and adults should do 60 minutes or more of physical activity each day. Implementing physical exercise in the school system and ensuring an environment in which children can reduce barriers to maintain a healthy lifestyle is essential.

Exercise Trends

Worldwide there has been a large shift towards less physically demanding work. This has been accompanied by increasing use of mechanized transportation, a greater prevalence of labor saving technology in the home, and fewer active recreational pursuits. Personal lifestyle changes however can correct the lack of physical exercise.

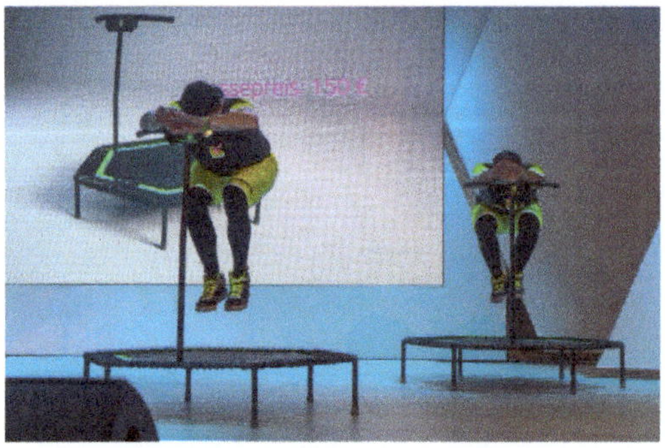

Jumping fitness exercise

Research in 2015 indicates integrating mindfulness to physical exercise interventions increases exercise adherence, self-efficacy and also has positive effects both psychologically and physiologically.

Nutrition and Recovery

Proper nutrition is as important to health as exercise. When exercising, it becomes even more important to have a good diet to ensure that the body has the correct ratio of macronutrients while providing ample micronutrients, in order to aid the body with the recovery process following strenuous exercise.

Active recovery is recommended after participating in physical exercise because it removes lactate from the blood more quickly than inactive recovery. Removing lactate from circulation allows for an easy decline in body temperature, which can also benefit the immune system, as an individual may be vulnerable to minor illnesses if the body temperature drops too abruptly after physical exercise.

History

The benefits of exercise have been known since antiquity. Marcus Cicero, around 65 BCE, stated: "It is exercise alone that supports the spirits, and keeps the mind in vigor."

Several mass exercise movements were started in the early twentieth century to realise the benefits of exercise. The first and most significant of these in the UK was the Women's League of Health and Beauty founded in 1930 by Mary Bagot Stack that had 166,000 members in 1937.

However, the link between physical health and exercise (or lack of it) was only discovered in 1949 and reported in 1953 by a team led by Jerry Morris. Dr. Morris noted that men of similar social class and occupation (bus conductors versus bus drivers) had markedly different rates of heart attacks, depending on the level of exercise they got: bus drivers had a sedentary occupation and a higher incidence of heart disease, while bus conductors were forced to move continually and had a lower incidence of heart disease. This link had not previously been noted and was later confirmed by other researchers.

Other Animals

Physical exercise has been shown to benefit a wide range of other mammals, as well as salmon, juvenile crocodiles, and at least one species of bird.

However, several studies have shown that lizards display no benefit from exercise, leading them to be termed "metabolically inflexible". Indeed, damage from overtraining may occur following weeks of forced treadmill exercise in lizards.

A number of studies of both rodents and humans have demonstrated that individual differences in both ability and propensity for exercise (i.e., voluntary exercise) have some genetic basis.

Several studies of rodents have demonstrated that maternal or juvenile access to wheels that allow voluntary exercise can increase the propensity to run as adults. These studies further suggest that physical activity may be more "programmable" than food intake.

Aerobic Exercise

Aerobic exercise (also known as cardio) is physical exercise of low to high intensity that depends primarily on the aerobic energy-generating process. Aerobic literally means "relating to, involving, or requiring free oxygen", and refers to the use of oxygen to adequately meet energy demands during exercise via aerobic metabolism. Generally, light-to-moderate intensity activities that are sufficiently supported by aerobic metabolism can be performed for extended periods of time.

When practiced in this way, examples of cardiovascular/aerobic exercise are medium to long distance running/jogging, swimming, cycling, and walking, according to the first extensive research on aerobic exercise, conducted in the 1960s on over 5,000 U.S. Air Force personnel by Dr. Kenneth H. Cooper.

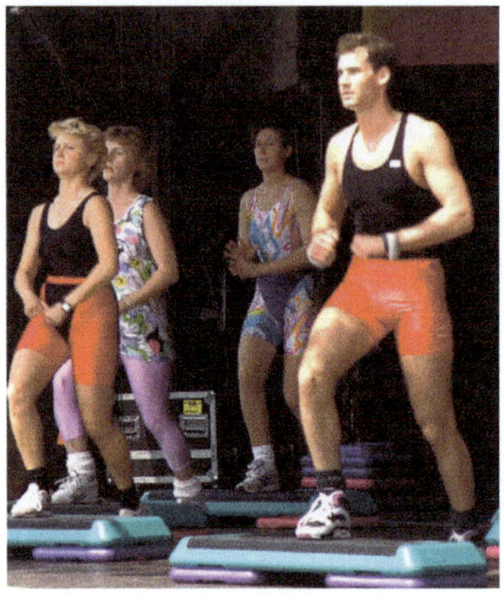

Cardio

History

Kenneth Cooper was the first person to introduce the concept of aerobic exercise. In the 1960s, Cooper started research into preventive medicine. He became intrigued by the belief that exercise can preserve one's health. In 1970 he created his own institute (the Cooper Institute) for non-profit research and education devoted to preventive medicine. He sparked millions into becoming active and is now known as the "father of aerobics".

Aerobic Versus Anaerobic Exercise

EXERCISE ZONES

BEATS PER MINUTE / AGE	20	25	30	35	40	45	50	55	65	70
100%	200	195	190	185	180	175	170	165	155	150
VO2 Max (Maximum effort)										
90%	180	176	171	167	162	158	153	149	140	135
Anaerobic (Hardcore training)										
80%	160	156	152	148	144	140	136	132	124	126
Aerobix (Cardio training / Endurance)										
70%	140	137	133	130	126	123	119	116	109	105
Weight control (Fitness / Fat burn)										
60%	120	117	114	111	108	105	102	99	93	90
Moderate activity (Maintenance / Warm up)										
50%	100	98	95	93	90	88	85	83	78	75

Fox and Haskell formula showing the split between aerobic (light orange) and anaerobic (dark orange) exercise and heart rate

Aerobic exercise and fitness can be contrasted with anaerobic exercise, of which strength training and short-distance running are the most salient examples. The two types of exercise differ by the duration and intensity of muscular contractions involved, as well as by how energy is generated within the muscle.

New research on the endocrine functions of contracting muscles has shown that both aerobic and anaerobic exercise promote the secretion of myokines, with attendant benefits including growth of new tissue, tissue repair, and various anti-inflammatory functions, which in turn reduce the risk of developing various inflammatory diseases. Myokine secretion in turn is dependent on the amount of muscle contracted, and the duration and intensity of contraction. As such, both types of exercise produce endocrine benefits.

In almost all conditions, anaerobic exercise is accompanied by aerobic exercises because the less efficient anaerobic metabolism must supplement the aerobic system due to energy demands that exceed the aerobic system's capacity. What is generally called aerobic exercise might be better termed "solely aerobic", because it is designed to be low-intensity enough not to generate lactate via pyruvate fermentation, so that all carbohydrate is aerobically turned into energy.

Initially during increased exertion, muscle glycogen is broken down to produce glucose, which undergoes glycolysis producing pyruvate which then reacts with oxygen (Krebs cycle, Chemiosmosis) to produce carbon dioxide and water and releases energy. If there is a shortage of oxygen (anaerobic exercise, explosive movements), carbohydrate is consumed more rapidly because the pyruvate ferments into lactate. If the intensity of the exercise exceeds the rate with which the cardiovascular system can supply muscles with oxygen, it results in buildup of lactate and quickly makes it impossible to continue the exercise. Unpleasant effects of lactate buildup initially include the burning sensation in the muscles, and may eventually include nausea and even vomiting if the exercise is continued without allowing lactate to clear from the bloodstream.

As glycogen levels in the muscle begin to fall, glucose is released into the bloodstream by the liver, and fat metabolism is increased so that it can fuel the aerobic pathways. Aerobic exercise may be fueled by glycogen reserves, fat reserves, or a combination of both, depending on the intensity. Prolonged moderate-level aerobic exercise at 65% VO2 max (the heart rate of 150 bpm for a 30-year-old human) results in the maximum contribution of fat to the total energy expenditure. At this level, fat may contribute 40% to 60% of total, depending on the duration of the exercise. Vigorous exercise above 75% VO2max (160 bpm) primarily burns glycogen.

Major muscles in a rested, untrained human typically contain enough energy for about 2 hours of vigorous exercise. Exhaustion of glycogen is a major cause of what marathon runners call "hitting the wall". Training, lower intensity levels, and carbohydrate loading may allow postponement of the onset of exhaustion beyond 4 hours.

Aerobic exercise comprises innumerable forms. In general, it is performed at a moderate level of intensity over a relatively long period of time. For example, running a long distance at a moderate pace is an aerobic exercise, but sprinting is not. Playing singles tennis, with near-continuous motion, is generally considered aerobic activity, while golf or two person team tennis, with brief bursts of activity punctuated by more frequent breaks, may not be predominantly aerobic. Some sports are thus inherently "aerobic", while other aerobic exercises, such as fartlek training or aerobic dance classes, are designed specifically to improve aerobic capacity and fitness. It is most common for aerobic exercises to involve the leg muscles, primarily or exclusively. There are some exceptions. For example, rowing to distances of 2,000 m or more is an aerobic sport that exercises several major muscle groups, including those of the legs, abdominals, chest, and arms. Common kettlebell exercises combine aerobic and anaerobic aspects.

Benefits

Among the recognized benefits of doing regular aerobic exercise are:

- Strengthening the muscles involved in respiration, to facilitate the flow of air in and out of the lungs
- Strengthening and enlarging the heart muscle, to improve its pumping efficiency and reduce the resting heart rate, known as aerobic conditioning
- Improving circulation efficiency and reducing blood pressure
- Increasing the total number of red blood cells in the body, facilitating transport of oxygen
- Improved mental health, including reducing stress and lowering the incidence of depression, as well as increased cognitive capacity.
- Reducing the risk for diabetes. One meta-analysis has shown, from multiple conducted studies, that aerobic exercise does help lower Hb A_{1C} levels for type 2 diabetics.

As a result, aerobic exercise can reduce the risk of death due to cardiovascular problems. In addition, high-impact aerobic activities (such as jogging or using a skipping rope) can stimulate bone growth, as well as reduce the risk of osteoporosis for both men and women.

In addition to the health benefits of aerobic exercise, there are numerous performance benefits:

- Increased storage of energy molecules such as fats and carbohydrates within the muscles, allowing for increased endurance
- Neovascularization of the muscle sarcomeres to increase blood flow through the muscles
- Increasing speed at which aerobic metabolism is activated within muscles, allowing a greater portion of energy for intense exercise to be generated aerobically
- Improving the ability of muscles to use fats during exercise, preserving intramuscular glycogen
- Enhancing the speed at which muscles recover from high intensity exercise
- Neurobiological effects: improvements in brain structural connections and increased gray matter density, new neuron growth, improved cognitive function (cognitive control and various forms of memory), and improvement or maintenance of mental health

Some drawbacks of aerobic exercise include:

- Overuse injuries because of repetitive, high-impact exercise such as distance running.
- Is not an effective approach to building muscle.

- Only effective for fat loss when used consistently.

Both the health benefits and the performance benefits, or "training effect", require a minimum duration and frequency of exercise. Most authorities suggest at least twenty minutes performed at least three times per week.

Aerobic Capacity

Aerobic capacity describes the functional capacity of the cardiorespiratory system, (the heart, lungs and blood vessels). Aerobic capacity refers to the maximum amount of oxygen consumed by the body during intense exercises, in a given time frame. It is a function both of cardiorespiratory performance and the maximum ability to remove and utilize oxygen from circulating blood. To measure maximal aerobic capacity, an exercise physiologist or physician will perform a VO_2 max test, in which a subject will undergo progressively more strenuous exercise on a treadmill, from an easy walk through to exhaustion. The individual is typically connected to a respirometer to measure oxygen consumption, and the speed is increased incrementally over a fixed duration of time. The higher the measured cardiorespiratory endurance level, the more oxygen has been transported to and used by exercising muscles, and the higher the level of intensity at which the individual can exercise. More simply put, the higher the aerobic capacity, the higher the level of aerobic fitness. The Cooper and multi-stage fitness tests can also be used to assess functional aerobic capacity for particular jobs or activities.

The degree to which aerobic capacity can be improved by exercise varies very widely in the human population: while the average response to training is an approximately 17% increase in VO_2max, in any population there are "high responders" who may as much as double their capacity, and "low responders" who will see little or no benefit from training. Studies indicate that approximately 10% of otherwise healthy individuals cannot improve their aerobic capacity with exercise at all. The degree of an individual's responsiveness is highly heritable, suggesting that this trait is genetically determined.

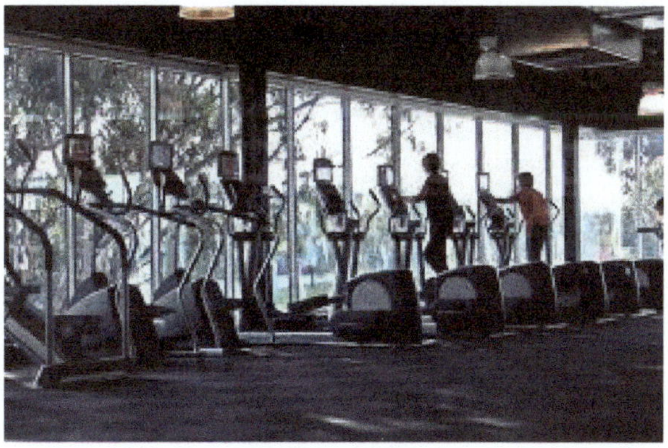

Aerobic workout

Alternatives

Higher intensity exercise, such as High-intensity interval training (HIIT), increases the resting metabolic rate (RMR) in the 24 hours following high intensity exercise, ultimately burning more calories than lower intensity exercise; low intensity exercise burns more calories during the exercise, due to the increased duration, but fewer afterwards.

Commercial Success

Aerobic exercise has long been a popular approach to achieving weight loss and physical fitness, often taking a commercial form.

- In the 1970s Judi Sheppard Missett helped create the market for commercial aerobics with her Jazzercise program
- In the 1980s Richard Simmons hosted an aerobic exercise show on television, and also released a series of exercise videos
- In the 1990s Billy Blanks's Tae Bo helped popularize cardio-boxing workouts that incorporated martial arts movements

Common Aerobic Exercises

Cycling

Cycling, also called bicycling or biking, is the use of bicycles for transport, recreation, exercise or sport. Persons engaged in cycling are referred to as "cyclists", "bikers", or less commonly, as "bicyclists". Apart from two-wheeled bicycles, "cycling" also includes the riding of unicycles, tricycles, quadracycles, recumbent and similar human-powered vehicles (HPVs).

Bicycles were introduced in the 19th century and now number approximately one billion worldwide. They are the principal means of transportation in many parts of the world.

Cycling is widely regarded as a very effective and efficient mode of transportation optimal for short to moderate distances.

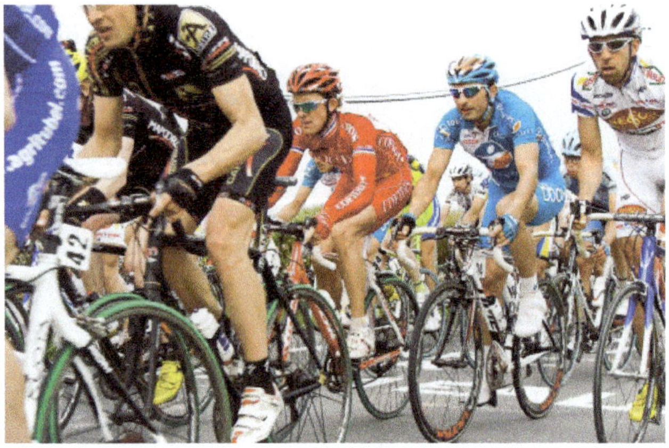

Tro-Bro Léon racing, 2009.

Bicycles provide numerous benefits in comparison with motor vehicles, including the sustained physical exercise involved in cycling, easier parking, increased maneuverability, and access to roads, bike paths and rural trails. Cycling also offers a reduced consumption of fossil fuels, less air or noise pollution, and much reduced traffic congestion. These lead to less financial cost to the user as well as to society at large (negligible damage to roads, less road area required). By fitting bicycle racks on the front of buses, transit agencies can significantly increase the areas they can serve.

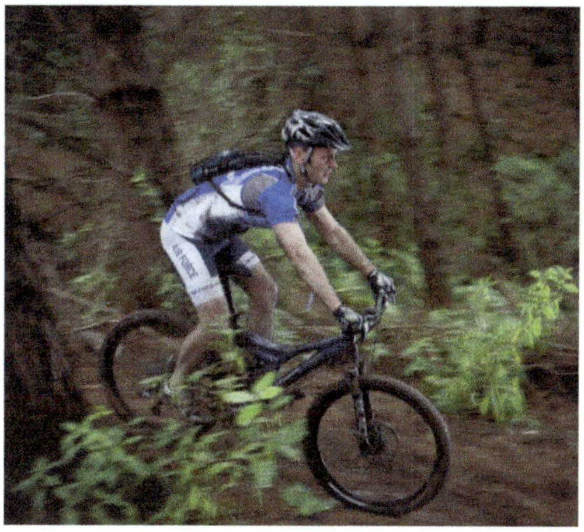

Mountain biking.

Among the disadvantages of cycling are the requirement of bicycles (excepting tricycles or quadracycles) to be balanced by the rider in order to remain upright, the reduced protection in crashes in comparison to motor vehicles, longer travel time (except in densely populated areas), vulnerability to weather conditions, difficulty in transporting passengers, and the fact that a basic level of fitness is required for cycling moderate to long distances.

Equipment

In many countries, the most commonly used vehicle for road transport is a utility bicycle. These have frames with relaxed geometry, protecting the rider from shocks of the road and easing steering at low speeds. Utility bicycles tend to be equipped with accessories such as mudguards, pannier racks and lights, which extends their usefulness on a daily basis. As the bicycle is so effective as a means of transportation various companies have developed methods of carrying anything from the weekly shop to children on bicycles. Certain countries rely heavily on bicycles and their culture has developed around the bicycle as a primary form of transport. In Europe, Denmark and the Netherlands have the most bicycles per capita and most often use bicycles for everyday transport.

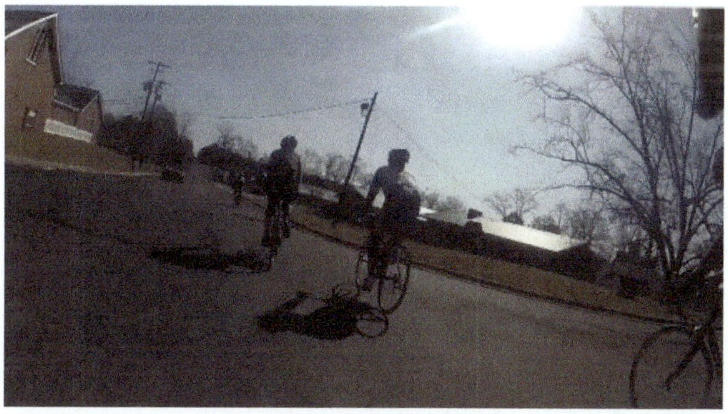

Cycling in Alabama

Road bikes tend to have a more upright shape and a shorter wheelbase, which make the bike more mobile but harder to ride slowly. The design, coupled with low or dropped handlebars, requires the rider to bend forward more, making use of stronger muscles (particularly the gluteus maximus) and reducing air resistance at high speed.

The price of a new bicycle can range from US$50 to more than US$20,000 (the highest priced bike in the world is the custom Madone by Damien Hirst, sold at $500,000 USD), depending on quality, type and weight (the most exotic road bicycles can weigh as little as 3.2 kg (7 lb)). However, UCI regulations stipulate a legal race bike cannot weigh less than 6.8 kg (14.99 lbs). Being measured for a bike and taking it for a test ride are recommended before buying.

The drivetrain components of the bike should also be considered. A middle grade dérailleur is sufficient for a beginner, although many utility bikes are equipped with hub gears. If the rider plans a significant amount of hillclimbing a triple-chainrings crankset gear system may be preferred. Otherwise, the relatively lighter and less expensive double chainring may be better. Much simpler fixed wheel bikes are also available.

Many road bikes, along with mountain bikes, include clipless pedals to which special shoes attach, via a cleat, enabling the rider to pull on the pedals as well as push. Other possible accessories for the bicycle include front and rear lights, bells or horns, child carrying seats, cycling computers with GPS, locks, bar tape, fenders (mud-guards), baggage racks, baggage carriers and pannier bags, water bottles and bottle cages.

For basic maintenance and repairs cyclists can carry a pump (or a CO_2 cartridge), a puncture repair kit, a spare inner tube, and tire levers and a set of allen keys. Cycling can be more efficient and comfortable with special shoes, gloves, and shorts. In wet weather, riding can be more tolerable with waterproof clothes, such as cape, jacket, trousers (pants) and overshoes and high-visibility clothing is advisable to reduce the risk from motor vehicle users.

Items legally required in some jurisdictions, or voluntarily adopted for safety reasons, include bicycle helmets, generator or battery operated lights, reflectors, and audible signalling devices such as a bell or horn. Extras include studded tires and a bicycle computer.

Bikes can also be heavily customized, with different seat designs and handle bars, for example.

Skills

Many schools and police departments run educational programs to instruct children in bicycle handling skills and introduce them to the rules of the road as they apply to cyclists. In different countries these may be known as bicycle rodeos or operated as schemes such as Bikeability. Education for adult cyclists is available from organizations such as the League of American Bicyclists.

Beyond simply riding, another skill is riding efficiently and safely in traffic. One popular approach to riding in motor vehicle traffic is vehicular cycling, occupying road space as car does. Alternately, in countries such as Denmark and the Netherlands, where cycling is popular, cyclists are sometimes segregated into bike lanes at the side of, or separate from, main highways and roads. Many primary schools participate in the national road test in which children individually complete a circuit on roads near the school while being observed by testers.

Infrastructure

Cyclists, pedestrians and motorists make different demands on road design which may lead to conflicts. Some jurisdictions give priority to motorized traffic, for example setting up one-way street systems, free-right turns, high capacity roundabouts, and slip roads. Others share priority with cyclists so as to encourage more cycling by applying varying combinations of traffic calming measures to limit the impact of motorized transport, and by building bike lanes, bike paths and cycle tracks.

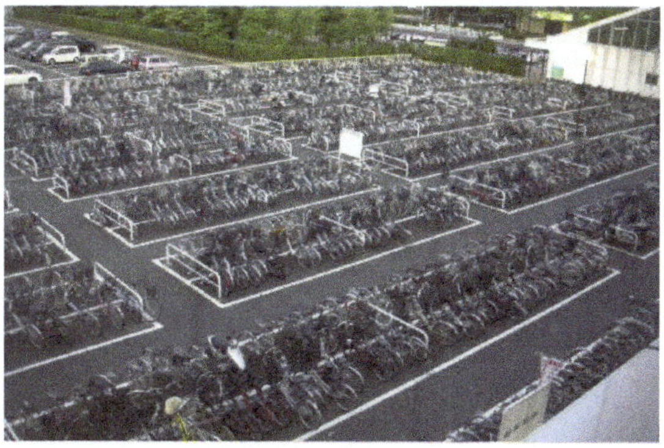

A parking lot for bicycles in Niigata, Niigata, Japan.

In jurisdictions where motor vehicles were given priority, cycling has tended to decline while in jurisdictions where cycling infrastructure was built, cycling rates have remained steady or increased. Occasionally, extreme measures against cycling may occur. In Shanghai, where bicycles were once the dominant mode of transport, bicycle travel on a few city roads was banned temporarily in December 2003.

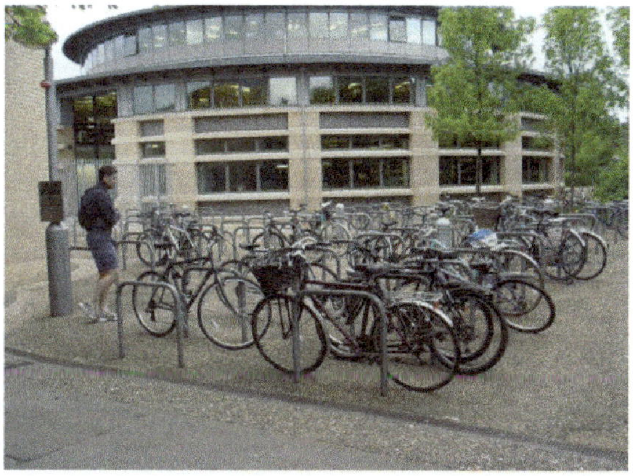

Bicycle stands outside the Centre for Mathematical Sciences at the University of Cambridge. Many students at the university opt to travel by bicycle.

In areas in which cycling is popular and encouraged, cycle-parking facilities using bicycle stands, lockable mini-garages, and patrolled cycle parks are used in order to reduce theft. Local governments promote cycling by permitting bicycles to be carried on public transport or by providing external attachment devices on public transport vehicles. Conversely, an absence of secure cycle-parking is a recurring complaint by cyclists from cities with low modal share of cycling.

Extensive cycling infrastructure may be found in some cities. Such dedicated paths in some cities often have to be shared with in-line skaters, scooters, skateboarders, and pedestrians. Dedicated cycling infrastructure is treated differently in the law of every jurisdiction, including the question of liability of users in a collision. There is also some debate about the safety of the various types of separated facilities.

Bicycles are considered a sustainable mode of transport, especially suited for urban use and relatively shorter distances when used for transport (compared to recreation). Case studies and good practices (from European cities and some worldwide examples) that promote and stimulate this kind of functional cycling in cities can be found at Eltis, Europe's portal for local transport.

A number of cities, including Paris, London and Barcelona, now have successful bike hire schemes designed to help people cycle in the city. Typically these feature utilitarian city bikes which lock into docking stations, released on payment for set time periods. In London this can cost as little as 12 Pence per day, with all journeys less than 30 minutes then free.

Types

Utility

Utility cycling refers both to cycling as a mode of daily commuting transport as well as the use of a bicycle in a commercial activity, mainly to transport goods, mostly accomplished in an urban environment.

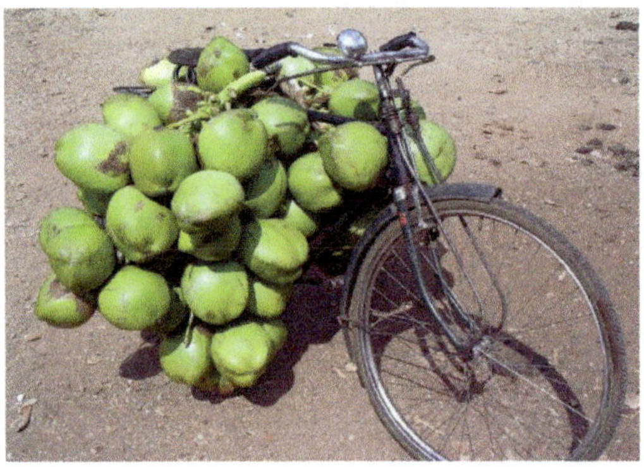

A bicycle loaded with tender coconuts for sale. Karnataka, India.

The postal services of many countries have long relied on bicycles. The British Royal Mail first started using bicycles in 1880; now bicycle delivery fleets include 37,000 in the UK, 25,700 in Germany, 10,500 in Hungary and 7000 in Sweden. In Australia, Australia Post has also reintroduced bicycle postal deliveries on some routes due to an inability to recruit sufficient licensed riders willing to use their uncomfortable motorbikes. The London Ambulance Service has recently introduced bicycling paramedics, who can often get to the scene of an incident in Central London more quickly than a motorized ambulance.

Late in the 20th century, urban police bicycles became more common, as the mobility of car-borne officers was increasingly limited by traffic congestion and pedestrianisation.

Bicycles enjoy substantial use as general delivery vehicles in many countries. In the UK and North America, as their first jobs, generations of teenagers have worked at delivering newspapers by bicycle. London has many delivery companies that use bicycles with trailers. Most cities in the West, and many outside it, support a sizeable and visible industry of cycle couriers who deliver documents and small packages. In India, many of Mumbai's Dabbawalas use bicycles to deliver home cooked lunches to the city's workers. In Bogotá, Colombia the city's largest bakery recently replaced most of its delivery trucks with bicycles. Even the car industry uses bicycles. At the huge

Mercedes-Benz factory in Sindelfingen, Germany workers use bicycles, color-coded by department, to move around the factory.

Recreational

Bicycle Touring

Bicycles are used for recreation at all ages. Bicycle touring, also known as cyclotourism, involves touring and exploration or sightseeing by bicycle for leisure. A brevet or randonnée is an organized long-distance ride.

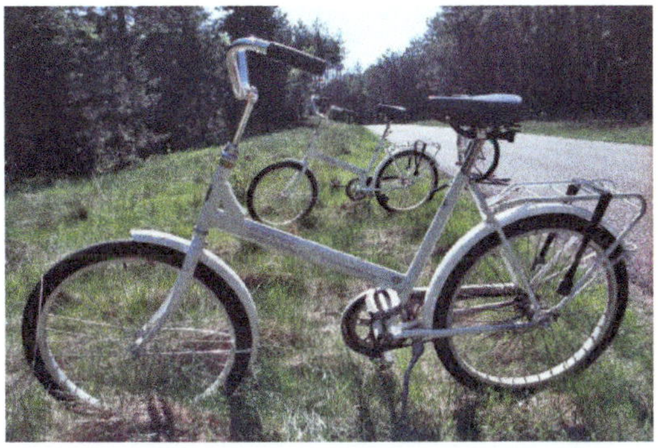

In the Netherlands, bicycles are freely available for use in the Hoge Veluwe National Park.

One popular Dutch pleasure is the enjoyment of relaxed cycling in the countryside of the Netherlands. The land is very flat and full of public bicycle trails and cycle tracks where cyclists are not bothered by cars and other traffic, which makes it ideal for cycling recreation. Many Dutch people subscribe every year to an event called *fietsvierdaagse* — four days of organised cycling through the local environment. Paris–Brest–Paris (PBP), which began in 1891, is the oldest bicycling event still run on a regular basis on the open road, covers over 1,200 km (746 mi) and imposes a 90-hour time limit. Similar if smaller institutions exist in many countries.

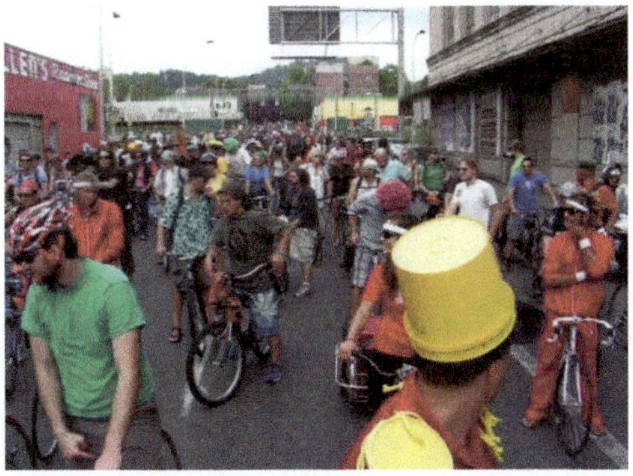

Tour de Fat group ride in Portland, Oregon

Organized Rides

Many cycling clubs hold organized rides in which bicyclists of all levels participate. The typical organized ride starts with a large group of riders, called the mass, bunch or even peloton. This will thin out over the course of the ride. Many riders choose to ride together in groups of the same skill level to take advantage of drafting.

Most organized rides, for example cyclosportives (or gran fondos), Challenge Rides or reliability trials, and hill climbs include registration requirements and will provide information either through the mail or online concerning start times and other requirements. Rides usually consist of several different routes, sorted by mileage, and with a certain number of rest stops that usually include refreshments, first aid and maintenance tools. Routes can vary by as much as 100 miles (160 km).

Mountain

Mountain biking began in the 1970s, originally as a downhill sport, practised on customized cruiser bicycles around Mount Tamalpais. Most mountain biking takes place on dirt roads, trails and in purpose-built parks. Downhill mountain biking has just evolved in the recent years and is performed at places such as Whistler Mountain Bike Park. Slopestyle, a form of downhill, is when riders do tricks such as tailwhips, 360s, backflips and front flips. There are several disciplines of mountain biking besides downhill. Cross country, often referred to as XC, all mountain, trail, free ride, and newly popular enduro.

Other

The Marching and Cycling Band HHK from Haarlem (the Netherlands) is one of the few marching bands around the world which also performs on bicycles.

Racing

Shortly after the introduction of bicycles, competitions developed independently in many parts of the world. Early races involving boneshaker style bicycles were predictably fraught with injuries. Large races became popular during the 1890s "Golden Age of Cycling", with events across Europe, and in the U.S. and Japan as well. At one point, almost every major city in the US had a velodrome or two for track racing events, however since the middle of the 20th century cycling has become a minority sport in the US whilst in Continental Europe it continues to be a major sport, particularly in the United Kingdom, France, Belgium, Italy and Spain. The most famous of all bicycle races is the Tour de France. This began in 1903, and continues to capture the attention of the sporting world.

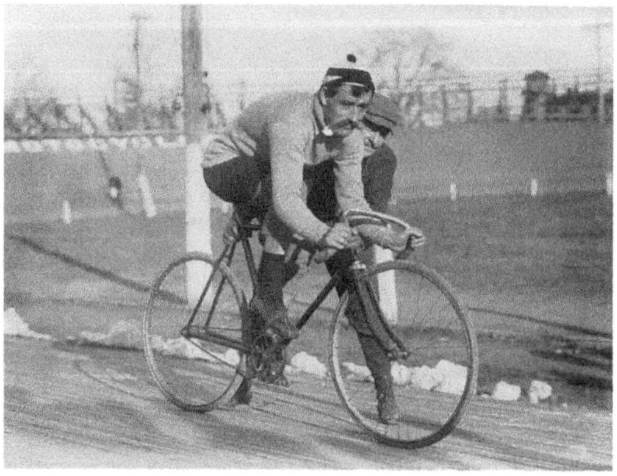

Bicycle racing in 1909.

In 1899, Charles Minthorn Murphy became the first man to ride his bicycle a mile in under a minute (hence his nickname, Mile-a-Minute Murphy), which he did by drafting a locomotive at New York's Long Island.

As the bicycle evolved its various forms, different racing formats developed. Road races may involve both team and individual competition, and are contested in various ways. They range from the one-day road race, criterium, and time trial to multi-stage events like the Tour de France and its sister events which make up cycling's Grand Tours. Recumbent bicycles were banned from bike races in 1934 after Marcel Berthet set a new hour record in his *Velodyne streamliner* (49.992 km on November 18, 1933). Track bicycles are used for track cycling in Velodromes, while cyclo-cross races are held on outdoor terrain, including pavement, grass, and mud. Cyclocross races feature man-made features such as small barriers which riders either bunny hop over or dismount and walk over. Time trial races, another form of road racing require a rider to ride against the clock. Time trials can be performed as a team or as a single rider. Bikes are changed for time trial races, using aero bars. In the past decade, mountain bike racing has also reached international popularity and is even an Olympic sport.

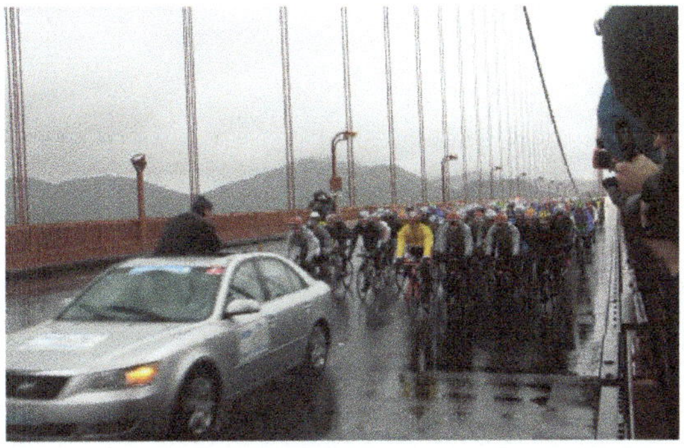

A peloton of professional bicycle racers on the Golden Gate Bridge

Professional racing organizations place limitations on the bicycles that can be used in the races that they sanction. For example, the Union Cycliste Internationale, the governing body of international cycle sport (which sanctions races such as the Tour de France), decided in the late 1990s to create additional rules which prohibit racing bicycles weighing less than 6.8 kilograms (14.96 pounds). The UCI rules also effectively ban some bicycle frame innovations (such as the recumbent bicycle) by requiring a double triangle structure.

War

The bicycle is not suited for combat, but it has been used as a method of reconnaissance as well as transporting soldiers and supplies to combat zones. In this it has taken over many of the functions of horses in warfare. In the Second Boer War, both sides used bicycles for scouting. In World War I, France, Germany, Australia and New Zealand used bicycles to move troops. In its 1937 invasion of China, Japan employed some 50,000 bicycle troops, and similar forces were instrumental in Japan's march or "roll" through Malaya in World War II. Germany used bicycles again in World War II, while the British employed airborne "Cycle-commandos" with folding bikes.

In the Vietnam War, communist forces used bicycles extensively as cargo carriers along the Ho Chi Minh Trail.

The last country known to maintain a regiment of bicycle troops was Switzerland, which disbanded its last unit in 2003.

Activism

Two broad and correlated themes run in bicycle activism: one is about advocating the bicycle as an alternative mode of transport, and the other is about the creation of conditions to permit and/or encourage bicycle use, both for utility and recreational cycling. Although the first, which emphasizes the potential for energy and resource conservation and health benefits gained from cycling versus automobile use, is relatively undisputed, the second is the subject of much debate.

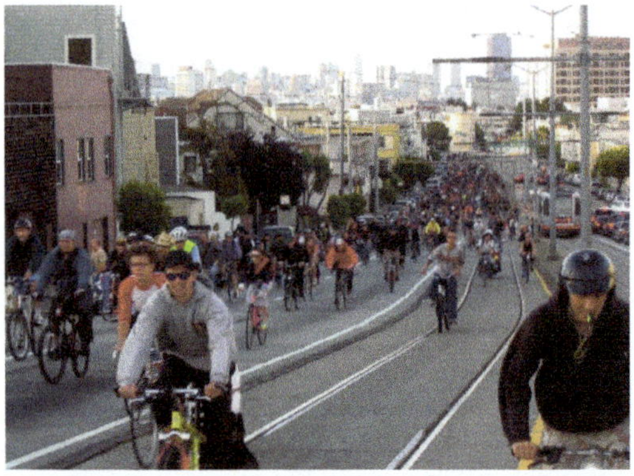

San Francisco Critical Mass, April 29, 2005.

It is generally agreed that improved local and inter-city rail services and other methods of mass transportation (including greater provision for cycle carriage on such services) create conditions to encourage bicycle use. However, there are different opinions on the role of various types of cycling infrastructure in building bicycle-friendly cities and roads.

Some bicycle activists (including some traffic management advisers) seek the construction of bike paths, cycle tracks and bike lanes for journeys of all lengths and point to their success in promoting safety and encouraging more people to cycle. Some activists, especially those from the vehicular cycling tradition, view the safety, practicality, and intent of such facilities with suspicion. They favor a more holistic approach based on the 4 'E's; *education* (of everyone involved), *encouragement* (to apply the education), *enforcement* (to protect the rights of others), and *engineering* (to facilitate travel while respecting every person's equal right to do so). Some groups offer training courses to help cyclists integrate themselves with other traffic.

Critical Mass is an event typically held on the last Friday of every month in cities around the world where bicyclists take to the streets *en masse*. While the ride was originally founded with the idea of drawing attention to how unfriendly the city was to bicyclists, the leaderless structure of Critical Mass makes it impossible to assign it any one specific goal. In fact, the purpose of Critical Mass is not formalized beyond the direct action of meeting at a set location and time and traveling as a group through city streets.

There is a long-running cycle helmet debate among activists. The most heated controversy surrounds the topic of compulsory helmet use.

Associations

Cyclists form associations, both for specific interests (trails development, road maintenance, bike maintenance, urban design, racing clubs, touring clubs, etc.) and for more global goals (energy conservation, pollution reduction, promotion of fitness). Some bicycle clubs and national associations became prominent advocates for improvements to roads and highways. In the United States, the League of American Wheelmen lobbied for the improvement of roads in the last part of the 19th century, founding and leading the national Good Roads Movement. Their model for political organization, as well as the paved roads for which they argued, facilitated the growth of the automobile.

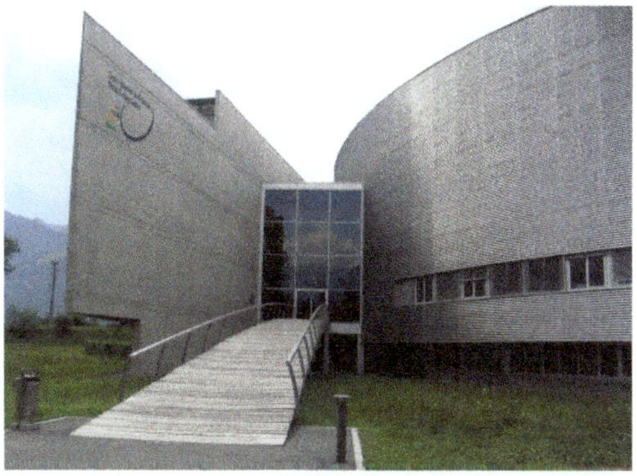

Headquarters of the Union Cycliste Internationale in Switzerland

As a sport, cycling is governed internationally by the Union Cycliste Internationale in Switzerland, USA Cycling (merged with the United States Cycling Federation in 1995) in the United States, (for upright bicycles) and by the International Human Powered Vehicle Association (for other HPVs, or human-powered vehicles). Cycling for transport and touring is promoted on a European level by the European Cyclists' Federation, with associated members from Great Britain, Japan and elsewhere. Regular conferences on cycling as transport are held under the auspices of Velo City; global conferences are coordinated by Velo Mondial.

Health Effects

The health benefits of cycling outweigh the risks, when cycling is compared to a sedentary lifestyle. A Dutch study found that cycling can extend lifespans by up to 14 months, but the risks equated to a reduced lifespan of 40 days or less. Cycling in the Netherlands is much safer than in other parts of the world. Overall, benefits of cycling or walking have been shown to exceed risks by ratios of 9:1 to 96:1 when compared with no exercise at all. These studies do not compare cycling with other forms of cardiovascular conditioning that do not come with cycling's inherent risks.

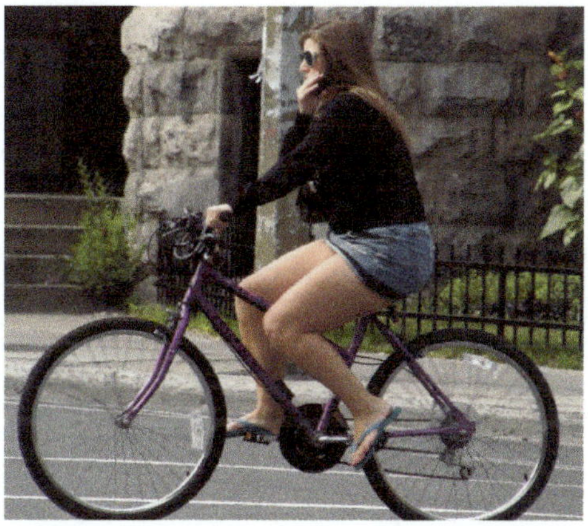

Woman doing casual cycling in Canada

Exercise

The physical exercise gained from cycling is generally linked with increased health and well-being. According to the World Health Organization, physical inactivity is second only to tobacco smoking as a health risk in developed countries, and this is associated with many tens of billions of dollars of healthcare costs. The WHO's report suggests that increasing physical activity is a public health 'best buy', and that cycling is a 'highly suitable activity' for this purpose. The charity Sustrans reports that investment in cycling provision can give a 20:1 return from health and other benefits. It has been estimated that, on average, approximately 20 life-years are gained from the health benefits of road bicycling for every life-year lost through injury.

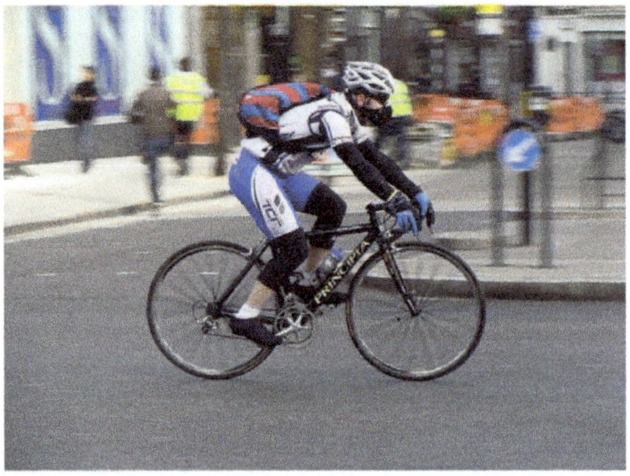

Heavily equipped London cyclist: specialist cycle clothing, pollution mask, dark glasses and helmet.

Bicycles are often used by people seeking to improve their fitness and cardiovascular health. In this regard, cycling is especially helpful for those with arthritis of the lower limbs who are unable to pursue sports that cause impact to the knees and other joints. Since cycling can be used for the practical purpose of transportation, there can be less need for self-discipline to exercise.

Cycling while seated is a relatively non-weight bearing exercise that, like swimming, does little to promote bone density. Cycling up and out of the saddle, on the other hand, does a better job by transferring more of the rider's body weight to the legs. However, excessive cycling while standing can cause knee damage It used to be thought that cycling while standing was less energy efficient, but recent research has proven this not to be true. Other than air resistance, there is no wasted energy from cycling while standing, if it is done correctly.

Cycling on a stationary cycle is frequently advocated as a suitable exercise for rehabilitation, particularly for lower limb injury, owing to the low impact which it has on the joints. In particular, cycling is commonly used within knee rehabilitation programs.

As a response to the increased global sedentarity and consequent overweight and obesity, one response that has been adopted by many organizations concerned with health and environment is the promotion of Active travel, which seeks to promote walking and cycling as safe and attractive alternatives to motorized transport. Given that many journeys are for relatively short distances, there is considerable scope to replace car use with walking or cycling, though in many settings this may require some infrastructure modification, particularly to attract the less experienced and confident.

Bicycle Safety

Cycling suffers from a perception that it is unsafe. This perception is not always backed by hard numbers, because of under reporting of accidents and lack of bicycle use data (amount of cycling, kilometers cycled) which make it hard to assess the risk and monitor changes in risks. In the UK, fatality rates per mile or kilometre are slightly less than those for walking. In the US, bicycling fatality rates are less than 2/3 of those walking the same distance. However, in the UK for example the fatality and serious injury rates *per hour of travel* are just over *double* for cycling than those for walking. Thus if a person is, for example, about to undertake a ten kilometre journey to a given destination it may on average be safer to undertake this journey by bicycle than on foot. However, if a person is intending, for example, to undertake an hour's exercise it is likely to be considerably *more* dangerous to take that exercise by cycling rather than by walking.

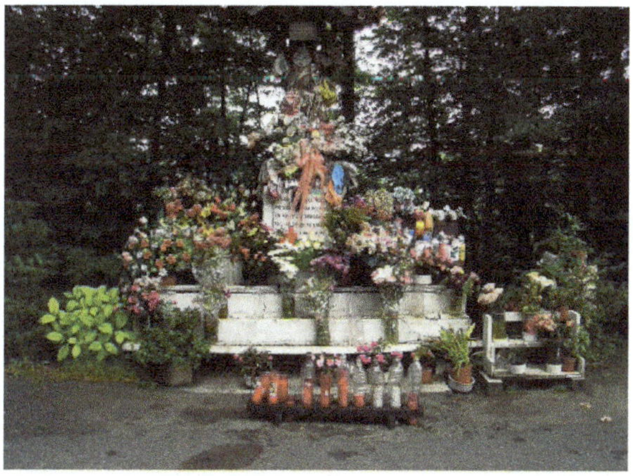

Virgin Mary venerated as the holy protector of bicyclists on the roads of the mountainous Basque Country

Despite the risk factors associated with bicycling, cyclists have a lower overall mortality rate when compared to other groups. A Danish study in 2000 found that even after adjustment for other risk factors, including leisure time physical activity, those who did not cycle to work experienced a 39% higher mortality rate than those who did.

Injuries (to cyclists, from cycling) can be divided into two types:

- Physical trauma (extrinsic)
- Overuse (intrinsic).

Physical Trauma

Acute physical trauma includes injuries to the head and extremities resulting from falls and collisions. Most cycle deaths result from a collision with a car or heavy goods vehicle, both motorist and cyclist having been found responsible for collisions. A third of collisions between motorists and cyclists are caused by car dooring. However, around a fifth of non-fatal injuries to cyclists do not involve any other person or vehicle.

Since a large percentage of the collisions between motor and pedal vehicles occur at night, bicycle lighting is recommended for safety when bicycling at night.

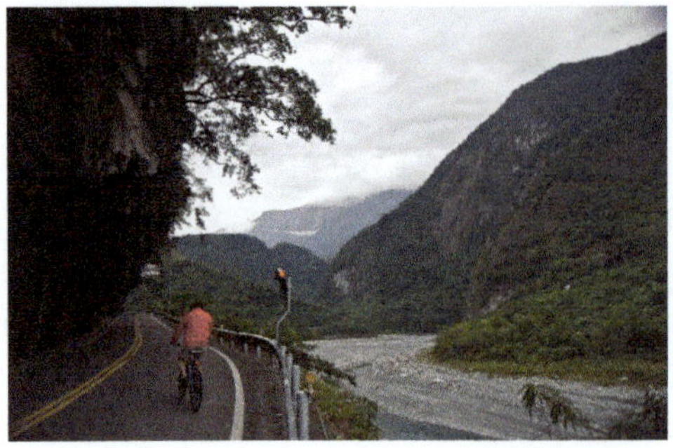

Bicyclist pedals uphill at the Taroko Gorge in Taiwan

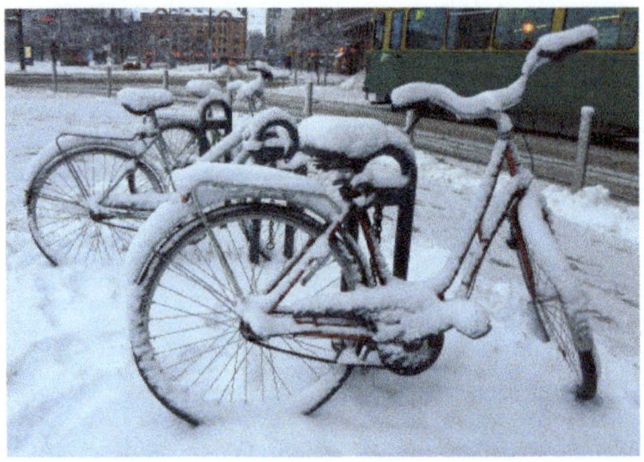

Bicycles in Helsinki (Finland)

Overuse Injuries

Of a study of 518 cyclists, a large majority reported at least one overuse injury, with over one third requiring medical treatment. The most common injury sites were the neck (48.8%) and the knees (41.7%), as well as the groin/buttocks (36.1%), hands (31.1%), and back (30.3%). Women were more likely to suffer from neck and shoulder pain than men.

Many cyclists suffer from overuse injuries to the knees, affecting cyclists at all levels. These are caused by many factors:

- Incorrect bicycle fit or adjustment, particularly the saddle.
- Incorrect adjustment of clipless pedals.
- Too many hills, or too many miles, too early in the training season.
- Poor training preparation for long touring rides.
- Selecting too high a gear. A lower gear for uphill climb protects the knees, even though muscles may be well able to handle a higher gear.

Excessive saddle height can cause posterior knee pain, while setting the saddle too low can cause pain in the anterior of the knee. An incorrectly fitted saddle may eventually lead to muscle imbalance. A 25 to 35 degree knee angle is recommended to avoid an overuse injury.

Overuse injuries, including chronic nerve damage at weight bearing locations, can occur as a result of repeatedly riding a bicycle for extended periods of time. Damage to the ulnar nerve in the palm, carpal tunnel in the wrist, the genitourinary tract or bicycle seat neuropathy may result from overuse. Recumbent bicycles are designed on different ergonomic principles and eliminate pressure from the saddle and handlebars, due to the relaxed riding position.

Note that overuse is a relative term, and capacity varies greatly between individuals. Someone starting out in cycling must be careful to increase length and frequency of cycling sessions slowly, starting for example at an hour or two per day, or a hundred miles or kilometers per week. Bilateral muscular pain is a normal by-product of the training process, whereas unilateral pain may reveal "exercise-induced arterial endofibrosis". Joint pain and numbness are also early signs of overuse injury.

Cycling has been linked to sexual impotence due to pressure on the perineum from the seat, but fitting a proper sized seat prevents this effect. In extreme cases, pudendal nerve entrapment can be a source of intractable perineal pain. Some cyclists with induced pudendal nerve pressure neuropathy gained relief from improvements in saddle position and riding techniques.

The National Institute for Occupational Safety and Health (NIOSH) has investigated the potential health effects of prolonged bicycling in police bicycle patrol units, including the possibility that some bicycle saddles exert excessive pressure on the urogenital area of cyclists, restricting blood flow to the genitals. Their study found that using bicycle seats without protruding noses reduced pressure on the groin by at least 65% and significantly reduced the number of cases of urogenital paresthesia. A follow-up found that 90% of bicycle officers who tried the no-nose seat were using it six months later. NIOSH recommends that riders use a no-nose bicycle seat for workplace bicycling.

A Spanish study of top triathletes found those who cover more than 186 miles (300 km) a week on their bikes have less than 4% normal looking sperm, where normal adult males would be expected to have from 15% to 20%.

Despite rumors to the contrary, there is no scientific evidence linking cycling with testicular cancer.

Exposure to Air Pollution

One concern is that riding in traffic may expose the cyclist to higher levels of air pollution, especially if he or she travels on or along busy roads. Some authors have claimed this to be untrue, showing that the pollutant and irritant count within cars is consistently higher, presumably because of limited circulation of air within the car and due to the air intake being directly in the stream of other traffic. Other authors have found small or inconsistent differences in concentrations but claim that exposure of cyclists is higher due to increased minute ventilation and is associated with minor biological changes. The significance of the associated health effect, if any, is unclear but probably much smaller than the health impacts associated with accidents and the health benefits derived from additional physical activity.

Burpee (Exercise)

The burpee, or squat thrust, is a full body exercise used in strength training and as an aerobic exercise. The basic movement is performed in four steps and known as a "four-count burpee":

1. Begin in a standing position.
2. Drop into a squat position with your hands on the ground. (count 1)
3. Kick your feet back into a plank position, while keeping your arms extended. (count 2)
4. Immediately return your feet to the squat position. (count 3)
5. from the squat position (count 4)

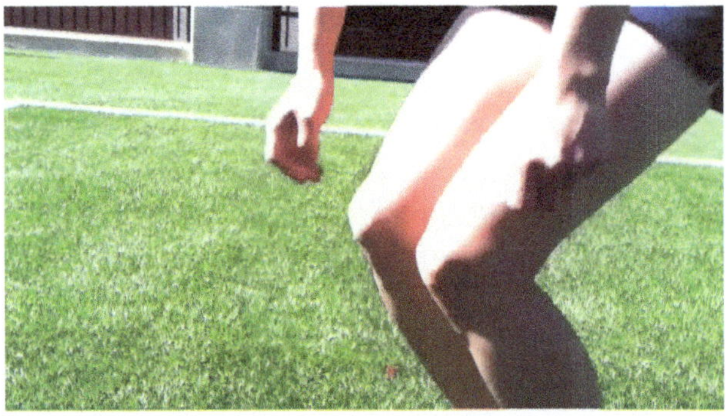

See how to do a basic burpee (the squat thurst version - with the fifth step (count 4) replaced with standing up rather than jumping up).

Origin

According to Oxford Dictionaries Online, the exercise was named in the 1930s for American physiologist Royal H. Burpee, who developed the *burpee test*. He earned a PhD in applied physiology from Columbia University in 1940 and created the "burpee" exercise as part of his PhD thesis as a quick and simple way to assess fitness. The exercise was popularized when the United States Armed Services adopted it as a way to assess the fitness level of recruits when the US entered WWII. Consisting of a series of the exercises performed in rapid succession, the test was meant to be a quick measure of agility, coordination and strength.

Variants

Box-jump burpee

The athlete jumps onto a box, rather than straight up and down.

Burpee broad jump

A burpee followed by a stationary two footed distance jump.

Burpee push up (also known as a "bastardo")

The athlete performs one push-up after assuming the push-up position.

Dumbbell burpee

The athlete holds a pair of dumbbells while performing the exercise.

Eight-count push up or Double burpee

The athlete performs two push-ups after assuming the plank position. This cancels the drive from landing after the jump and makes the next jump harder. Each part of the burpee might be repeated to make it even harder.

Hindu push up burpee

Instead of a regular push up, do a Hindu push up.

Jump-over burpee

The athlete jumps over an obstacle between burpees.

Burpee

The athlete jumps straight up as high as possible at the end of the movement, before beginning the next burpee.

Knee push-up burpee

The athlete bends their knees and rests them on the ground before performing the push up.

Long-jump burpee

The athlete jumps forward, not upward.

Muscle-up burpee

Combine a muscle-up (a variation of a pull-up) with the jump or do a muscle-up instead of the jump.

One-armed burpee

The athlete uses only one arm for the whole exercise including the pushup.

One leg burpee

The athlete stands on one leg, bends at the waist and puts hands on ground so they are aligned with shoulders. Next jump back with the standing leg to plank position. Jump forward with the one leg that was extended, and do a one-leg jump. Repeat on opposite side.

Parkour burpee

Following one burpee on the ground, the athlete jumps upon a table and performs the second burpee on the table, then jumps back to the initial position.

Pull-up burpee

Combine a pull-up with the jump or do a pull-up instead of the jump.

Side burpee

The athlete bends at waist and places hand shoulder-width apart to the side of right or left foot. Jump both legs out to side and land on the outer and inner sides of your feet. Jump back in, jump up, and repeat on opposite side.

Squat Thrust

Same as a four-count burpee except the fourth count is only standing up from the squat instead of jumping.

Tuck-jump burpee

The athlete pulls their knees to their chest (tucks) at the peak of the jump.

Burpee pull and push up (body blaster)

The athlete performs a push up when in the plank position of the burpee for 30 seconds to a minute depending on what they would like, then jumps and finishes with a pull-up, and repeats.

World Records

At 4 pm on May 17, 2014, in Greenwood, SC, Cameron Dorn broke two burpee world records: the most burpees performed in 12 hours with 5,657 and the most burpees completed in 24 hours with 10,105.

At 6 am on October 21, 2013, in Portland, OR, Lloyd Weema broke the burpee world record: the most chest to ground burpees performed in 72 hours with 9,480.

Skipping Rope

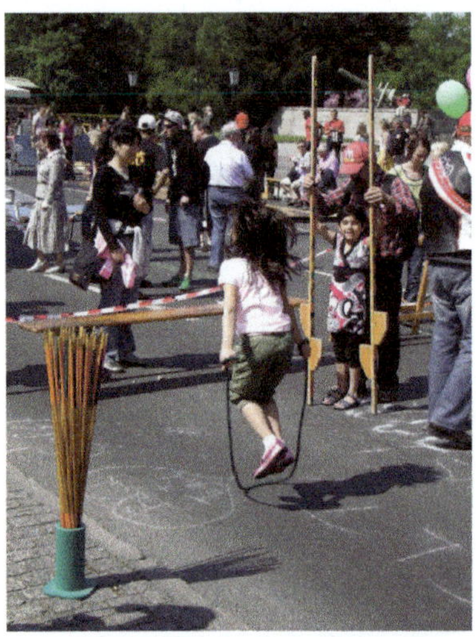

A young girl playing on a skipping rope.

A skipping rope (British English) or jump rope (American English) is a tool used in the activity of skipping played by children and many young adults, where one or more participants jump over a rope swung so that it passes under their feet and over their heads. There are three main variations of the activity. The most basic involves a single participant turning and jumping the rope. *Long rope* involves a minimum of three participants, two of whom turn the rope while one or more jump. The most difficult version, often called Double Dutch, also involves three or more participants, but uses two ropes turned in opposite directions. Rhymes are often chanted during the activity.

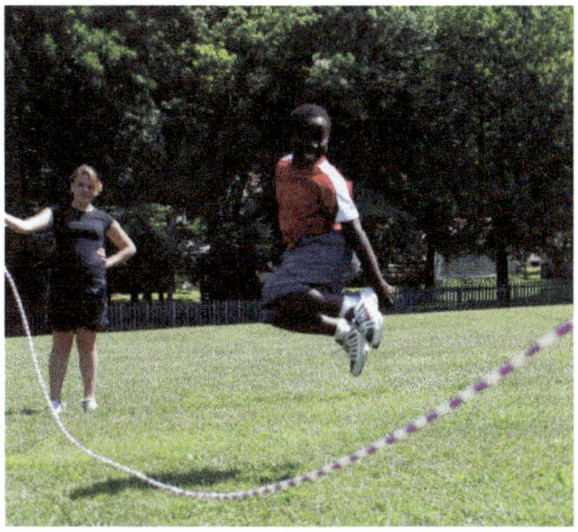

Boy jumps *Long rope* in Virginia

Skipping Rope Techniques

There are many techniques which can be used when using a skipping rope. These can be used individually, or combined in a series.

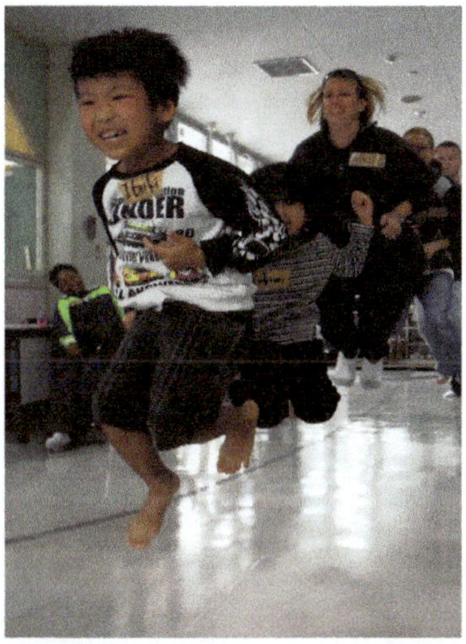

Several simultaneous jumpers, jumping a single rope

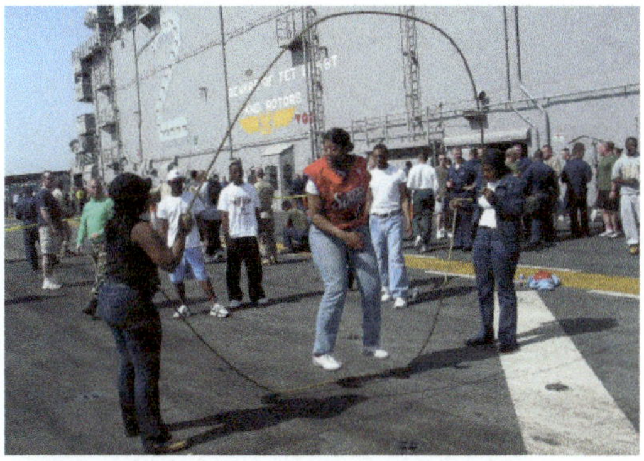

Double Dutch - Competition during a steel beach picnic on the ship USS *Saipan* (LHA-2)

Solo Participants

Basic Jump or Easy Jump

Jump with both feet slightly apart over the rope. Beginners usually master this technique first before moving onto more advanced techniques.

Alternate Foot Jump (Speed Step)

Use alternate feet to jump off the ground. This technique can be used to effectively double the number of skips per minute as compared to the above technique. This step can be used for speed events.

Criss-cross

Perform the basic jump whilst crossing arms in front of the body.

Side Swing

The rope is passed by the side of the participant's body, without jumping it.

EB (Front-back Cross)

Perform the criss-cross whilst crossing one arm behind the back.

Double Under

A high basic jump, turning the rope twice under the feet. Turning the rope three times is called a triple under. In competitions, participants may attempt quadruple (quads) and quintuple unders (quins) using the same method.

Toad

Perform the criss-cross with one arm crossing under the opposite leg from the inside.

Leg Over

A basic jump with one arm hooked under the adjacent leg.

Awesome Annie

Alternates between a leg over and a toad without a jump in between.

Inverse Toad

Perform the toad whilst one arm crosses the adjacent leg from the outside.

Elephant

A cross between the inverse toad and the toad, with both arms crossing under one leg.

Frog or Donkey Kick

The participant does a handstand, returns to their feet and turns the rope under them. A more advanced version turns the rope during the return to the ground.

The James Hirst

The participant performs a backflip into a split and then back to a skip in the upright position.

Competition Techniques

In competitions, participants are required to demonstrate competence using specific techniques. The selection required depend on the judging system and country in which the tournament is held.

Health Effects

Skipping as Exercise

Skipping may be used for a cardiovascular workout, similar to jogging or bicycle riding. This aerobic exercise can achieve a "burn rate" of up to 700 calories per hour of vigorous activity, with about 0.1 calories consumed per jump. Ten minutes of skipping is roughly the equivalent of running an eight-minute mile. Jumping rope for 15–20 minutes is enough to burn off the calories from a candy bar.

Weighted skipping ropes are available for such athletes to increase the difficulty and effectiveness of such exercise. Individuals or groups can participate in the exercise, and learning proper techniques is relatively simple compared to many other athletic activities. The exercise is also appropriate for a wide range of ages and fitness levels.

Competition

United States

Historically in the United States there were two competing jump rope organizations: the International Rope Skipping Organization (IRSO), and the World Rope Skipping Federation (WRSF). IRSO focused on stunt-oriented and gymnastic/athletic type moves, while the WRSF appreciated the aesthetics and form of the exercise. In 1995 these two organizations merged to form The United States Amateur Jump Rope Federation (USAJRF). USAJRF hosts annual national tournaments, as well as camps, workshops, and clinics on instruction. Jump rope is also part of the Amateur Athletic Union and participates in their annual AAU Junior Olympic Games.

Jumping Jack

A jumping jack (Canada & US) or star jump (UK and other Commonwealth nations), also called side-straddle hop in the US military, is a physical jumping exercise performed by jumping to a position with the legs spread wide and the hands touching overhead, sometimes in a clap, and then returning to a position with the feet together and the arms at the sides. The jumping jack name comes from the traditional toy of the same name, while "star jump" refers to the person's appearance with legs and arms spread.

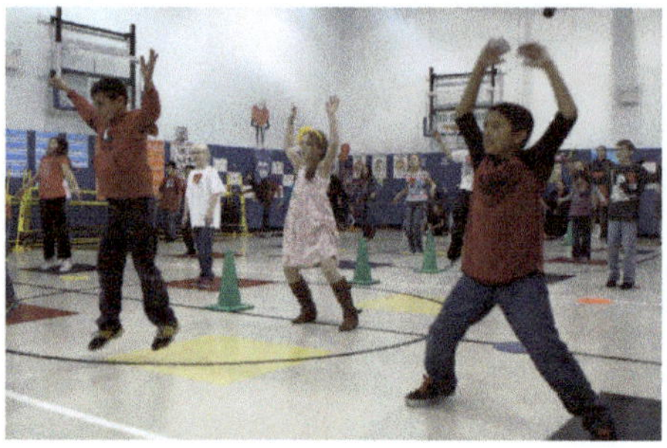

Schoolchildren in the US performing jumping jacks

Variations

More intensive versions of this jump include bending down (over) and touching the floor in between each jump.

Power JacksPower Jacks are similar to jumping jacks, except a person squats lower and jumps as high as possible during each repetition.

A similar jump exercise is called half-jacks, which were created to prevent rotator cuff injuries, which have been linked to the repetitive movements of the exercise. They are like regular jumping jacks but the arms go halfway above the head instead of all the way above it. The arms also hit the sides to help tighten the jump.

Although he played no part in inventing the exercise, the late fitness expert Jack LaLanne was given credit for popularizing it in the United States. LaLanne used the jumping exercise during routines he promoted in decades of television fitness programming.

Ashrita Furman set the Guinness World Record for number of star jumps (jumping jacks) in one minute at 61, on May 17, 2008. Raymond Butler set a new record of 77 on September 18, 2013. In 2010, National Geographic Kids organized an event in 1050 locations as a part of Michelle Obama's "Let's Move!" exercise campaign in which 300,365 people were measured doing jumping jacks (for one minute) in a 24-hour period.

Jogging

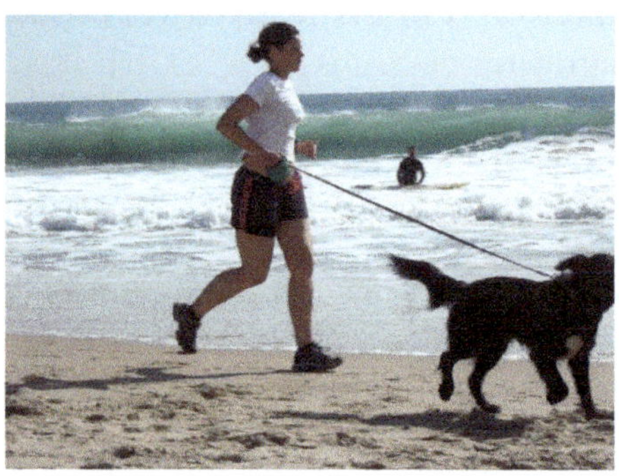

Woman jogging with a dog on Carcavelos Beach

Jogging is a form of trotting or running at a slow or leisurely pace. The main intention is to increase physical fitness with less stress on the body than from faster running, or to maintain a steady speed for longer periods of time. Performed over long distances, it is a form of aerobic endurance training.

Definition

Jogging is running at a gentle pace. The definition of jogging as compared with running is not standard. One definition describes jogging as running slower than 6 miles per hour (10 km/h).

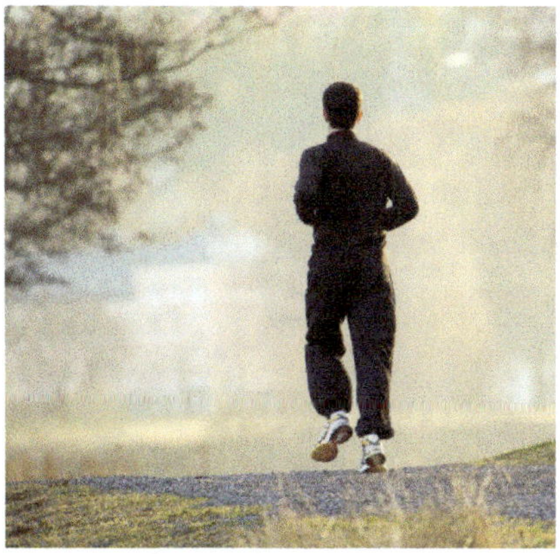

Evening jogger in Skien, Norway.

Jogging is also distinguished from running by having a wider lateral spacing of foot strikes, creating side-to-side movement that likely adds stability at slower speeds or when coordination is lacking.

History

The word *jog* originated in England in the mid-16th century. The etymology of the word is unknown, but it may be related to *shog* or have been a new invention. In 1593, William Shakespeare wrote in *Taming of the Shrew*, "you may be jogging whiles your boots are green". At that point, it usually meant to leave. The term *jog* was often used in English and North American literature to describe short quick movements, either intentional or unintentional. It is also used to describe a quick, sharp shake or jar. Richard Jefferies, an English naturalist, wrote of "joggers", describing them as quickly moving people who brushed others aside as they passed. This usage became common throughout the British Empire, and in his 1884 novel *My Run Home*, the Australian author Rolf Boldrewood wrote, "Your bedroom curtains were still drawn as I passed on my morning jog".

In the United States jogging was called "roadwork" when athletes in training, such as boxers, customarily ran several miles each day as part of their conditioning. In New Zealand during the 1960s or 1970s, the word "roadwork" was mostly supplanted by the word "jogging", promoted by coach Arthur Lydiard, who is credited with popularizing jogging. The idea of jogging as an organised activity was mooted in a sports page article in the *New Zealand Herald* in February 1962, which told of a group of former athletes and fitness enthusiasts who would meet once a week to run for "fitness and sociability". Since they would be jogging, the newspaper suggested that the club "may be called the Auckland Joggers' Club"—which is thought to be the first use of the noun "jogger". University of Oregon track coach Bill Bowerman, after jogging with Lydiard in New Zealand in 1962, published the book *Jogging* in 1966, popularizing jogging in the United States.

Burundi Jogging Ban

In March 2014, jogging was banned in Burundi due to "fears it was being used as a cover for subversion". According to the BBC, "The tradition of Saturday morning runs started during Burundi's long years of ethnic conflict", as residents in the city of Bujumbura, where the surrounding hills were home to armed militants before 2005, "would try to vent their fear and frustration and claustrophobia, by running, often in a group".

Exercise

Jogging may also be used as a warm up or cool down for runners, preceding or following a workout or race. It is often used by serious runners as a means of active recovery during interval training. For example, a runner who completes a fast 400 metre repetition at a sub-5-minute mile pace may drop to an 8-minute mile jogging pace for a recovery lap.

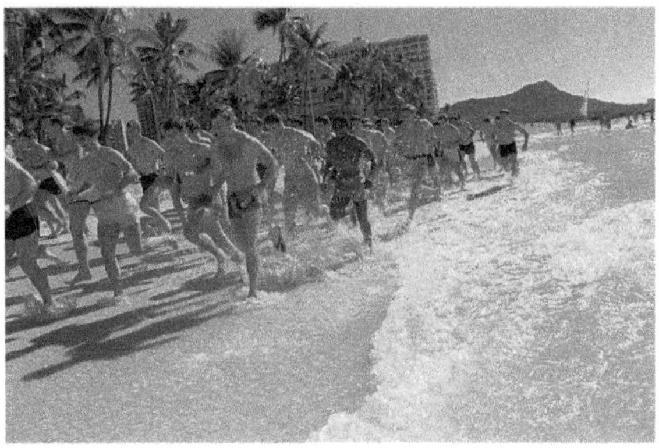

Members of the United States Air Force Academy American football team jog on Waikiki beach, Hawaii.

Jogging can be used as a method to increase endurance or to provide a means of cardiovascular exercise but with less stress on joints or demand on the circulatory system.

Benefits

According to a study by Stanford University School of Medicine, jogging is effective in increasing human lifespan, and decreasing the effects of aging, with benefits for the cardiovascular system. Jogging is useful for fighting obesity and staying healthy.

The National Cancer Institute has performed studies that suggest jogging and other types of aerobic exercise can reduce the risk of lung, colon, breast and prostate cancers, among others. It is suggested by the American Cancer Society that jogging for at least 30 minutes five days a week can help in cancer prevention.

While jogging on a treadmill will provide health benefits such as cancer prevention, and aid in weight loss, a study published in BMC Public Health reports that jogging outdoors can have the additional benefits of increased energy and concentration. Jogging outdoors is a better way to improve energy levels and advance mood than using a treadmill at the gym.

Jogging also prevents muscle and bone damage that often occurs with age, improves heart performance and blood circulation and assists in preserving a balanced weight gain.

A Danish study released in 2015 reported that "light" and "moderate" jogging were associated with reduced mortality compared to both non-jogging and "strenuous" jogging. The optimal amount per week was 1 to 2.4 hours, the optimal frequency was 2–3 times per week, and the optimal speed was "slow" or "average".

Strength Training

Strength training is a type of physical exercise specializing in the use of resistance to induce muscular contraction which builds the strength, anaerobic endurance, and size of skeletal muscles.

When properly performed, strength training can provide significant functional benefits and improvement in overall health and well-being, including increased bone, muscle, tendon and ligament strength and toughness, improved joint function, reduced potential for injury, increased bone density, increased metabolism, increased fitness, improved cardiac function, and improved lipoprotein lipid profiles, including elevated HDL ("good") cholesterol. Training commonly uses the technique of progressively increasing the force output of the muscle through incremental weight increases and uses a variety of exercises and types of equipment to target specific muscle groups. Strength training is primarily an anaerobic activity, although some proponents have adapted it to provide the benefits of aerobic exercise through circuit training.

Sports where strength training is central are bodybuilding, weightlifting, powerlifting, strongman, Highland games, shotput, discus throw, and javelin throw. Many other sports use strength training as part of their training regimen, notably American football, wrestling, track and field, rowing, lacrosse, basketball, pole dancing, hockey, professional wrestling, rugby union, rugby league and soccer. Strength training for other sports and physical activities is becoming increasingly popular.

Uses

The benefits of weight training include greater muscular strength, improved muscle tone and appearance, increased endurance and enhanced bone density.

Increased Physical Attractiveness

Many people take up weight training to improve their physical attractiveness. There is evidence that a body type consisting of broad shoulders and a narrow waist, attainable through strength training, is the most physically attractive male attribute according to women participating in the research. Most men can develop substantial muscles; most women lack the testosterone to do it, but they can develop a firm, "toned" physique, and they can increase their strength by the same proportion as that achieved by men (but usually from a significantly lower starting point). An individual's genetic make-up dictates the response to weight training stimuli to a significant extent, training can not exceed a muscle's intrinsic genetically determined qualities, but clearly polymorphic expression of Myosin heavy chains is possible.

Workouts elevate metabolism for up to 14 hours following 45-minutes of vigorous exercise.

Increased General Physical Health

Strength training also provides functional benefits. Stronger muscles improve posture, provide better support for joints, and reduce the risk of injury from everyday activities. Older people who take up weight training can prevent some of the loss of muscle tissue that normally accompanies aging—and even regain some functional strength—and by doing so become less frail. They may be able to avoid some types of physical disability. Weight-bearing exercise also helps to prevent osteoporosis and to improve bone strength in those with osteoporosis. The benefits of weight training for older people have been confirmed by studies of people who began engaging in it even in their 80s and 90s.

Though strength training can stimulate the cardiovascular system, many exercise physiologists, based on their observation of maximal oxygen uptake, argue that aerobics training is a better cardiovascular stimulus. Central catheter monitoring during resistance training reveals increased cardiac output, suggesting that strength training shows potential for cardiovascular exercise. However, a 2007 meta-analysis found that, though aerobic training is an effective therapy for heart failure patients, combined aerobic and strength training is ineffective.

Strength training may be important to metabolic and cardiovascular health. Recent evidence suggests that resistance training may reduce metabolic and cardiovascular disease risk. Overweight individuals with high strength fitness exhibit metabolic/cardiovascular risk profiles similar to normal-weight, fit individuals rather than overweight unfit individuals.

For Rehabilitation or to Address an Impairment

For many people in rehabilitation or with an acquired disability, such as following stroke or orthopaedic surgery, strength training for weak muscles is a key factor to optimise recovery. For people with such a health condition, their strength training is likely to need to be designed by an appropriate health professional, such as a physiotherapist or an occupational therapist.

Increased Sports Performance

Stronger muscles improve performance in a variety of sports. Sport-specific training routines are used by many competitors. These often specify that the speed of muscle contraction during weight training should be the same as that of the particular sport.

For the Pleasure of the Activity

One side effect of any intense exercise is increased levels of dopamine, serotonin, and norepinephrine, which can help to improve mood and counter feelings of depression.

Developing research has demonstrated that many of the benefits of exercise are mediated through the role of skeletal muscle as an endocrine organ. That is, contracting muscles release multiple substances known as myokines which promote the growth of new tissue, tissue repair, and various anti-inflammatory functions, which in turn reduce the risk of developing various inflammatory diseases.

Technique

The basic principles of strength training involve a manipulation of the number of repetitions (reps), sets, tempo, exercises and force to cause desired changes in strength, endurance or size by overloading of a group of muscles. The specific combinations of reps, sets, exercises, resistance and force depend on the purpose of the individual performing the exercise: to gain size and strength multiple (4+) sets with fewer reps must be performed using more force. A wide spectrum of regimens can be adopted to achieve different results, but the classic formula recommended by the American College of Sports Medicine reads as follows:

- 8 to 12 repetitions of a resistance training exercise for each major muscle group at an intensity of 40% to 80% of a one-repetition max (RM) depending on the training level of the participant.
- Two to three minutes of rest is recommended between exercise sets to allow for proper recovery.
- Two to four sets are recommended for each muscle group

Typically failure to use good form during a training set can result in injury or an inability to meet training goals – since the desired muscle group is not challenged sufficiently, the threshold of overload is never reached and the muscle does not gain in strength. There are cases when cheating is beneficial, as is the case where weaker groups become the weak link in the chain and the target muscles are never fully exercised as a result.

The benefits of strength training include increased muscle, tendon and ligament strength, bone density, flexibility, tone, metabolic rate and postural support.

Terminology

Strength training has a variety of specialized terms used to describe parameters of strength training:

- Exercise – different movements which involve rotating joints in specific patterns to challenge muscles in different ways.
- Form – each exercise has a specific form, a topography of movement designed to maximize safety and muscle strength gains.
- Rep – short for repetition, a rep is a single cycle of lifting and lowering a weight in a controlled manner, moving through the form of the exercise.
- Set – a set consists of several repetitions performed one after another with no break between them with the number of reps per set and sets per exercise depending on the goal of the individual. The number of repetitions one can perform at a certain weight is called the Rep Maximum (RM). For example, if one could perform ten reps at 75 lbs, then their RM for that weight would be 10RM. 1RM is therefore the maximum weight that someone can lift in a given exercise – i.e. a weight that they can only lift once without a break.

- Tempo – the speed with which an exercise is performed; the tempo of a movement has implications for the weight that can be moved and the effects on the muscle.

Realization of Training Goals

For developing endurance, gradual increases in volume and gradual decreases in intensity is the most effective program. Sets of thirteen to twenty repetitions develop anaerobic endurance, with some increases to muscle size and limited impact on strength.

It has been shown that for beginners, multiple-set training offers minimal benefits over single-set training with respect to either strength gain or muscle mass increase, but for the experienced athlete multiple-set systems are required for optimal progress. However, one study shows that for leg muscles, three sets are more effective than one set.

Beginning weight-trainers are in the process of training the neurological aspects of strength, the ability of the brain to generate a rate of neuronal action potentials that will produce a muscular contraction that is close to the maximum of the muscle's potential.

Variable	Training goal				
	Strength	Power	Hypertrophy	Endurance	Speed
Load (% of 1RM)	90–80	60–45	80–60	60–40	30
Reps per set	1–5	1–5	6–12	13–60	1–5
Sets per exercise	4–7	3–5	4–8	2–4	3–5
Rest between sets (mins)	2–6	2–6	2–5	1–2	2–5
Duration (seconds per set)	5–10	4–8	20–60	80–150	20–40
Speed per rep (% of max)	60–100	90–100	60–90	60–80	100
Training sessions per week	3–6	3–6	5–7	8–14	3–6
Table reproduced from Siff, 2003					

Weights for each exercise should be chosen so that the desired number of repetitions can just be achieved.

Progressive Overload

In one common method, weight training uses the principle of progressive overload, in which the muscles are overloaded by attempting to lift at least as much weight as they are capable. They respond by growing larger and stronger. This procedure is repeated with progressively heavier weights as the practitioner gains strength and endurance.

However, performing exercises at the absolute limit of one's strength (known as one rep max lifts) is considered too risky for all but the most experienced practitioners. Moreover, most individuals wish to develop a combination of strength, endurance and muscle size. One repetition sets are not well suited to these aims. Practitioners therefore lift lighter (sub-maximal) weights, with more repetitions, to fatigue the muscle and all fibres within that muscle as required by the progressive overload principle.

Commonly, each exercise is continued to the point of momentary muscular failure. Contrary to widespread belief, this is not the point at which the individual thinks they cannot complete any more repetitions, but rather the first repetition that fails due to inadequate muscular strength. Training to failure is a controversial topic with some advocating training to failure on all sets while others believe that this will lead to overtraining, and suggest training to failure only on the last set of an exercise. Some practitioners recommend finishing a set of repetitions just before reaching a personal maximum at a given time. Adrenaline and other hormones may promote additional intensity by stimulating the body to lift additional weight (as well as the neuro-muscular stimulations that happen when in "fight-or-flight" mode, as the body activates more muscle fibres), so getting "psyched up" before a workout can increase the maximum weight lifted.

Weight training can be a very effective form of strength training because exercises can be chosen, and weights precisely adjusted, to safely exhaust each individual muscle group after the specific numbers of sets and repetitions that have been found to be the most effective for the individual. Other strength training exercises lack the flexibility and precision that weights offer.

Split Training

Split training involves working no more than three muscle groups or body parts per day, instead spreading the training of specific body parts throughout a training cycle of several days. It is commonly used by more advanced practitioners due to the logistics involved in training all muscle groups maximally. Training all the muscles in the body individually through their full range of motion in a single day is generally not considered possible due to caloric and time constraints. Split training involves fully exhausting individual muscle groups during a workout, then allowing several days for the muscle to fully recover. Muscles are worked roughly twice per week and allowed roughly 72 hours to recover. Recovery of certain muscle groups is usually achieved on days while training other groups, i.e. a 7-day week can consist of a practitioner training trapezius, side shoulders and upper shoulders to exhaustion on one day, the following day the arms to exhaustion, the day after that the rear, front shoulders and back, the day after that the chest. In this way all mentioned muscle groups are allowed the necessary recovery.

Intensity, Volume, and Frequency

Three important variables of strength training are intensity, volume, and frequency. Intensity refers to the amount of work required to achieve the activity, and is proportional to the mass of the weights being lifted. Volume refers to the number of muscles worked, exercises, sets and reps during a single session. Frequency refers to how many training sessions are performed per week.

These variables are important because they are all mutually conflicting, as the muscle only has so much strength and endurance, and takes time to recover due to microtrauma. Increasing one by any significant amount necessitates the decrease of the other two, e.g. increasing weight means a reduction of reps, and will require more recovery time and therefore fewer workouts per week. Trying to push too much intensity, volume and frequency will result in overtraining, and eventually lead to injury and other health issues such as chronic soreness and general lethargy, illness or even acute trauma such as avulsion fractures. A high-medium-low formula can be used to avoid overtraining, with either intensity, volume, or frequency being high, one of the others being medium, and the other being low. One example of this training strategy can be found in the following chart:

Type	High	Med	Low
Intensity (% of 1RM)	80–100%	50–70%	10–40%
Volume (per muscle)	1 exercise	2 exercises	3+ exercises
Sets	1 set	2–3 sets	4+ sets
Reps	1–6 reps	8–15 reps	20+ reps
Session frequency	1 p/w	2–3 p/w	4+ p/w

A common training strategy is to set the volume and frequency the same each week (e.g. training 3 times per week, with 2 sets of 12 reps each workout), and steadily increase the intensity (weight) on a weekly basis. However, to maximize progress to specific goals, individual programs may require different manipulations, such as decreasing the weight, and increase volume or frequency.

Making program alterations on a daily basis (daily undulating periodization) seems to be more efficient in eliciting strength gains than doing so every 4 weeks (linear periodization), but for beginners there are no differences between different periodization models.

Periodization

There are many complicated definitions for periodization, but the term simply means the division of the overall training program into periods which accomplish different goals.

Periodization is the modulating of volume, intensity, and frequency over time, to both stimulate gains and allow recovery.

In some programs for example; volume is decreased during a training cycle while intensity is increased. In this template, a lifter would begin a training cycle with a higher rep range than he will finish with.

For this example, the lifter has a 1 rep max of 225 lb:

Week	Set 1	Set 2	Set 3	Set 4	Set 5	Volume Lbs.	% Exertion(Last Set)	% of 1 Rep Max(Last Set)
1	125 lb x 8reps	130 lb x 8reps	135 lb x 8reps	140 lb x 8reps	145 lb x 8reps	5,400	78%	64%
2	135 lb x 7reps	140 lb x 7reps	145 lb x 7reps	150 lb x 7reps	155 lb x 7reps	5,075	81%	69%
3	145 lb x 6reps	150 lb x 6reps	155 lb x 6reps	160 lb x 6reps	165 lb x 6reps	4,650	84%	73%
4	155 lb x 5reps	160 lb x 5reps	165 lb x 5reps	170 lb x 5reps	175 lb x 5reps	4,125	87%	78%
5	165 lb x 4reps	170 lb x 4reps	175 lb x 4reps	180 lb x 4reps	185 lb x 4reps	3,500	90%	82%
6	175 lb x 3reps	180 lb x 3reps	185 lb x 3reps	190 lb x 3reps	195 lb x 3reps	2,775	92%	87%

This is an example of periodization where the number of repetitions decreases while the weight increases.

Practice of Weight Training

Methods and Equipment

There are many methods of strength training. Examples include weight training, circuit training, isometric exercise, gymnastics, plyometrics, Parkour, yoga, Pilates, Super Slow.

Strength training may be done with minimal or no equipment, for instance bodyweight exercises. Equipment used for strength training includes barbells and dumbbells, weight machines and other exercise machines, weighted clothing, resistance bands, gymnastics apparatus, Swiss balls, wobble boards, indian clubs, pneumatic exercise equipment, hydraulic exercise equipment.

Aerobic Exercise Versus Anaerobic Exercise

Strength training exercise is primarily anaerobic. Even while training at a lower intensity (training loads of ~20-RM), anaerobic glycolysis is still the major source of power, although aerobic metabolism makes a small contribution. Weight training is commonly perceived as anaerobic exercise, because one of the more common goals is to increase strength by lifting heavy weights. Other goals such as rehabilitation, weight loss, body shaping, and bodybuilding often use lower weights, adding aerobic character to the exercise.

Except in the extremes, a muscle will fire fibres of both the aerobic or anaerobic types on any given exercise, in varying ratio depending on the load on the intensity of the contraction. This is known as the energy system continuum. At higher loads, the muscle will recruit all muscle fibres possible, both anaerobic ("fast-twitch") and aerobic ("slow-twitch"), in order to generate the most force. However, at maximum load, the anaerobic processes contract so forcefully that the aerobic fibers are completely shut out, and all work is done by the anaerobic processes. Because the anaerobic muscle fibre uses its fuel faster than the blood and intracellular restorative cycles can resupply it, the maximum number of repetitions is limited. In the aerobic regime, the blood and intracellular processes can maintain a supply of fuel and oxygen, and continual repetition of the motion will not cause the muscle to fail.

Circuit weight training is a form of exercise that uses a number of weight training exercise sets separated by short intervals. The cardiovascular effort to recover from each set serves a function similar to an aerobic exercise, but this is not the same as saying that a weight training set is itself an aerobic process.

Exercises for Specific Muscle Groups

Weight trainers commonly divide the body's individual muscles into ten major muscle groups. These do not include the hip, neck and forearm muscles, which are rarely trained in isolation. The most common exercises for these muscle groups are listed below. (Videos of these and other exercises are available at exrx.net and from the University of Wisconsin-La Crosse.)

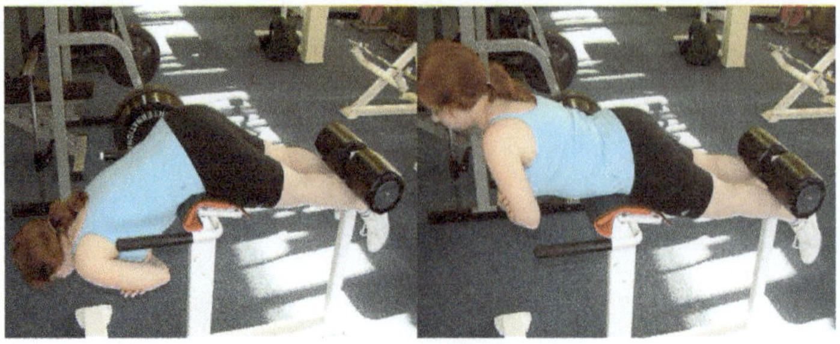

A *back extension*.

The sequence shown below is one possible way to order the exercises. The large muscles of the lower body are normally trained before the smaller muscles of the upper body, because these first exercises require more mental and physical energy. The core muscles of the torso are trained before the shoulder and arm muscles that assist them. Exercises often alternate between "pushing" and "pulling" movements to allow their specific supporting muscles time to recover. The stabilising muscles in the waist should be trained last.

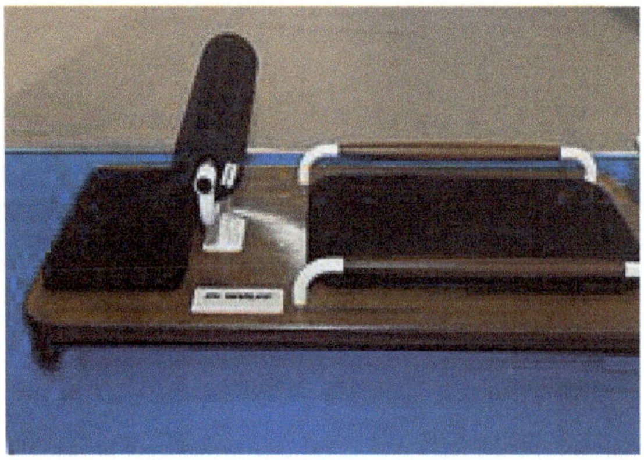

Back Exercise Faszienkurs

Advanced Techniques

A number of techniques have been developed to make weight training exercises more intense, and thereby potentially increase the rate of progress. Many weight lifters use these techniques to bring themselves past a plateau, a duration where a weightlifter may be unable to do more lifting repetitions, sets, or use higher weight resistance.

Set Structure

Drop sets

> Drop sets do not end at the point of momentary muscular failure, but continue with progressively lighter weights.

Pyramid sets

> Pyramid sets are weight training sets in which the progression is from lighter weights with a greater number of repetitions in the first set, to heavier weights with fewer repetitions in subsequent sets.

A reverse pyramid is the opposite in which the heavier weights are used at the beginning and progressively lightened.

Burnouts

Burnouts combine pyramids and drop sets, working up to higher weights with low reps and then back down to lower weights and high reps.

Diminishing set

The diminishing set method is where a weight is chosen that can be lifted for 20 reps in one set, and then 70 repetitions are performed in as few sets as possible.

Rest-pause (heavy singles)

Rest-pause heavy singles are performed at or near 1RM, with ten to twenty seconds of rest between each lift. The lift is repeated six to eight times. It is generally recommended to use this method infrequently.

Giant set

The Giant set, is a form of training that targets one muscle group (e.g. the triceps) with four separate exercises performed in quick succession, often to failure and sometimes with the reduction of weight halfway through a set once muscle fatigue sets in. This form of intense training 'shocks' the muscles and as such, is usually performed by experienced trainers and should be used infrequently.

Combined Sets

Supersets

Supersets combine two or more exercises with similar motions to maximize the amount of work of an individual muscle or group of muscles. The exercises are performed with no rest period between the exercises. An example would be doing bench press, which predominantly works the pectoralis and triceps muscles, and then moving to an exercise that works just the triceps such as the triceps extension or the pushdown.

Push-pull supersets

Push-pull supersets are similar to regular supersets, but exercises are chosen which work opposing muscle groups. This is especially popular when applied to arm exercises, for example by combining biceps curls with the triceps pushdown. Other examples include the shoulder press and lat pulldown combination, and the bench press and wide grip row combination.

Pre-exhaustion

Pre-exhaustion combines an isolation exercise with a compound exercise for the same muscle group. The isolation exercise first exhausts the muscle group, and then the compound exercise uses the muscle group's supporting muscles to push it further than would otherwise be possible. For example, the triceps muscles normally help the pectorals perform their function. But in the "bench press" the weaker triceps often fails first, which limits the impact on the pectorals. By preceding the bench press with the pec fly, the pectorals can be pre-exhausted so that both muscles fail at the same time, and both benefit equally from the exercise.

Breakdowns

Breakdowns were developed by Fredrick Hatfield and Mike Quinn to work the different types of muscle fibers for maximum stimulation. Three different exercises that work the same muscle group are selected, and used for a superset. The first exercise uses a heavy weight (~85% of 1 rep max) for around five reps, the second a medium weight (~70% of 1 rep max) for around twelve reps, and finally the third exercise is performed with a light weight (~50% of 1 rep max) for twenty to thirty reps, or even lighter (~40% of 1 rep max) for forty or more reps. (Going to failure is discouraged.) The entire superset is performed three times.

Beyond Failure

Forced reps

Forced reps occur after momentary muscular failure. An assistant provides just enough help to get the weight trainer past the sticking point of the exercise, and allow further repetitions to be completed. Weight trainers often do this when they are spotting their exercise partner. With some exercises forced reps can be done without a training partner. For example, with one-arm *biceps curls* the other arm can be used to assist the arm that is being trained.

Cheat reps

Cheating is a deliberate compromise of form to maximize reps. Cheating has the advantage that it can be done without a training partner, but compromises safety. A typical example of cheat reps occurs during biceps curls when, beginning with the load at the waist, the exerciser swings the barbell or dumbbell forward and up during the concentric phase utilizing momentum to assist their bicep muscles in moving the load to a shortened muscle position. Momentum assistance during the concentric phase allows them to move greater loads during the more difficult concentric phase. The objective can be to position greater loads of resistance to the biceps in preparation of performing the eccentric phase than the more difficult concentric phase would otherwise allow. Replacing a typical function of a training partner with a solo exerciser performing cheat reps facilitates forced reps or negative reps when training alone.

Rest-pause (post-failure)

After a normal set of 6–8 reps (to failure), the weight is re-racked and the trainer takes 10–15 deep breaths, and then performs one more repetition. This process can be repeated for two further repetitions. The twenty-rep squat is another, similar approach, in that it follows a 12–15 rep set of squats with individual rest-pause reps, up to a total of 20 reps.

Weight stripping a.k.a. Number Setting

Weight stripping is a technique used after failure with a normal resistance in certain exercises, particularly with easily adjustable machines, whereby the weight trainer or a partner gradually reduces the resistance after a full set is taken to failure. With each reduction in resistance, as many possible reps are completed and the resistance is then reduced again. This is continued until the resistance is approximately half the original resistance.

Negative reps

Negative reps are performed with much heavier weights. Assistants lift the weight, and then the weight trainer attempts to resist its downward progress through an eccentric contraction. Alternatively, an individual can use an exercise machine for negatives by lifting the weight with both arms or legs, and then lowering it with only one. Or they can simply lower weights more slowly than they lift them: for example, by taking two seconds to lift each weight and four seconds to lower it.

Partial reps

Partial reps, as the name implies, involves movement through only part of the normal path of an exercise. Partial reps can be performed with heavier weights. Usually, only the easiest part of the repetition is attempted.

Burns

Burns involve mixing partial reps into a set of full range reps in order to increase intensity. The partials can be performed at any part of the exercise movement, depending on what works best for the particular exercise. Also, the partials can either be added after the end of a set or in some alternating fashion with the full range reps. For example, after performing a set of *biceps curls* to failure, an individual would cheat the bar back to the most contracted position, and then perform several partial reps.

Other Techniques

Progressive movement training

Progressive movement training attempts to gradually increase the range of motion throughout a training cycle. The lifter will start with a much heavier weight than they could handle in the full range of motion, only moving through the last 3–5" of the movement. Throughout the training cycle, the lifter will gradually increase the range of motion until the joint moves through the full range of the exercise. This is a style that was made popular by Paul Anderson.

Super slow

Super slow repetitions are performed with lighter weights. The lifting and lowering phases of each repetition take 10 seconds or more.

Timed rests

By strictly controlling the rest periods between reps and sets a trainer can reduce their level of blood oxygenation, which helps to increase the stress on the muscles.

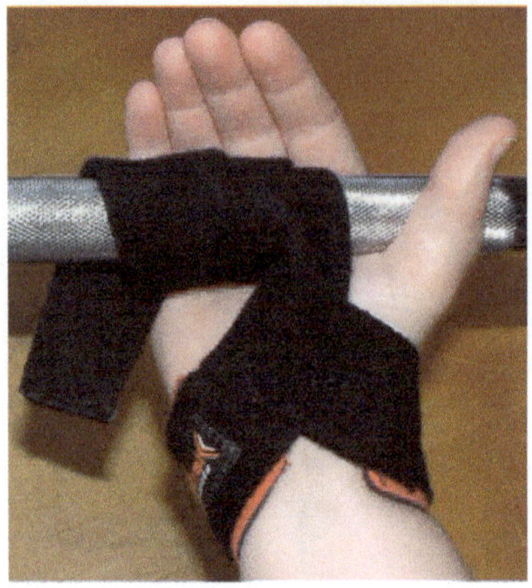

Using a wrist strap.

Wrist straps

Wrist straps (lifting straps) are sometimes used to assist in gripping very heavy weights. Wrist straps can be used to isolate muscle groups like in "lat pull-downs", where the trainee would primarily use the latissimus dorsi muscles of the back rather than the biceps. They are particularly useful for the *deadlift*. Some lifters avoid using wrist straps to develop their grip strength, just as some go further by using thick bars. Wrist straps can allow a lifter initially to use more weight than they might be able to handle safely for an entire set, as unlike simply holding a weight, if it is dropped then the lifter must descend with it or be pulled down. Straps place stress on the bones of the wrist which can be potentially harmful if excessive.

Risks and Concerns

Strength training is a safe form of exercise when the movements are controlled, and carefully defined. Or some safety measures can also be taken before the training. However, as with any form of exercise, improper execution and the failure to take appropriate precautions can result in injury. A helmet, boots, gloves, and back belt can aide in injury prevention. Principles of weight training safety apply to strength training.

Bodybuilding

Bodybuilding is a sport in which the goal is to increase muscle size and definition. Bodybuilding increases the endurance of muscles, as well as strength, though not as much as if it were the primary goal. Bodybuilders compete in bodybuilding competitions, and use specific principles and methods of strength training to maximize muscular size and develop extremely low levels of body fat. In contrast, most strength trainers train to improve their strength and endurance while not giving special attention to reducing body fat below normal. Strength trainers tend to focus on compound exercises to build basic strength, whereas bodybuilders often use isolation exercises to visually separate their muscles, and to improve muscular symmetry. Pre-contest training for bodybuilders is different again, in that they attempt to retain as much muscular tissue as possible while undergoing severe dieting. However, the bodybuilding community has been the source of many strength training principles, techniques, vocabulary, and customs.

Nutrition

It is widely accepted that strength training must be matched by changes in diet in order to be effective. Although aerobic exercise has been proven to have an effect on the dietary intake of macronutrients, strength training has not and an increase in dietary protein is generally believed to be required for building skeletal muscle with popular sources advising weight trainers to consume a high-protein diet with from 1.4 to 1.8 g of protein per kg of body weight per day (0.6 to 0.8 g per pound). Protein that is neither needed for cell growth and repair nor consumed for energy is converted into urea mainly through the deamination process and is excreted by the kidneys. It was once thought that a high-protein diet entails risk of kidney damage, but studies have shown that kidney problems only occur in people with previous kidney disease. However failure to properly hydrate can put an increased strain on the kidney's ability to function. An adequate supply of carbohydrates (5–7 g per kg) is also needed as a source of energy and for the body to restore glycogen levels in muscles.

A light, balanced meal prior to the workout (usually one to two hours beforehand) ensures that adequate energy and amino acids are available for the intense bout of exercise. The type of nutrients consumed affects the response of the body, and nutrient timing whereby protein and carbohydrates are consumed prior to and after workout has a beneficial impact on muscle growth. Water is consumed throughout the course of the workout to prevent poor performance due to dehydration. A protein shake is often consumed immediately following the workout, because both protein uptake and protein usage are increased at this time. Glucose (or another simple sugar) is often consumed as well since this quickly replenishes any glycogen lost during the exercise period. To maximise muscle protein anabolism, recovery drink should contain glucose (dextrose), protein (usually whey) hydrosylate containing mainly dipeptides and tripeptides, and leucine. Some weight trainers also take ergogenic aids such as creatine or steroids to aid muscle growth. However, the effectiveness of some products is disputed and others are potentially harmful.

Sex Differences in Mass Gains

Due to the androgenic hormonal differences between males and females, the latter are generally unable to develop large muscles regardless of the training program used. Normally the most that can be achieved is a look similar to that of a fitness model. Muscle is denser than fat, so someone who builds muscle while keeping the same body weight will occupy less volume; if two people weigh the same (and are the same height) but have different lean body mass percentages, the one with more muscle will appear thinner.

In addition, though bodybuilding uses the same principles as strength training, it is with a goal of gaining muscle bulk. Strength trainers with different goals and programs will not gain the same mass as a professional bodybuilder.

Muscle Toning

Some weight trainers perform light, high-repetition exercises in an attempt to "tone" their muscles without increasing their size.

The word tone derives from the Latin "tonus" (meaning "tension"). In anatomy and physiology, as well as medicine, the term "muscle tone" refers to the continuous and passive partial contraction of the muscles, or the muscles' resistance to passive stretching during resting state as determined by a deep tendon reflex. Muscle tonus is dependent on neurological input into the muscle. In medicine, observations of changes in muscle tonus can be used to determine normal or abnormal states which can be indicative of pathology. The common strength training term "tone" is derived from this use.

What muscle builders refer to as a *toned physique* or "muscle firmness" is one that combines reasonable muscular size with moderate levels of body fat, qualities that may result from a combination of diet and exercise.

Muscle tone or firmness is derived from the increase in actin and myosin cross filaments in the sarcomere. When this occurs the same amount of neurological input creates a greater firmness or tone in the resting continuous and passive partial contraction in the muscle.

Exercises of 6–12 reps cause hypertrophy of the sarcoplasm in slow-twitch and high-twitch muscle fibers, contributing to overall increased muscle bulk. Both however can occur to an extent during this rep range. *Even though most are of the opinion that higher repetitions are best for producing the desired effect of muscle firmness or tone, it is not.* Low volume strength training of 5 repetitions or fewer will increase strength by increasing actin and myosin cross filaments thereby increasing muscle firmness or tone. The low volume of this training will inhibit the hypertrophy effect.

Lowered-calorie diets have no positive effect on muscle hypertrophy for muscle of any fiber type. They may, however, decrease the thickness of subcutaneous fat (fat between muscle and skin), through an overall reduction in body fat, thus making muscle striations more visible.

Weight Loss

Exercises like sit-ups, or abdominal crunches, performs less work than whole-body aerobic exercises thereby expending fewer calories during exercise than jogging, for example.

Hypertrophy serves to maintain muscle mass, for an elevated basal metabolic rate, which has the potential to burn more calories in a given period compared to aerobics. This helps to maintain a higher metabolic rate which would otherwise diminish after metabolic adaption to dieting, or upon completion of an aerobic routine.

Weight loss also depends on the type of strength training used. Weight training is generally used for bulking, but the bulking method will more than likely not increase weight because of the diet involved. However, when resistance or circuit training is used, because they are not geared towards bulking, women tend to lose weight more quickly. Lean muscles require calories to maintain themselves at rest, which will help reduce fat through an increase in the basal metabolic rate.

History

Until the 20th century, the history of strength training was very similar to the history of weight training. With the advent of modern technology, materials and knowledge, the methods that can be used for strength training have multiplied significantly.

Hippocrates explained the principle behind strength training when he wrote "that which is used develops, and that which is not used wastes away", referring to muscular hypertrophy and atrophy. Progressive resistance training dates back at least to Ancient Greece, when legend has it that wrestler Milo of Croton trained by carrying a newborn calf on his back every day until it was fully grown. Another Greek, the physician Galen, described strength training exercises using the halteres (an early form of dumbbell) in the 2nd century. Ancient Persians used the *meels*, which became popular during the 19th century as the Indian club, and has recently made a comeback in the form of the clubbell.

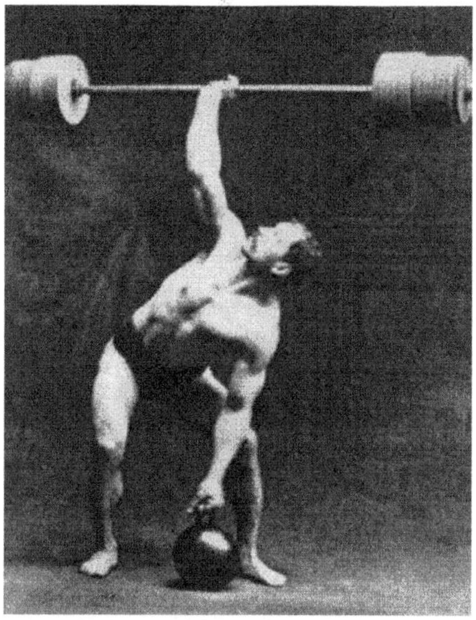

Arthur Saxon performing a Two Hands Anyhow with an early kettlebell and plate-loaded barbell.

The dumbbell was joined by the barbell in the latter half of the 19th century. Early barbells had hollow globes that could be filled with sand or lead shot, but by the end of the century these were replaced by the plate-loading barbell commonly used today.

Strength training with isometric exercise was popularised by Charles Atlas from the 1930s onwards. The 1960s saw the gradual introduction of exercise machines into the still-rare strength training gyms of the time. Strength training became increasingly popular in the 1980s following the release of the bodybuilding movie *Pumping Iron* and the subsequent popularity of Arnold Schwarzenegger.

Special Populations

Safety Concerns Related to Children

Orthopaedic specialists used to recommend that children avoid weight training because the growth plates on their bones might be at risk. The very rare reports of growth plate fractures in children who trained with weights occurred as a result of inadequate supervision, improper form or excess weight, and there have been no reports of injuries to growth plates in youth training programs that followed established guidelines. The position of the National Strength and Conditioning Association is that strength training is safe for children if properly designed and supervised.

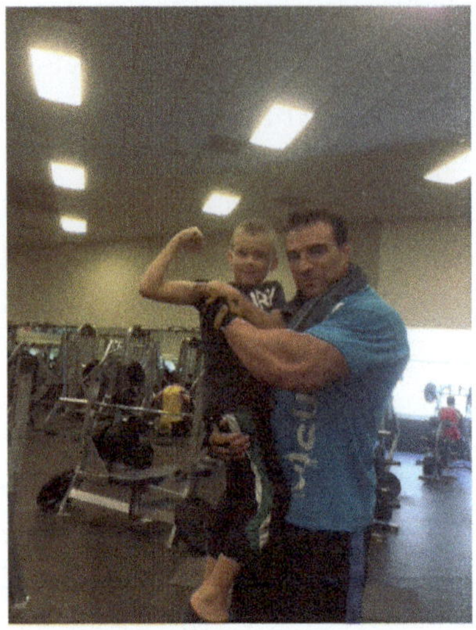

Properly supervised strength training for children.

Younger children are at greater risk of injury than adults if they drop a weight on themselves or perform an exercise incorrectly; further, they may lack understanding of, or ignore the safety precautions around weight training equipment. As a result, supervision of minors is considered vital to ensuring the safety of any youth engaging in strength training.

Australia's Stance on Pre-Adolescence Strength Training

Strength training is the fourth most popular form of fitness in Australia. Due to its popularity amongst all ages, there is great scepticism on what the appropriate age to commence strength training in young athletes is. Some points of the opposing view of strength training in young adolescence are stunted growth, health and bone problems in later stages of life and unhealthy eating habits. Studies by Australian experts that have been recognised by the Australian Institute of Sport (AIS) have debunked these myths. There is no link between any prolonged health risks and strength training in pre-adolescence if the procedures of strength training are followed correctly and under suitable supervision. Strength training for pre-adolescents should focus on skills and techniques. Children should only work on strengthening all the big muscle groups, using free weight and body weight movements with relatively light loads. The benefits of these practices include increased strength performance, injury prevention and learning good training principles.

For Older Adults

Older adults are prone to loss of muscle strength. With more strength older adults have better health, better quality of life, and fewer falls. In cases in which an older person begins strength training, their doctor or health care provider may neglect to emphasize a strength training program which results in muscle gains. Under-dosed strength training programs should be avoided in favor of a program which matches the abilities and goals of the person exercising.

In setting up an exercise program for an older adult, they should go through a baseline fitness assessment to determine their current limits. Any exercise program for older adults should match the intensity, frequency, and duration of exercise that the person can perform. The program should have a goal of increased strength as compared to the baseline measurement.

Recommended training for older adults is three times a week of light strength training exercises. Exercise machines are a commonly used equipment in a gym setting, including treadmills with exercises such as walking or light jogging. Home-based exercises should usually consist of body weight or elastic band exercises that maintain a low level of impact on the muscles. Weights can also be used by older adults if they maintain a lighter weight load with an average amount of repetitions (10–12 REPS) with suitable supervision. It is important for older adults to maintain a light level of strength training with low levels of impact to avoid injuries.

Common Strength Training Exercises

Bench Press

The bench press is an upper body strength training exercise that consists of pressing a weight upwards from a supine position. The exercise works the pectoralis major as well as supporting chest, arm, and shoulder muscles such as the anterior deltoids, serratus anterior, coracobrachialis, scapulae fixers, trapezii, and the triceps. A barbell is generally used to hold the weight, but a pair of dumbbells can also be used.

The barbell bench press is one of three lifts in the sport of powerlifting and is used extensively in weight training, bodybuilding, and other types of training to develop the chest muscles.

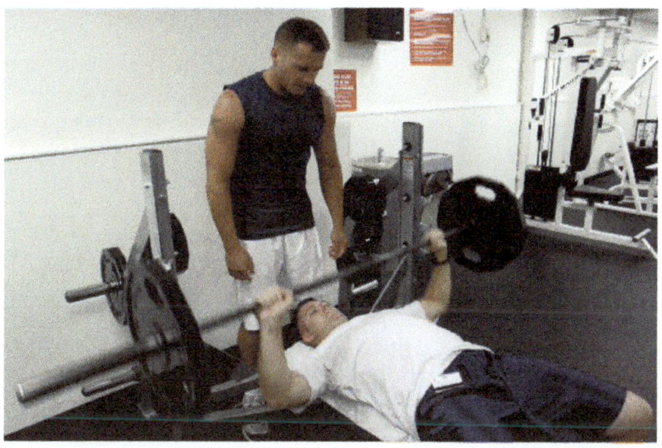

A man performs a barbell bench press while another spots him.

Movement

The person performing the exercise lies on their back with a weight grasped in both hands. They push the weight upwards until their arms are extended, not allowing the elbows to lock. They then lower the weight to chest level. This is one repetition (rep).

Powerlifting: take posture with body weight resting on buttocks and upper traps whilst driving feet into the floor. Movement requires the weight to be taken at full arms' length, lowered to upper torso, paused, and then lifted to starting position.

History

The bench press has evolved over the years, from floor, bridge, and belly toss variations to the methods used by bodybuilders and powerlifters today.

At first the strict floor press was the most popular method. In 1899, using a barbell with 48 centimetres (19 in) discs (plates), George Hackenschmidt, inventor of the barbell hack squat, rolled a barbell over his face (which was turned to the side) and performed a strict floor press with 164 kilograms (362 lb). This stood as a record for 18 years until Joe Nordquest broke it by 1 kilogram (2.2 lb) in 1916.

Around this time, new methods started gaining ground. Lifters started figuring out that strong glutes could help them get the bar from the ground to overhead. They would lie on the floor and position the bar over their abdomen, then perform an explosive glute bridge movement, catapulting the bar upwards and catching it at lockout.

Lifting techniques, training and drugs have improved over the years and the raw bench press record lift has grown from 164 kilograms (362 lb) to 335 kilograms (739 lb) in less than 100 years.

Muscles

A conventional bench press uses pectoralis major muscle, anterior deltoid, coracobrachialis to horizontally adduct the shoulder. It also uses predominantly triceps brachii and anconeous to extend the elbows. Wider hand spacing places a greater emphasis on shoulder flexion and narrower hand spacing utilizes more elbow extension. Because of this, wider hand spacing is associated with training the pectorals and narrower hand spacing is associated with training the triceps.

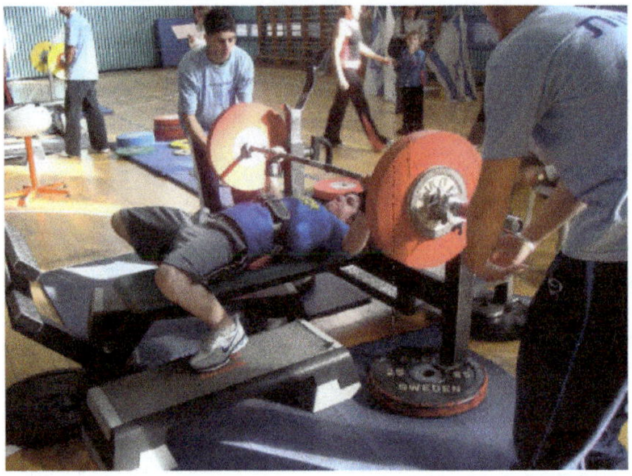

A female athlete performing a bench press at the IPA world championship 2007, in the "Bench Only" category

In addition to the major phasic (dynamic) muscles the bench press also uses tonic (stabilizing) muscles: scapular stabilizers (serratus anterior, middle and inferior trapezius), humeral head stabilizers (rotator cuff muscles), and core (transverse abdominis, obliques, multifidus, erector spinae, quadratus lumborum)

Variations

Variations of the bench press involve different groups of muscles, or involve the same muscles in different ways:

- The flat bench press involves both portions of the pectoralis major muscle but focuses on the lower (sternal) head as well as the anterior deltoid muscle. The term 'bench press' on its own is assumed to refer to a flat bench press.

- An incline elevates the shoulders and lowers the pelvis as if reclining in a chair; this variation emphasizes anterior deltoids with little emphasis at the upper (clavicular) head of the pectoralis major. This variation is called the incline bench press.
- A decline bench press elevates the pelvis and lowers the head, and emphasizes the lower portion of the pectoralis major.
- A reverse grip bench press utilizes an underhand (supinated) grip on the bar. A supinated grip externally rotates the humerus, which puts the shoulders in a much more favorable position for the lift, decreasing injury potential without compromising range of motion. It emphasises the clavicular head of the pectoralis major more than an incline bench press. On the eccentric phase of the lift, the bar path will create a larger arc and eventually touch a point on the chest that is lower compared to the regular bench press, because the upper arms and elbows are closer to the body and the angle between the humerus and the torso is smaller.
- A bench press performed with the hands close together ("close grip") relies on the triceps to complete the pressing motion. Called the close grip bench press, this variation is best performed with arms in a near-vertical position to reduce strain placed upon the wrists, elbows and shoulders.
- A bench press performed with the hands far apart ("wide grip") shortens the range of motion, lessening the contribution of the triceps.
- A lifter can elect to lower the bar to nipple level, to the xiphoid process, or even further, to the abdomen. On the other hand, a lifter may lower the bar to a very high point on the chest, or even to the neck; the latter variation is called a guillotine press and emphasizes the upper pectorals.
- The bench press can be performed with various modifications to make the lifter or the weight less stable. Examples include lifting on a Swiss ball, using dumbbells instead of a barbell, or lifting with the legs on the bench or in the air

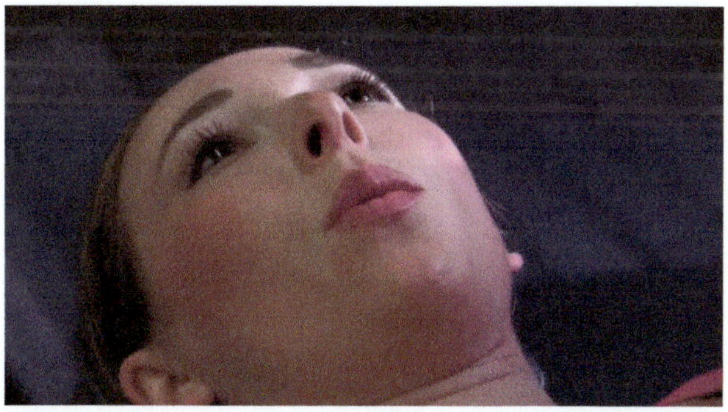

A woman explains how to properly perform the dumbbell bench press and the dumbbell incline bench press.

- The bench press can be performed with chains and bands, which are used to strengthen the top end of the range of motion in the movement (the 'lockout') and develop explosive power in the bench press.
- An 'equipped' bench press is performed with a stiff, supportive shirt that allows greater weights to be used. The materials and cut of the bench shirt, as well as the skill of the

lifter and the rules of performance, will determine how much additional weight can be pressed in the shirt as opposed to without it. The contrast between equipped, and unequipped (raw) bench press weights is illustrated in the progression of the bench press world records, with the record equipped lift exceeding the unequipped lift by hundreds of pounds.

Possible Injuries

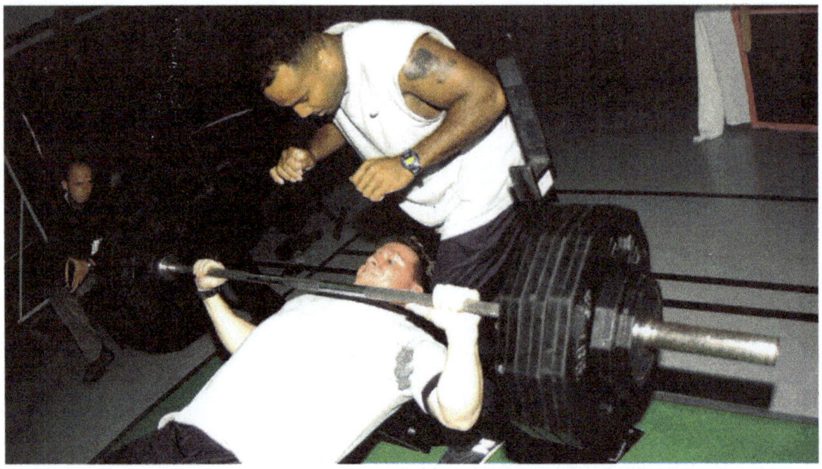

A man (lying down) performs a bench press with a spotter using a potentially dangerous thumbless grip.

Performing the bench press can contribute to multiple types of injuries:

- Torn ligaments/tendons in shoulders.
- Injuries to the trapezius muscle.
- Elbow/wrist strains.
- Cracked or broken ribs, usually the result of bouncing the bar off of the chest to add momentum to the lift or a loss of strength causing the bar to fall onto the chest.
- Distal clavicular osteolysis: bone spur or erosion at the end of the clavicle. Athletes suffering from this condition should avoid doing bench presses.
- Torn or damaged rotator cuff.
- Pectoral muscle tear.
- Death by asphyxiation by being trapped under the bar (several each year).

Isometric Exercise

Isometric exercise or isometrics are a type of strength training in which the joint angle and muscle length do not change during contraction (compared to concentric or eccentric contractions, called dynamic/isotonic movements). Isometrics are done in static positions, rather than being dynamic through a range of motion. Plank is one of the most popular isometric exercise, as it challenges all core muscles.

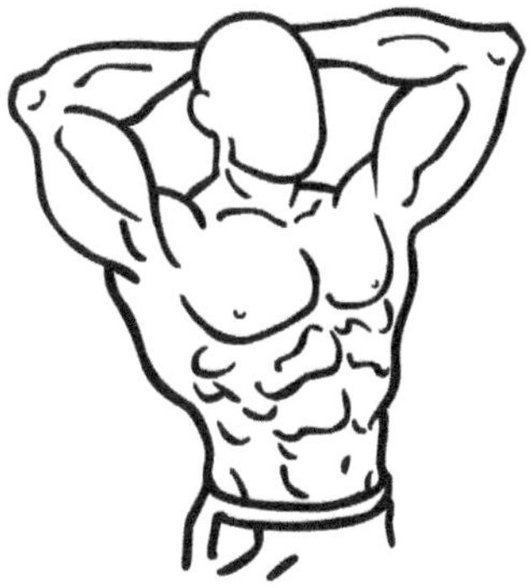

Front-and-back-neck-isometric-2.

Overcoming Versus Yielding

In an overcoming isometric, the joint and muscle work against an immovable object. In contrast, in a yielding isometric, the joint and muscle are held in a static position while opposed by resistance.

In the context of the bench press, an example of a yielding isometric would be holding the bar at a given place even though it could be pressed higher, and an overcoming isometric would be pressing the bar up into the safety guards of a squat cage that prevent pushing the bar any higher.

The distinction is that in a yielding isometric, one is pressing roughly the exact amount of pressure needed to negate the resistance, neither dropping or lifting it. Whereas in an overcoming isometric, one can be exerting more force and simply unable to move it. The yielding wavers slightly into concentric and eccentric actions due to inexact control, whereas the overcoming isometric is more purely isometric and can involve more variation in the force used, since one can press harder without the bar moving.

Unweighted

20available effort as strength is depleted, allowing longer time under (maximum volitional) tension. This is thought by experts such as Ken Hutchins and Drew Baye to be best for building muscle. However, subjects depend on a subjective perception of effort and progress, unless a metered system is available.

Weighted

Yielding isometrics allow measurable progress. Free-weight enthusiasts tend to believe the "back pressure" of real weight is superior for building strength, possibly triggering a productive "fight or flight" response. However, the extremely heavy weights needed by advanced subjects can be an inconvenience, and present a risk of injury.

Definition

An isometric exercise is a form of exercise involving the static contraction of a muscle without any visible movement in the angle of the joint. The term "isometric" combines the Greek words "Isos" (equal) and "metria" (measuring), meaning that in these exercises the length of the muscle and the angle of the joint do not change, though contraction strength may be varied. This is in contrast to *isotonic contractions*, in which the contraction strength does not change, though the muscle length and joint angle do.

Isometric Resistance

Resistance in isometric exercises typically involves contractions of the muscle using:

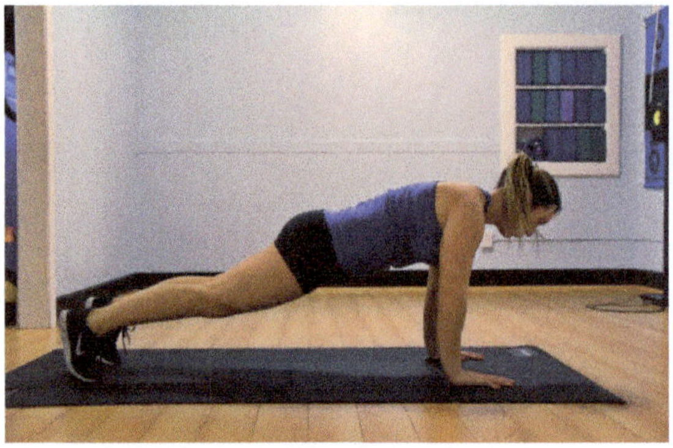

Plank.jpg

- The body's own structure and ground
- Structural items (e.g., pushing against a fence)
- Free weights, weight machines, or elastic equipment (e.g., holding a weight in a fixed position)
- Pressure-plate-type equipment that has a digital display of maximal force.

Depending on the goal of the exercise, the exertion can be maximal or sub-maximal.

History

Isometric exercises are thousands of years old, with examples listed from the static holds in certain branches of yoga or oriental martial arts.

Isometric exercises were first brought to the modern public's attention in the early days of physical culture, the precursor to bodybuilding. Many of the great bodybuilders of the day incorporated isometric exercises into their training regimens.

Many of today's training protocols incorporate isometric exercises, which are often made into parts of normal, isotonic exercises. For example, during a set of seated rows, a subject can hold their position when the handles are closest to their chest in order to "squeeze" the muscle, in an effort to further strain the muscle.

Contrary to popular opinion, The Charles Atlas "Dynamic tension" Course did not use any true isometric exercises, but rather dynamic self-resistance, that is, pitting one muscle group against another and calisthenics.

Medical Uses

Isometric exercises can also be used at the bedside to differentiate various heart murmurs; the murmur of mitral regurgitation gets louder as compared to the quieter murmur of aortic stenosis. They can also be used to prevent disuse syndrome in a limb that has been immobilized by a cast following a fracture.

Seated Isometric Exercises

One benefit of isometric exercise is that it can be done pretty much anywhere using your own body weight. According to *Sit Sense,* a book on seated exercises, you can get a significant workout with seated isometric exercises and significantly lower your blood pressure. Seated isometric exercise is ideal for geriatrics or rehabilitation.

Comparison With Dynamic Exercises

Isometric training maximally increases strength over all joint angles the exercises are performed at, similar to how dynamic exercises increase strength throughout the full range of motion, but with less risk of injury than weight training (no weights). More recent research has confirmed the finding that every skill has a specific strength component that must be practiced with the skill itself. When a subject performs a dynamic resistance movement, supportive muscle groups can work isometrically. For example, the abdominal musculature during a squat and the muscles of the forearm when gripping a dumbbell or barbell.

NASA Studies

NASA has researched the use of isometrics in preventing muscle atrophy experienced by astronauts as a result of living in a zero gravity environment. Isometrics, muscle lengthening and muscle shortening exercises were studied and compared. The outcome showed that while all three exercise types did indeed promote muscle growth, isometrics failed to prevent a decrease in the amount of contractile proteins found in the muscle tissue. The result was muscle degradation at a molecular level. As contractile proteins are what cause muscles to contract and give them their physical strength, NASA concluded that isometrics may not be the best way for astronauts to maintain muscle tissue.

Deadlift

The deadlift is a weight training exercise in which a loaded barbell is lifted off the ground to the hips, then lowered back to the ground. It is one of the three powerlifting exercises, along with the squat and bench press.

Deadlift Phases

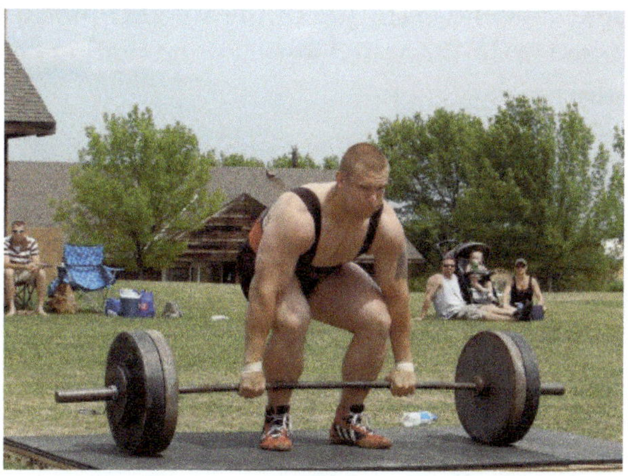

Phase 1

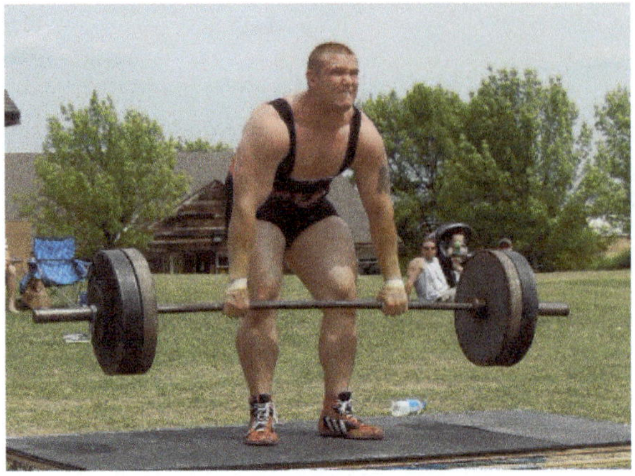

Phase 2

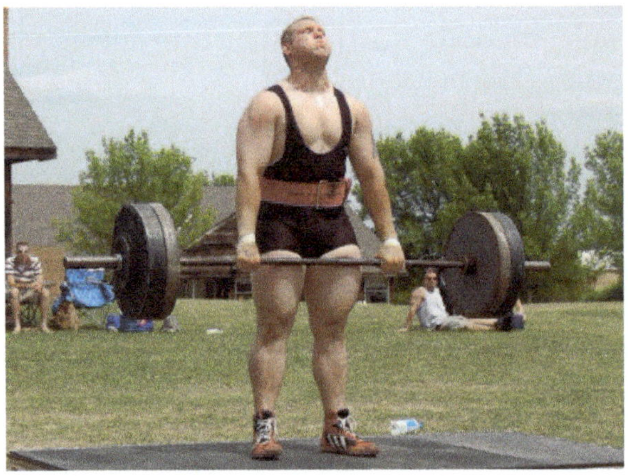

Phase 3

Overview

Deadlift refers to the lifting of dead (without momentum) weight, such as weights lying on the ground. It is one of the few standard weight training exercises in which all repetitions begin with *dead* weight. There are two positions one can approach when doing the deadlift, which include the conventional deadlift and sumo-deadlift. In most other lifts there is an eccentric (lowering of the weight) phase followed by the concentric (lifting of the weight) phase. During these exercises, a small amount of energy is stored in the stretched muscles and tendons in the eccentric phase, if the lifter is not flexible beyond the range of motion.

Performing

Form

Conventional deadlift: The deadlift can be broken down into three parts: The setup, the initial pull or drive, and the lockout.

Setup: When performing a deadlift, a lifter will set up in a position that eccentrically loads the gluteus maximus, minimus, biceps femoris, semitendinosus, and semimembranosus while the muscles of the lumbar contract isometrically in an effort to stabilize the spine.

- Set up behind the bar with it touching or nearly touching the legs.
- Begin by hinging at the hips and knees, setting one's weight predominantly in the heels while maintaining flat feet.
- Spine stays long and straight as hips hinge back, taking care not to allow knees to track forward over one's toes.
- Gripping the bar either between the legs or on the outside, a lifter will depress their shoulders away from their ears in an effort to load the lats and generate force throughout their erectors.

Drive: The next section of the deadlift produces the highest amount of force. By pushing down through their heels while simultaneously pushing up and forward with their hips and maintaining depressed scapula and a long tense spine an individual can remain safe during this motion. This is considered the most difficult part of the entire movement due to the amount of work required to drive the bar off the ground initially.

- Keep the muscles of the back contracted tightly in order to maintain a safe posture throughout the motion.
- Drive up and forward with the hips and legs to move the bar up and oneself erect simultaneously.
- Take a deep diaphragmatic breath and hold it in during the movement. Thus creating an outward pressure on the core to further stabilize the lumbopelvic hip complex and core throughout the motion.

Lockout: The finish is the most critical aspect of the motion. This requires being totally erect with the spine and forceful hip extension to engage the muscles of the lumbar spine and abdomen in unison with the glutes.

- Finish by driving the hips completely into the bar and getting as tall as possible. Contract the glutes while shortening the rectus abdominus to finish the movement with the pelvis in a neutral position.
- Contracting the glutes as well as the abdominal muscles is critical towards low back health and safety.

Lowering the weight: Finishing a deadlift is simply performing these same steps, yet in reverse order. As the muscles of the back and core must remain tight throughout the motion, one should simply hinge at the hips and knees to bring the weight down. Lowering their chest towards their knees while keeping the bar close will be the safest way to ultimately complete the motion.

The stiff-legged deadlift is a variation whereby the knees are only slightly bent and not moved during the exercise.

- the Romanian deadlift is a variation on the stiff-legged named for Nicu Vlad. As it begins at the top and does not begin the concentric from a dead stop, it is alternatively called an undead lift.

The Sumo deadlift is a variation where one will approach the bar with the feet wider than shoulder-width apart and grip the bar with a close grip inside of one's legs and proceed with correct form. Compared to conventional deadlifts, the Sumo deadlift puts more emphasis on the glutes, hamstrings, hips, quads, and traps with less of an impact on spinal erectors and the posterior chain. Weightlifters with a history of back injuries may find that sumo deadlifts are a viable alternative. If allowed in competition, many lifters favor the Sumo deadlift due to shorter bar travel from floor to lockout.

Weights

Deadlifts can be performed using dumbbells, barbells, or kettlebells with one hand or two hands & with one leg or two legs. Variations are only limited by the athlete's imagination. Other variations are the side deadlift or suitcase deadlift, rack pulls, deadlift lockouts, deficit deadlift or deadlift from a box (pulling from the floor while standing on a built or improvised low platform).

Each of these variations is called for to address specific weaknesses in a lifter's overall deadlift. For instance if the athlete has difficulty breaking contact at max. weight, deficit deadlifts are performed to strengthen the gluteus maximus and hamstrings due to the greater range of motion required by standing on the low platform or low box. On the other hand, if the lifter has no problem with breaking contact with the floor but has difficulty locking out, they should perform rack pulls to strengthen their upper back, posterior deltoids, and trapezius muscles while de-emphasizing the gluteus and hamstrings.

The archaic "dead weight lift", or "dead weight lift with lifting bar" involved a T-bar with weight loaded on it while the lifter stood on sturdy chairs or other such platforms. A remarkably heavy amount of weight could be lifted in this manner due to its short range of motion; the main limitations are in the grip. This lift is similar to the modern day rack pulls, where a heavy amount of weight is lifted deadlift style a short distance in a power cage or squat rack.

Grips

Typically, there are two grips used: overhand (pronated) or a mixed overhand-underhand (supinated) (sometimes called "offset," "staggered," "alternating", or "mixed") grip. Depending on forearm strength, the overhand grip may result in the bar potentially rolling about. Mixed grip is capable of neutralizing this through the "physics of reverse torsion." The mixed grip allows more weight to be held for this reason.

In order to prevent the bar from rolling out of the hands, some lifters have been known to use an Olympic weightlifting technique known as the hook grip. This is similar to an overhand grip, but the thumbs are inside, allowing the lifter to "hook" onto them with the fingers. The hook grip can make it easier to hold heavier weights using less grip strength, and keeps both shoulders and elbows in a symmetrical position. While it theoretically takes much of the stress off of the joints which might be created by the twisting of a mixed grip it has the disadvantage of being extremely uncomfortable for the thumbs, something which those who advocate it says will pass once a lifter becomes accustomed to it. Another, but rarely used method is a combination of the mixed overhand-underhand grip and the hook grip, preferred by people who lift heavier weights than their grip can handle, but who don't want to rely on lifting straps or other supportive gear.

Many powerlifters adopt the overhand grip for their lower weight sets and move to the mixed grip to lift larger weights so they can achieve their one rep max.

The trapbar deadlift is a variation of the deadlift using a special U-shaped bar (a trapbar). This allows more clearance for the knees to pass "through" the bar. To perform the trapbar deadlift, one loads the bar, steps inside the hollow portion of the bar, bends down, grasps the handles, stands erect, then lowers the bar to the ground in the exact opposite path. This is very helpful for both the handgrip and the lifter's hips.

Muscles Involved

The deadlift is a compound movement that works a variety of muscles groups:

- The grip strength (finger flexors) and the lower back (erector spinae) work isometrically to keep the bar held in the hands and to keep the spine from rounding.
- The gluteus maximus and hamstrings work to extend the hip joint.
- The quadriceps work to extend the knee joint.
- The adductor magnus works to stabilize the legs.
- Core musculature remains braced to stabilize the spine.

The deadlift activates a large number of individual muscles:

- Torso
    - Front
        - Abdomen
            - Rectus abdominis (under aponeurosis)
            - Abdominal external oblique muscle
            - Abdominal internal oblique muscle
    - Back
        - Iliocostalis
        - Intertransversarii laterales lumborum
        - Latissimus dorsi
        - Levator scapulae
        - Longissimus
        - Quadratus lumborum
        - Rhomboideus major

        - Serratus posterior superior
        - Serratus posterior inferior
        - Splenius cervicis
        - Teres Major
        - Trapezius muscle
- Legs
    - Quadriceps
        - Rectus femoris
        - Vastus lateralis
        - Vastus intermedius
        - Vastus medialis
    - Hamstrings
        - Semitendinosus
        - Semimembranosus
        - Biceps Femoris
- Arms
    - Biceps brachii muscle
        - long head
        - short head
        - Semitendinosus
        - Semimembranosus
- Hips
    - Gluteal muscles
        - Gluteus maximus
        - Gluteus minimus
    - Piriformis
    - Superior gemellus
- Forearms

- Flexor digitorum profundus

Deadlift Suit

Deadlift suit is special power lifting assistance clothing. The suits are made from very tight material. The material tightens on the squat on the way down, storing energy, that gives an extra boost with the stored tension to lift up. Thus records are recorded with and without the suit. The starting position with a suit is slightly different to maximize use, so training with a suit is different. Wrist Wraps are sometimes used to provide support, not necessarily to increase lift, like a suit.

World Records

- The record for a raw deadlift (a deadlift performed without the aid of a deadlift suit, where only a weight belt is allowed) is 460 kg (1,014.1 lb) by Benedikt Magnusson.
- The record for an equipped deadlift (a deadlift performed using a deadlift suit using a standard bar and plates where straps are disallowed) is 457.5 kg (1,008.6 lb) by Andy Bolton.
- The world record deadlift (using a standard bar and plates but suit, straps and hitching allowed) is 500 kg (1,102.3 lb) by Eddie Hall.
- The world record long bar deadlift in strongman competitions (using straps and a long bar) is 465 kg (1,025.1 lb) by Eddie Hall.
- The world record in strongman competitions (partial deadlift with wrist straps from 18" off the floor with high bending bar) is 535 kg (1180 pounds) by Tom Magee in the 1983 World's Strongest Man competition.
- The record for the tire deadlift (a deadlift performed using hummer tires instead of weight-plates) is 524 kg (1155 lbs) by Žydrūnas Savickas.

Squat (Exercise)

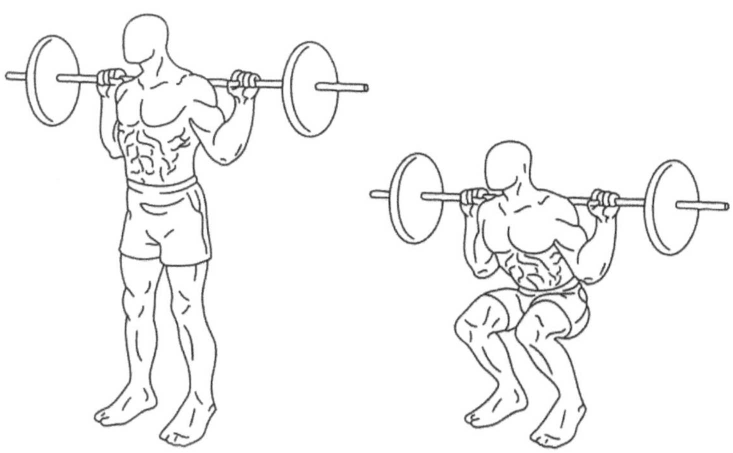

The parallel back squat

In strength training and fitness, the squat is a compound, full body exercise that trains primarily the muscles of the thighs, hips and buttocks, quadriceps (vastus lateralis, vastus medialis, vastus intermedius and rectus femoris), hamstrings, as well as strengthening the bones, ligaments and insertion of the tendons throughout the lower body. Squats are considered a vital exercise for increasing the strength and size of the legs and buttocks, as well as developing core strength. Isometrically, the lower back, the upper back, the abdominals, the trunk muscles, the costal muscles, and the shoulders and arms are all essential to the exercise and thus are trained when squatting with the proper form.

The squat is one of the three lifts in the strength sport of powerlifting, together with deadlifts and bench press.

Muscles Engaged

Primary Muscles

Gluteus Maximus (Glutes), Quadriceps (Quads)

Secondary Muscles (Synergists/Stabilizers)

- Erector spinae, transverse abdominus, gluteus medius/minimus (abductors), adductors, soleus, gastrocnemius, hamstrings

Form

The movement begins from a standing position. Weights are often used, either in the hand or as a bar braced across the trapezius muscle or rear deltoid muscle in the upper back. The movement is initiated by moving the hips back and bending the knees and hips to lower the torso and accompanying weight, then returning to the upright position. The shins and torso should remain vertical throughout the movement. An erect spine keeps the vertebra stacked directly on top of each other helping prevent low back injury.

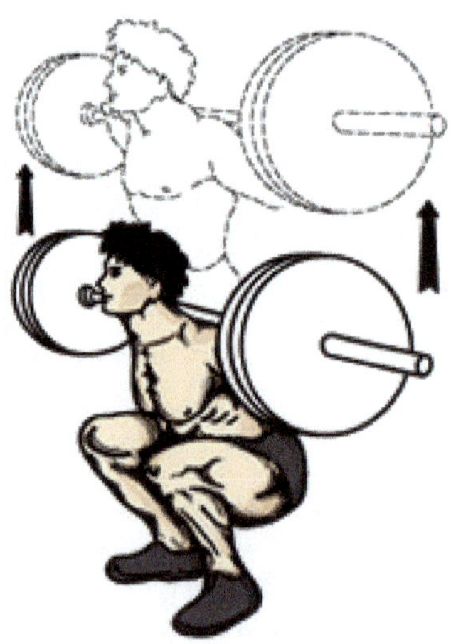

A deep squat

Squats can be performed to varying depths. The competition standard is for the crease of the hip (top surface of the leg at the hip joint) to fall below the top of the knee; this is colloquially known as "parallel" depth. Confusingly, many other definitions for "parallel" depth abound, none of which represents the standard in organized powerlifting. From shallowest to deepest, these other standards are: bottom of hamstring parallel to the ground; the hip joint itself below the top of the knee, or femur parallel to the floor; and the top of the upper thigh (i.e., top of the quadriceps) below the top of the knee.

Squatting below parallel qualifies a squat as deep while squatting above it qualifies as shallow. Some authorities caution against deep squats; though the forces on the ACL and PCL decrease at high flexion, compressive forces on the menisci and articular cartilages in the knee peak at these same high angles. This makes the relative safety of deep versus shallow squats difficult to determine.

As the body gradually descends, the hips and knees undergo flexion, the ankle extends ("dorsiflexes") and muscles around the joint contract eccentrically, reaching maximal contraction at the bottom of the movement while slowing and reversing descent. The muscles around the hips provide the power out of the bottom. If the knees slide forward or cave in then tension is taken from the hamstrings, hindering power on the ascent. Returning to vertical contracts the muscles concentrically, and the hips and knees undergo extension while the ankle plantarflexes. In a weight bearing squat, the heels should always maintain contact with the floor throughout the movement. Weight shifting forward on to the toes, and off the heels creates unnecessary stress on the knee joint. This added stress may lead to inflammation or other overuse injuries.

Two common errors include descending too rapidly and flexing the torso too far forward. Rapid descent risks being unable to complete the lift or causing injury. This occurs when the descent causes the squatting muscles to relax and tightness at the bottom is lost as a result. Over-flexing the torso greatly increases the forces exerted on the lower back, risking a spinal disc herniation.

Another error where health of the knee joint is concerned is when the knee is not aligned with the direction of the toes. If the knee is not tracking over the toes during the movement this results in twisting/shearing of the joint and unwanted torque affecting the ligaments which can soon result in injury. The knee should always follow the toe. Have your toes slightly pointed out in order to track the knee properly.

Equipment

Various types of equipment can be used to perform squats. A power cage can be used to reduce risk of injury and eliminate the need for a spotting partner. By putting the bar on a track, the Smith machine reduces the role of hip movement in the squat and in this sense resembles a leg press. Other equipment used can include a weight lifting belt to support the torso and boards to wedge beneath the ankles to improve stability and allow a deeper squat (weightlifting shoes also have wooden wedges built into the sole to achieve the same effect). Heel wedges and related equipment are discouraged by some as they are thought to worsen form over the long term. The barbell can also be cushioned with a special padded sleeve.

World Records

On October 8, 2011, Jonas Rantanen of Finland performed a squat with a weight of 575 kg (1268 lb) at the Bullfarm Powerlifting Championships in Helsinki, beating the previous record by Donnie Thompson (USA) of 573 kg (1265 lb).

The single-ply squat record is held by Dustin Slepicka (USA) at 500 kg (1102 lb).

The raw world record with knee wraps is 480 kg (1058 lb) done by Andrey Malanichev at the World Raw Powerlifting Federation World Championships meet in Almaty, Khazakstan on May 1, 2016.

The raw world record without knee wraps belongs to Ray Williams who lifted 966 lb (438 kg) on June 26, 2016 at IPF worlds in Killeen, Texas .

Variants

The squat has a number of variants, some of which can be combined:

Barbell

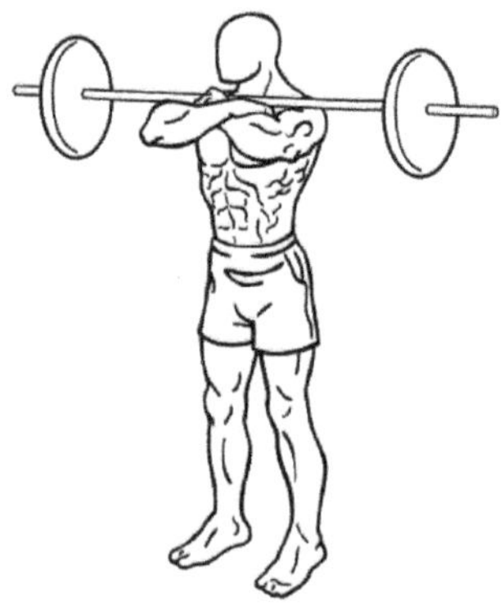

Starting position of a front squat, using the "California" or cross-armed grip.

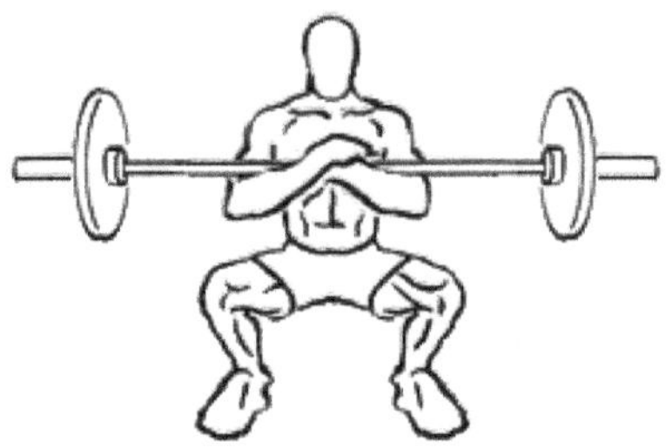

Zercher squat

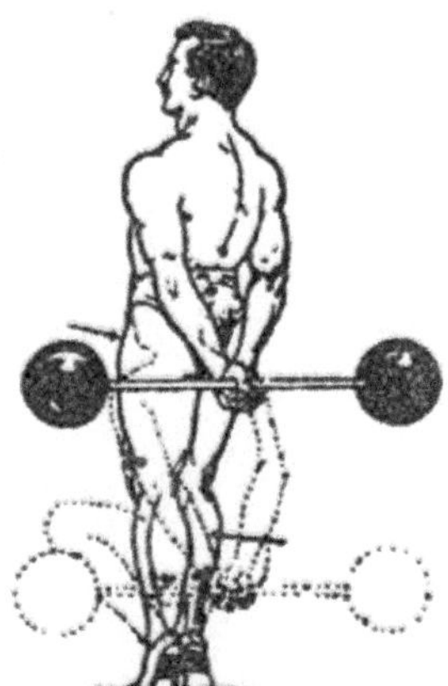

The Hack squat as pictured page 70 of George Hackenschmidt's book "The Way to Live" (1908)

- Back squat – the bar is held on the back of the body at the base of the neck or lower across the upper back. In powerlifting the barbell is often held in a lower position in order to create a lever advantage, while in weightlifting it is often held in a higher position which produces a posture closer to that of the clean and jerk. These variations are called low bar and high bar, respectively.
    - Box squat – at the bottom of the motion the squatter will sit down on a bench or other type of support then rise again. The box squat is commonly utilized by power lifters to train the squat. Pausing on the box creates additional stimulus in the hips and glutes. Some people believe this form of isometric training allows for greater gains in the squat compared to a traditional Olympic style squat, while others contend that the increased spinal loading creates more opportunity for injury.
- Sumo squat- The barbell is rested on the shoulders in the usual squat position. The legs should be slightly wider than shoulder width apart and the feet should be pointed outwards. when squatting, you should feel a stretch on the adductor longues and adductor magnus muscles which are found on the inner thigh.
- Front squat – the weight (usually a barbell) is held in front of the body across the clavicles and deltoids in either a clean grip, as is used in weightlifting, or with the arms crossed and hands placed on top of the barbell.
- Hack squat – the barbell is held in the hands just behind the legs; this exercise was first known as Hacke (heel) in Germany. According to European strength sports expert and Germanist Emmanuel Legeard this name was derived from the original form of the exercise where the heels were joined. The hack squat was thus a squat performed the way Prussian soldiers used to click their heels ("Hacken zusammen"). The hack squat was popularized in the English-speaking countries by early 1900s wrestler George Hackenschmidt. It is also called a "rear deadlift".
- Overhead squat – the barbell is held overhead in a wide-arm snatch grip; however, it is also possible to use a closer grip if balance allows.
- Zercher squat – the barbell is held in the crooks of the arms, on the inside of the elbow. One method of performing this is to deadlift the barbell, hold it against the thighs, squat into the lower portion of the squat, and then hold the bar on the thighs as you position the crook of your arm under the bar and then stand up. This sequence is reversed once the desired number of repetitions has been performed. Named after Ed Zercher, a 1930s strongman.

Lunge

- Split squat – an assisted one-legged squat where the non-lifting leg is rested on the ground a few 'steps' behind the lifter, as if it were a static lunge.
- Bulgarian squat – performed much like a split squat, but the foot of the non-lifting leg is rested on a knee-high platform behind the lifter.

Other

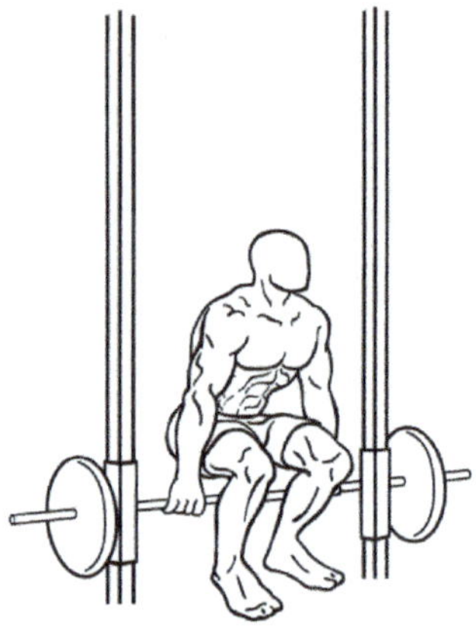

Hack squat with Smith machine

- Belt squat – is an exercise performed the same as other squat variations except the weight is attached to a hip belt i.e. a dip belt
- Goblet squat – a squat performed while holding a kettlebell next to one's chest and abdomen with both hands.
- Sissy squat – a squat with several sorts (dumbbell, weight plate, smith machine, barbell, bodyweight). In the most common variant, a dumbbell is held behind the legs while the heels are lifted off the ground and the torso remains flat while the lifter leans backwards; sometimes done with a plate held on the chest and one arm holding onto a chair or beam for support. Unlike most other squat variations, Vince Gironda promoted sissy squat as a rectus femoris isolation exercise.
- Smith squat – a squat using a smith machine. Hack squats can be done easily this way, as in the picture.
- Trap bar squat – a trap bar is held with hands at the sides.

Bodyweight

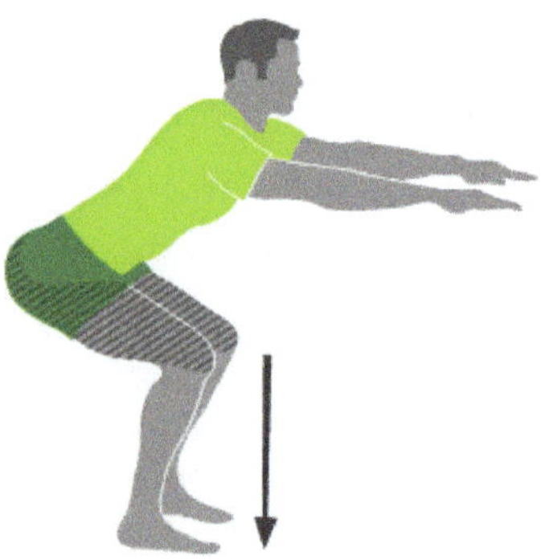

Bodyweight squat

- Bodyweight squat – done with no weight or barbell, often at higher repetitions than other variants.

- Overhead squat – a non-weight bearing variation of the squat exercise, with the hands facing each other overhead, biceps aligned with the ears, and feet hip-width apart. This exercise is a predictor of total-body flexibility, mobility, and possible lower body dysfunction.

- Face the wall squat – performed with or without weights. It is primarily to strengthen the vertebrae tissues. In the Chinese variant (面壁蹲墙) weights are not used. Toes, knees and nose line up almost touching the wall. Advanced forms include shoeless, wrists crossed behind the back, and fists in front of forehead, all performed with toes and knees closed and touching the wall.

- Hindu squat – done without weight where the heels are raised and body weight is placed on the toes; the knees track far past the toes.

- Jump squat – a plyometrics exercise where the squatter engages in a rapid eccentric contraction and jumps forcefully off the floor at the top of the range of motion.

- Pistol – a bodyweight single leg squat done to full depth, while the other leg is extended off the floor. Sometimes dumbbells, kettlebells or medicine balls are added for resistance.

- Shrimp squat - also called the *flamingo squat*, a version of the pistols squat where instead of extending the non-working leg out in front, it is bent and placed behind the working leg while squatting, perhaps held behind in a hand.

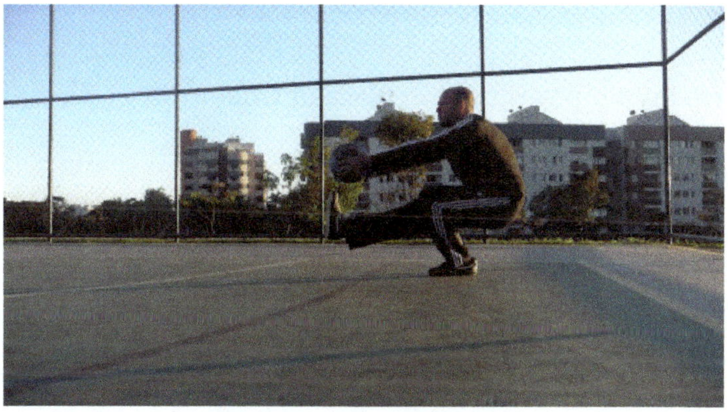

Medicine ball pistol squat

Injury Considerations

Although the squat has long been a basic element of weight training, it has in recent years been the subject of considerable controversy. Some trainers allege that squats are associated with injuries to the lumbar spine and knees. Others, however, continue to advocate the squat as one of the best exercises for building muscle and strength. Some coaches maintain that incomplete squats (those terminating above parallel) are both less effective and more likely to cause injury than a full squat (terminating with hips at or below knee level). A 2013 review concluded that deep squats performed with proper technique do not lead to increased rates of degenerative knee injuries and are an effective exercise. The same review also concluded that shallower squats may lead to degeneration in the lumbar spine and knees in the long-term.

Dip (Exercise)

The dip is an exercise used in strength training. Narrow, shoulder-width dips primarily train the triceps, with major synergists being the anterior deltoid, the pectoralis muscles (sternal, clavicular, and minor), and the rhomboid muscles of the back (in that order). Wide arm training places additional emphasis on the pectoral muscles, similar in respect to the way a wide grip bench press would focus more on the pectorals and less on the triceps.

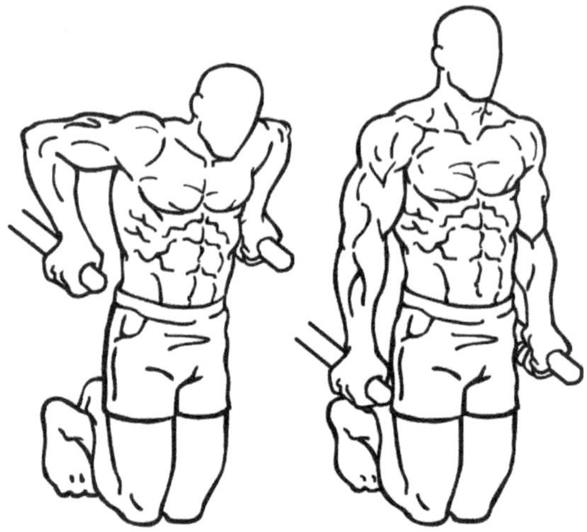

Dip exercise using a dip bar

Classic Meaning

In past decades, the term floor dip was used in place of what is now called a press-up or push-up.

Modern Meaning

To perform a dip, the exerciser hangs from a dip bar or from a set of rings with their arms straight down and shoulders over their hands, then lowers their body until their arms are bent to a 90 degree angle at the elbows, and then lifts their body up, returning to the starting position. Short people are able to cope better with a narrower grip, but not with a wider one.

Due to natural flexibility in the shoulder joints, it is important to try to "lock" them as much as possible during this exercise. Otherwise, the supporting rotator cuffs may become strained.

Variation

Usually dips are done on a dip bar, with the exerciser's hands supporting his or her entire body weight. For added resistance, weights can be added by use of a dip belt, weighted vest, or by wearing a backpack with weights in it. A dumbbell may also be held between the knees or ankles. For less resistance, an assisted dip/pull-up machine can be used which reduces the force necessary for the exerciser to elevate his body by use of a counterweight. One may also use resistance bands hooked under his feet to help if he lacks the strength to properly perform a dip.

In the absence of this equipment, a lighter variation of the dip can be performed called the "Bench Dip". The hands are placed on one bench directly underneath the shoulders or on two parallel benches. The legs are straightened and positioned horizontally; the feet rest on another bench in front of the exerciser. This variation trains the upper body muscles in a similar though not exact manner as the normal dip, whilst reducing the total weight lifted by a significant amount. This exercise can be done also off of the edge of a sofa, a kitchen counter, or any surface that supports the lifter.

Fly (Exercise)

A Cable fly or Cable flye is a strength training exercise in which the hand and arm move through an arc while the elbow is kept at a constant angle. Flies are used to work the muscles of the upper body. Because these exercises use the arms as levers at their longest possible length, the amount of weight that can be moved is significantly less than equivalent press exercises for the same muscles (the military press and bench press for the shoulder and chest respectively). Due to this leverage, fly exercises of all types have a large potential to damage the shoulder joint and its associated ligaments and the tendons of the muscles connecting to it. They should be done with caution and their effects first tested while using very light weights; which are gradually incremented after more strength is gained.

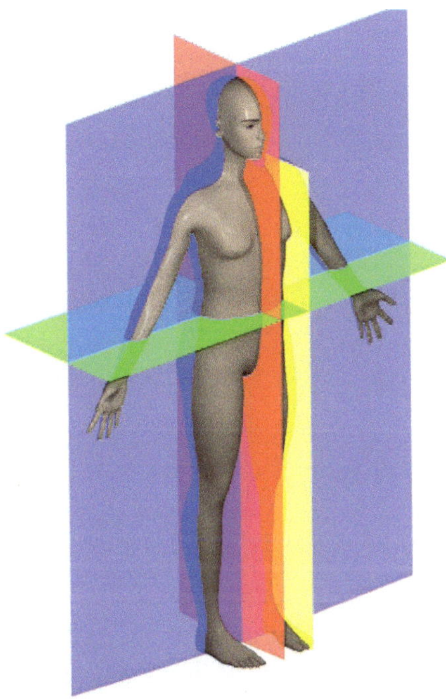

The main anatomical planes of the human body, including median (red), parasagittal (yellow), frontal or coronal plane (blue) and transverse or axial plane (green).

Equipment

Flies can be performed using any weight that can be held in the hand. The simplest equipment to use is a dumbbell, though the exercise can also be performed using a cable machine. Flies can be performed supine, sitting or standing upright. When using a cable machine, the hands and arms move through the same anatomical plane as the dumbbell version. Using dumbbells for pectoral flies requires the use of stabilizer muscles associated with performing flies, when compared to performing flies with a cable machine.

Chest Fly

The chest fly or pectoral fly (abbreviated to pec fly) primarily works the pectoralis major muscles to move the arms horizontally forward. If medially (internally) rotated, it is assisted in this by the anterior (front) head of the deltoideus in transverse flexion. If laterally (externally) rotated, the contribution of the deltoid is lessened and the pec major is strongly emphasized as the transverse adductor.

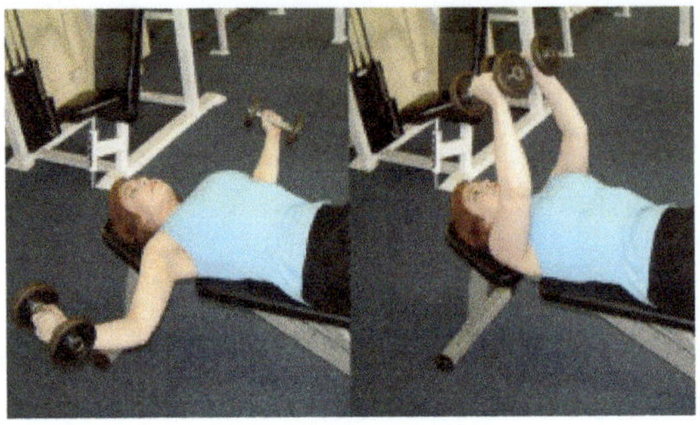

Dumbbell chest fly

The hands are usually brought out further than the elbows, in which case the flexors contract isometrically to inhibit undesired excess extension of the elbow. Muscles which do this are the biceps brachii, the brachialis and the brachioradialis. The biceps may also play a limited role in shoulder flexion. The straighter the elbow is, the more stretch in these muscles. For safety, many avoid locking out the joint.

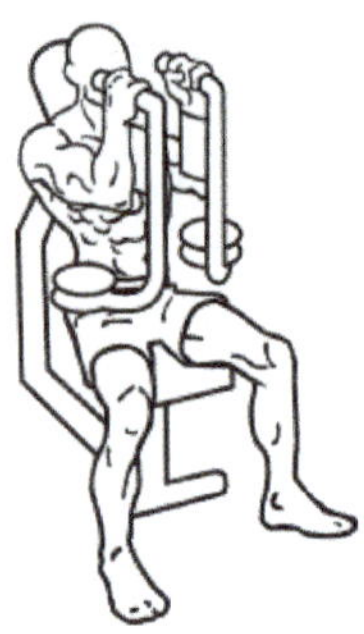

Butterfly machine fly (pec deck) end

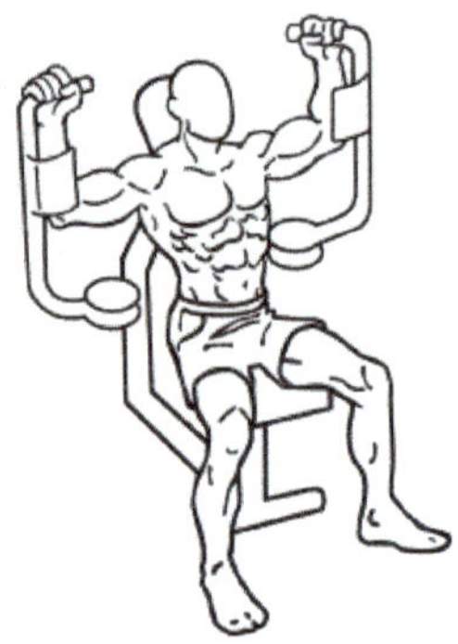

Butterfly machine fly (pec deck) start

This exercise can be done using other implements than dumbbells, such as kettlebells or weight plates. There are also machines such as the pec deck which perform a stabilized version of the movement while allowing people to sit upright.

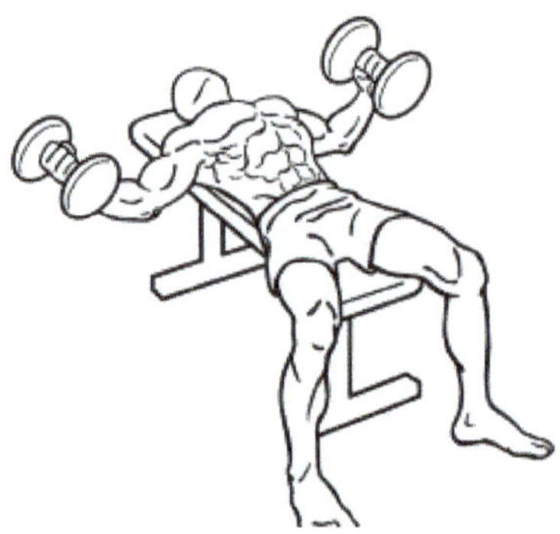

Dumbbell fly start

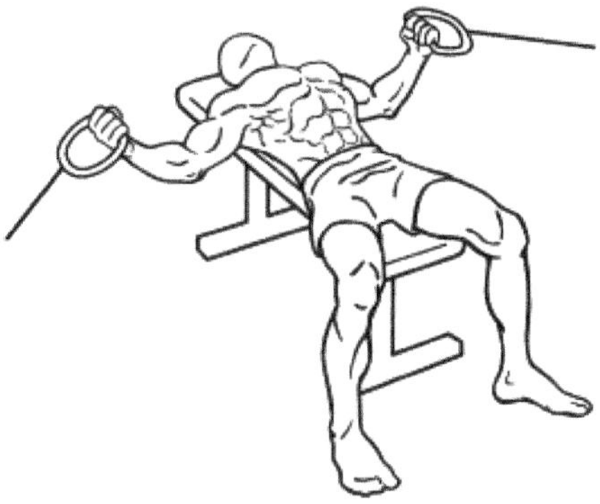

Lying cable fly start

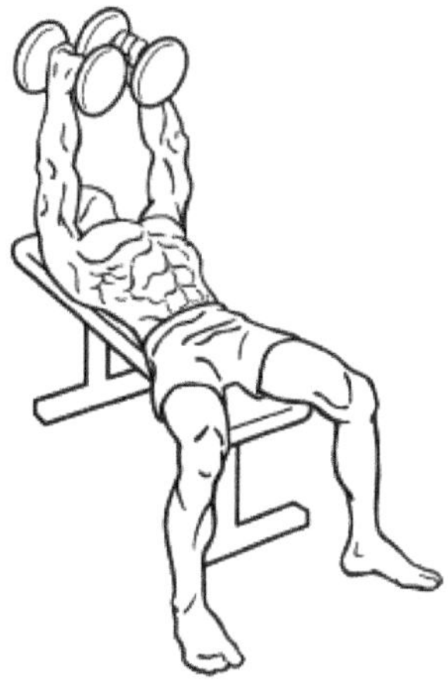

Dumbbell fly end

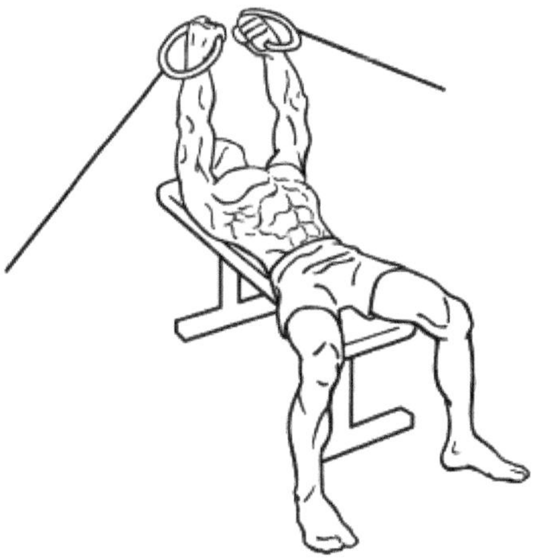

Lying cable fly end

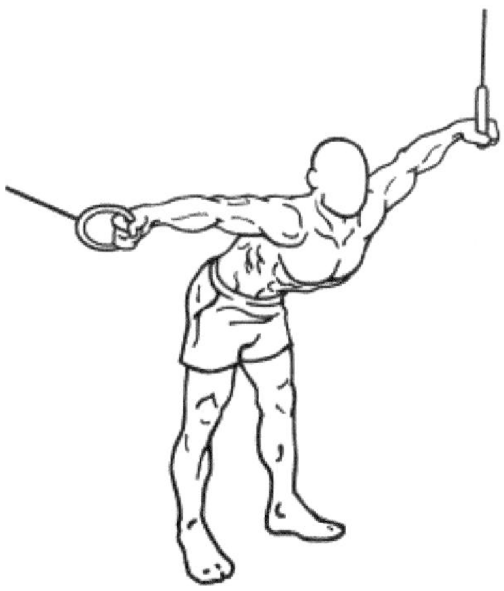

Cable crossover fly start

The movement is performed lying on the back on a bench, starting weights extended above the chest, meeting at the midsagittal plane. The arms are lowered through an arc passing through the transverse plane, terminating when the arm is roughly parallel to the floor, then returning to the starting position and repeating.

If using a cable machine, the body leans forward to counterbalance the weight moved, with the feet braced and the elbows are positioned slightly below shoulder height. The arms move the same arc as a bench fly, relative to the torso.

Incline

The clavicular portion of the pectoralis major is targeted through incline flies, when the arms rise upward as they adduct.

In flies the shoulders are sometimes externally (laterally) rotated to point the elbows down to shift emphasis away from use of the anterior deltoid as a transverse adductor. Recordsetter World Record holder Jason Faulkner (Incredible Faulk) is featured in a video Completing 47 lifts with 65 Lb. Dumbbells in 1 minute. This surpasses Eamonn Keane's Guinness Record by 1,200 Pounds for Most weight Incline fly lifted in 1 minute.

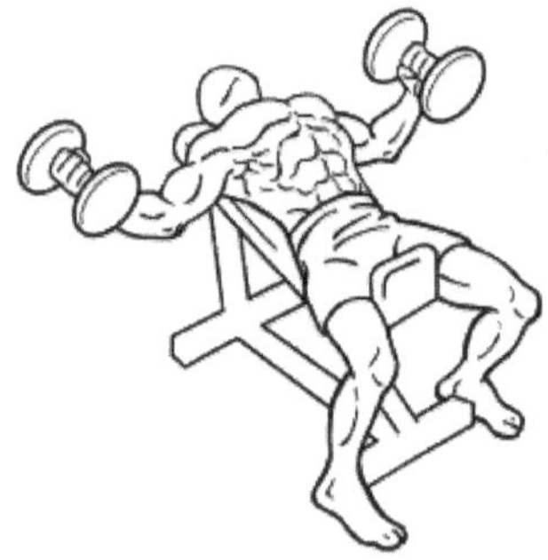

Incline dumbbell fly start

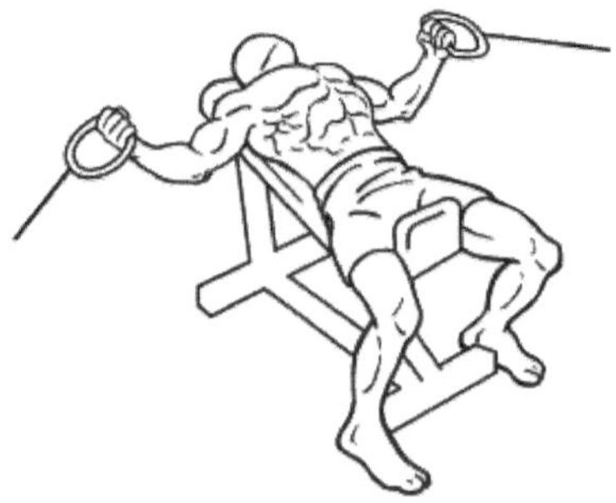

Incline cable fly start

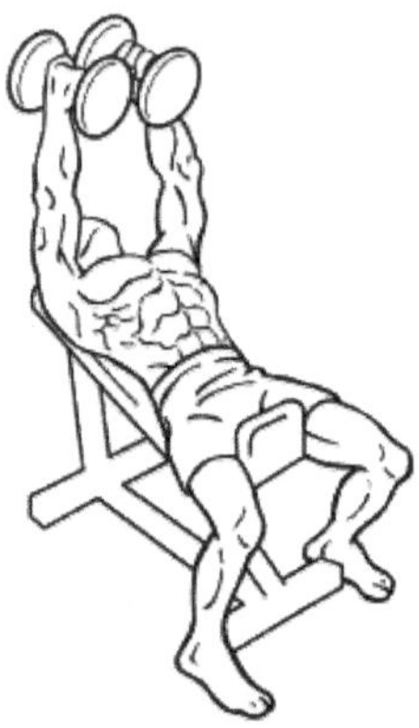

Incline dumbbell fly end

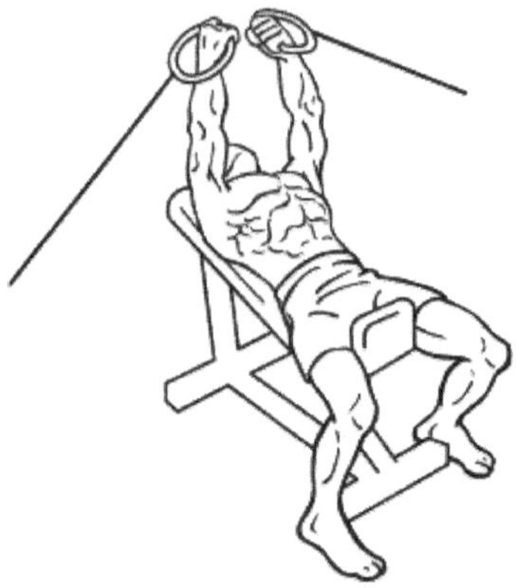

Incline cable fly end

Inverted Fly

The inverted fly (also known as a bent-over lateral raise, reverse fly or rear delt fly) works the posterior deltoid. This movement is the opposite of a chest fly. The exercise is performed with the torso parallel to the ground, facing down, with the hands in front of the face. Arms are moved through the transverse plane in an arc until parallel to the ground (or the limit of the range of motion of the shoulder is reached), then returned to the starting position and repeated.

In terms of glenohumeral movement, the posterior deltoid does not work alone, and is assisted by other muscles. If the shoulder is neutrally rotated (elbows pointing outward then towards the scapulae as they lift) the posterior deltoid will be assisted in this transverse extension by the lateral rotators of the rotator cuff: the infraspinatus and teres minor. If the shoulder is externally rotated (elbows pointing towards the hips) then it will be assisted in this transverse abduction by the middle deltoid head.

This fly, while it seems like an isolation movement, is actually a compound movement because it involves movement in a second joint: the scapulothoracic. The scapulae will retract (adduct) during this type of fly. The muscles that perform this function are the rhomboids and the trapezius.

If the lifter drops their elbows closer to their hips (rather than bringing them outward) the latissimus dorsi will come into play and deemphasize the use of the aforementioned muscles that cross both joints, as the lats bypass the scapulae and attach directly to the lumbar fascia.

A variation involves sitting upright and using a cable machine; the machine is next to the shoulder opposite the muscle being worked (in line with the coronal plane), and the hand moves through the transverse plane across the front of the body at approximately eye level.

Shoulder Fly

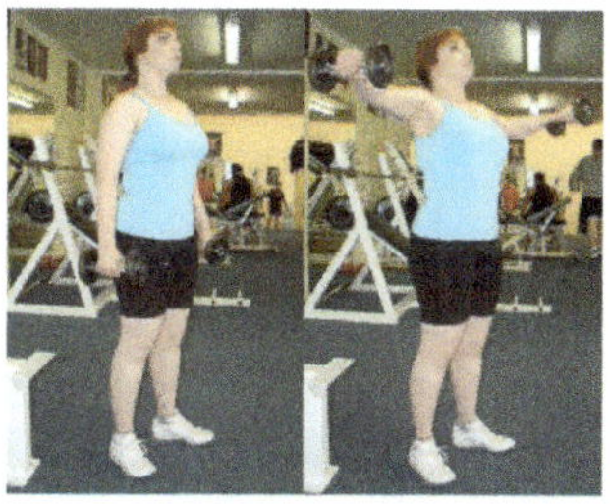

Dumbbell shoulder fly

The shoulder fly (also known as a lateral raise) works the deltoid muscle of the shoulder. The movement starts with the arms straight, and the hands holding weights at the sides or in front of the body. Arms are kept straight or slightly bent, and raised through an arc of movement in the coronal plane that terminates when the hands are at approximately shoulder height. Weights are lowered to the starting position, completing one "rep". When using a cable machine the individual stands with the coronal plane in line with the pulley, which is at or near the ground. The exercise can be completed one shoulder at a time (with the other hand used to stabilize the body against the weight moved), or with both hands simultaneously if two parallel pulleys are available.

This movement, when the shoulder is kept in neutral rotation, primarily targets the middle head of the deltoid. The anterior (front) and posterior (back) heads of the deltoid will also co-contract to aid in the abduction function. If the shoulder is laterally (externally, outwardly) rotated, the anterior deltoid becomes the prime mover of the glenohumeral joint, the posterior deltoid de-activates, and the middle head assists. By bending at the waist or leaning against a bench, the line of pull created allows the anterior deltoid to be isolated to a higher degree.

If repetitions are done explosively, it is possible for form to deteriorate and other muscles may come into play to do work instead of the deltoid, by generating upward and rotation momentum. The muscles which can be used to "cheat" in this movement are primarily the serratus anterior and the upper fibers of the trapezius, both of which elevate and upwardly rotate the scapulae.

Stretching

Stretching is a form of physical exercise in which a specific muscle or tendon (or muscle group) is deliberately flexed or stretched in order to improve the muscle's felt elasticity and achieve comfortable muscle tone. The result is a feeling of increased muscle control, flexibility, and range of motion. Stretching is also used therapeutically to alleviate cramps.

In its most basic form, stretching is a natural and instinctive activity; it is performed by humans and many other animals. It can be accompanied by yawning. Stretching often occurs instinctively after waking from sleep, after long periods of inactivity, or after exiting confined spaces and areas.

Increasing flexibility through stretching is one of the basic tenets of physical fitness. It is common for athletes to stretch before and after exercise in order to reduce risk of injury and increase performance.

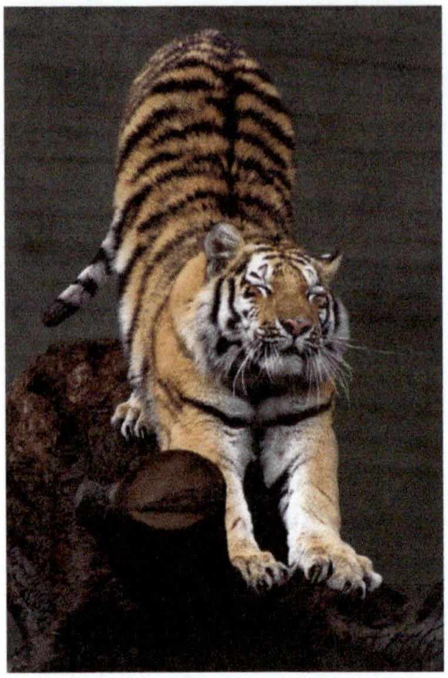

A stretching Siberian tiger

Stretching can be dangerous when performed incorrectly. There are many techniques for stretching in general, but depending on which muscle group is being stretched, some techniques may be ineffective or detrimental, even to the point of causing tears, hypermobility, instability, or permanent damage to the tendons, ligaments, and muscle fiber. The physiological nature of stretching and theories about the effect of various techniques are therefore subject to heavy inquiry.

Physiology

Studies have shed light on the function, in stretching, of a large protein within the myofibrils of skeletal muscles named titin. A study performed by Magid and Law demonstrated that the origin of passive muscle tension (which occurs during stretching) is actually within the myofibrils, not extracellularly as had previously been supposed. Due to neurological safeguards against injury, it is normally impossible for adults to stretch most muscle groups to their fullest length without training due to the activation of muscle antagonists as the muscle reaches the limit of its normal range of motion.

Types of Stretches

There are four different types of stretching: ballistic, dynamic, proprioceptive neuromuscular facilitation, and static stretching. Ballistic stretching is a rapid bouncing stretch in which a body part is moving with momentum that stretches the muscles to a maximum. Muscles respond to this type of stretching by contracting to protect itself from over extending. Dynamic stretching is a walking or movement stretch. By performing slow controlled movements through full range of motion, a person reduces risk of injury. Proprioceptive neuromuscular facilitation (PNF) is a type of stretch for a particular muscle and its specific job, so resistance should be applied, then the muscle should be relaxed. Static stretching is a type of stretch whereby a person stretches the muscle until a gentle tension is felt and then holds the stretch for thirty seconds or until a muscle release is felt, without any movement or bouncing.

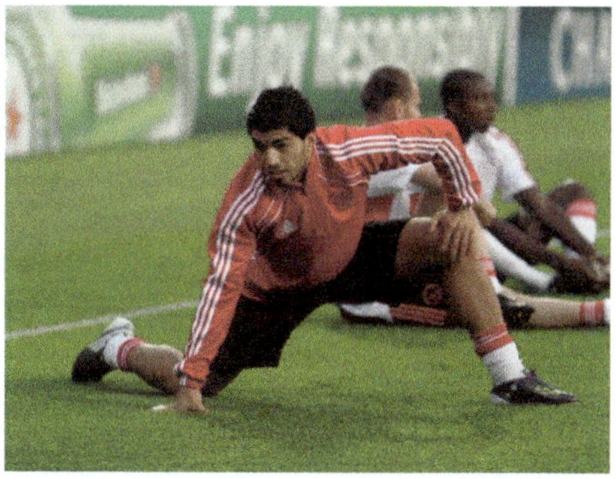

Football player Luis Suárez stretching prior to a match

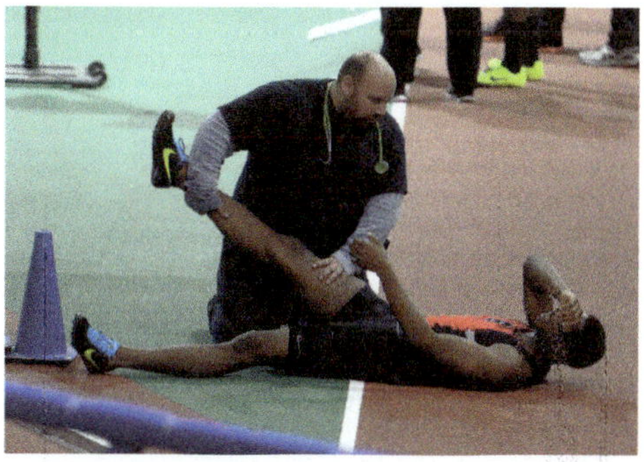

Assisted stretching may be performed when the athlete is unable to stretch optimally unassisted. For example, during cramp of the calf muscles assistance in stretching out the muscles may help.

Effectiveness

Although many people engage in stretching before or after exercise, the medical evidence has shown this has no meaningful benefit in preventing muscle soreness.

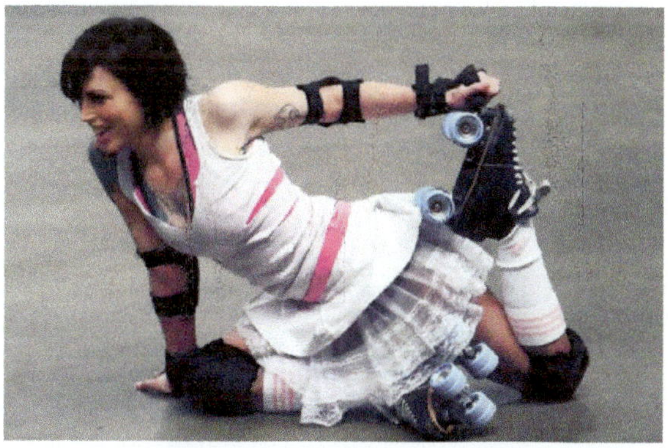

A roller derby athlete stretching.

Stretching does not appear to reduce the risk of injury during exercise, except perhaps for runners. There is some evidence that pre-exercise stretching may increase athletes' range of movement.

Flexibility

Some people are more flexible than others as defined by individual body flexibility score; this includes sex differences where females are generally more flexible than males. Stretching may not increase range of motion, but rather increase individual stretch tolerance, becoming detrimental to athletic performance. Among the factors these studies measure are capsular mobility, FlexiScore, and joint-muscle compliance.

Anaerobic Exercise

Anaerobic exercise is a physical exercise intense enough to cause lactate to form. It is used by athletes in non-endurance sports to promote strength, speed and power and by body builders to build muscle mass. Muscle energy systems trained using anaerobic exercise develop differently compared to aerobic exercise, leading to greater performance in short duration, high intensity activities, which last from mere seconds to up to about 2 minutes. Any activity lasting longer than about two minutes has a large aerobic metabolic component.

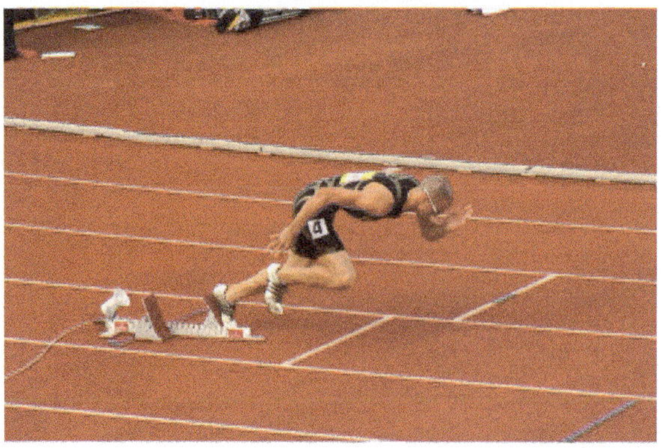

Anaerobic exercise

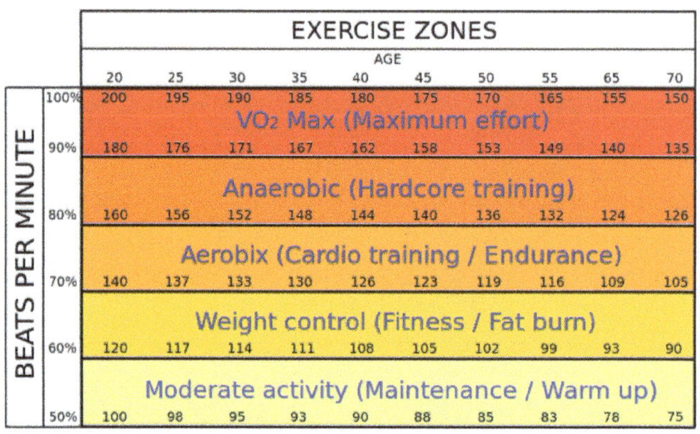

Fox and Haskell formula

Metabolism

Anaerobic metabolism, or anaerobic energy expenditure, is a natural part of whole-body metabolic energy expenditure. Fast twitch muscle (as compared to slow twitch muscle) operates using anaerobic metabolic systems, such that any recruitment of fast twitch muscle fibers leads to increased anaerobic energy expenditure. Intense exercise lasting upwards of about four minutes (e.g., a mile race) may still have a considerable anaerobic energy expenditure component. High-intensity interval training, although based on aerobic exercises like running, cycling and rowing, effectively becomes anaerobic when performed in excess of 90% maximum heart rate. Anaerobic energy expenditure is difficult to accurately quantify, although several reasonable methods to estimate the anaerobic component to exercise are available.

In contrast, aerobic exercise includes lower intensity activities performed for longer periods of time. Activities such as walking, long slow runs, rowing, and cycling require a great deal of oxygen to generate the energy needed for prolonged exercise (i.e., aerobic energy expenditure). In sports which require repeated short bursts of exercise however, the anaerobic system enables muscles to recover for the next burst. Therefore training for many sports demands that both energy producing systems be developed.

The two types of anaerobic energy systems are: 1) high energy phosphates, adenosine triphosphate and creatine phosphate; and 2) anaerobic glycolysis. The former is called *alactic anaerobic* and the latter *lactic anaerobic* system. High energy phosphates are stored in limited quantities within muscle cells. Anaerobic glycolysis exclusively uses glucose (and glycogen) as a fuel in the absence of oxygen, or more specifically when ATP is needed at rates that exceed those provided by aerobic metabolism. The consequence of such rapid glucose breakdown is the formation of lactic acid (or more appropriately, its conjugate base lactate at biological pH levels). Physical activities that last up to about thirty seconds rely primarily on the former, ATP-CP phosphagen system. Beyond this time both aerobic and anaerobic glycolysis-based metabolic systems begin to predominate.

The by-product of anaerobic glycolysis, lactate, has traditionally been thought to be detrimental to muscle function. However, this appears likely only when lactate levels are very high. Elevated lactate levels are only one of many changes that occur within and around muscle cells during intense exercise that can lead to fatigue. Fatigue, that is muscle failure, is a complex subject. Elevated muscle and blood lactate concentrations are a natural consequence of any physical exertion. The effectiveness of anaerobic activity can be improved through training.

Common Anaerobic Exercises

High-intensity Interval Training

High-intensity interval training (HIIT), also called high-intensity intermittent exercise (HIIE) or sprint interval training (SIT), is a form of interval training, an exercise strategy alternating short periods of intense anaerobic exercise with less-intense recovery periods. HIIT is a form of cardiovascular exercise. Usual HIIT sessions may vary from 4–30 minutes. These short, intense workouts provide improved athletic capacity and condition as well as improved glucose metabolism. Compared with other regimens, HIIT may not be as effective for treating hyperlipidemia and obesity, or improving muscle and bone mass. Some researchers also note that HIIT requires "an extremely high level of subject motivation," and question whether the general population could safely or practically tolerate the extreme nature of the exercise regimen.

Procedure

High-intensity interval training can be described as an exercise session composed entirely of HIIT techniques, or as a component of an exercise plan. HIIT exercise sessions generally consist of a warm up period, then several repetitions of high intensity exercise separated by medium intensity exercise for recovery, then a cool down period. The high intensity exercise should be done at near maximum intensity. The medium exercise should be about 50% intensity. The number of repetitions and length of each depends on the exercise, but may be as little as three repetitions with just 20 seconds of intense exercise The specific exercises performed during the high-intensity portions vary.

There is no specific formula to HIIT. Depending on one's level of cardiovascular development, the moderate-level intensity can be as slow as walking. A common formula involves a 2:1 ratio of work to recovery periods, for example, 30–40 seconds of hard sprinting alternated with 15–20 seconds of jogging or walking.

The entire HIIT session may last between four and thirty minutes, meaning that it is considered to be an excellent way to maximize a workout that is limited on time. Use of a clock or timer is recommended to keep accurate times, number of rounds and intensity.

Peter Coe regimen

A type of high-intensity interval training with short recovery periods was used in the 1970s by the athletics coach Peter Coe when setting sessions for his son Sebastian Coe. Inspired by the principles propounded by the German coach and university professor Woldemar Gerschler and the Swedish physiologist Per-Olof Åstrand, Coe set sessions involving repeated fast 200 metre runs with only 30 seconds recovery between each fast run.

Tabata Regimen

A version of HIIT was based on a 1996 study by Professor Izumi Tabata (田畑泉) et al. initially involving Olympic speedskaters. The study used 20 seconds of ultra-intense exercise (at an intensity of about 170% of VO_2max) followed by 10 seconds of rest, repeated continuously for 4 minutes (8 cycles). The exercise was performed on a mechanically braked cycle ergometer. Tabata called this the IE1 protocol. In the original study, athletes using this method trained 4 times per week, plus another day of steady-state training, and obtained gains similar to a group of athletes who did steady state training (70% VO_2max) 5 times per week. The steady state group had a higher VO_2max at the end (from 52 to 57 mL/(kg•min)), but the Tabata group had started lower and gained more overall (from 48 to 55 mL/(kg•min)). Also, only the Tabata group had gained anaerobic capacity benefits. It is important to note that in the original study from 1996, participants were disqualified if they could not keep a steady cycling pace of 85RPM for the full 20 seconds of work.

In popular culture, "Tabata training" has now come to refer to a wide variety of HIIT protocols and exercise regimens that may or may not have similar benefits to those found in Tabata's original study.

Gibala Regimen

Professor Martin Gibala and his team at McMaster University in Canada have been researching high-intensity exercise for several years. Their 2009 study on students uses 3 minutes for warming up, then 60 seconds of intense exercise (at 95% of VO_2max) followed by 75 seconds of rest, repeated for 8–12 cycles (sometimes referred to as "The Little Method"). Subjects using this method trained 3 times per week obtained gains similar to what would be expected from subjects who did steady state (50–70% VO_2max) training five times per week. While still a demanding form of training, this exercise protocol could be used by the general public with nothing more than an average exercise bike.

Gibala's group published a less intense version of their regimen in a 2011 paper in *Medicine & Science in Sports & Exercise*. This was intended as a gentler option for sedentary people who had done no exercise for over a year. It included 3 minutes of warm-up, 10 repetitions of 60-second bursts at 60% peak power (80- 95% of heart rate reserve) each followed by 60 seconds of recovery, and then a 5-minute cool-down.

Zuniga Regimen

Jorge Zuniga, assistant professor of exercise science at Creighton University, set out to determine how to fit the highest volume of work and oxygen consumption into the smallest amount of time. He found that intervals of 30 seconds at 90% of maximum power output followed by 30 seconds of rest allowed a for the highest VO_2 consumption and the longest workout duration at specified intensity. Alternative protocols considered included 100% of maximum power output on the same interval schedule, similar to the Coe Regimen, and 90% of maximum power output for three minutes, similar to traditional interval training.

Zuniga's protocol has been implemented to great success by his students participating in Creighton's Army ROTC program. Cadets completing the protocol twice a week saw greater improvements in APFT scores than in years past.

Timmons Regimen

Jamie Timmons, professor of systems biology at the University of Loughborough, is a proponent of a few short bursts of flat-out intensity. In a BBC *Horizon* programme in February 2012, he put Michael Mosley on an exercise bike regimen consisting of three sets of about 2 minutes of gentle pedaling followed by 20 second bursts of cycling at maximum effort. This was done three times a week for a total of 21 minutes of exercise per week (3 minutes of intense exercise), plus warm-up and recovery time.

Health Effects

Cardiovascular Fitness

A 2015 systematic review and meta-analysis of randomized controlled trials found that HIIT training and traditional endurance training both lead to significantly improved cardiovascular fitness in healthy adults ages 18–45 but greater improvements in VO_2 max were seen in those participating in the HIIT exercise regimen. Another analysis also found that HIIT regimens of one month or longer effectively improve cardiovascular fitness in adolescents and lead to moderate improvements in body composition. Furthermore, a separate systematic review and meta-analysis of seven small randomized controlled trials found that HIIT (defined as four intervals of four minutes at 85-95% of max heart rate with three-minute intervals at 60-70% of max heart rate) was more effective than moderate-intensity continuous training at improving blood vessel function and markers of blood vessel health.

Cardiovascular Disease

A 2015 meta-analysis comparing HIIT to moderate intensity continuous training (MICT) in people with coronary artery disease found that HIIT leads to greater improvements in VO_2 max but that MICT leads to greater reductions in body weight and heart rate. A 2014 meta-analysis found that the cardiorespiratory fitness, as measured by VO_2 max, of individuals with lifestyle-induced chronic cardiovascular or metabolic diseases (including high blood pressure, obesity, heart failure, coronary artery disease, or metabolic syndrome) who completed a HIIT exercise program was nearly double that of individuals who completed a MICT exercise program.

Metabolic Effects

HIIT significantly lowers insulin resistance compared to continuous training or control conditions and leads to modestly decreased fasting blood glucose levels and weight loss compared to those who do not undergo a physical activity intervention.

References

- Komanoff, Charles (2004). "Bicycling". In Cleveland, Cutler J. Encyclopedia of Energy. Elsevier. pp. 141–50. doi:10.1016/B0-12-176480-X/00185-6. ISBN 978-0-12-176480-7.
- Furness, Zack (2010). One Less Car: Bicycling and the Politics of Automobility. Philadelphia: Temple University Press. ISBN 978-1-59213-613-1.
- Hillman, Mayhew; Morgan, David; British Medical Association (1992). Cycling: Towards Health and Safety. Oxford University Press. ISBN 0-19-286151-4.
- Shaw, I..; Shaw, B.S. (2014). Resistance Training and the Prevention of Sports Injuries. In: Hopkins, G. (Ed.). Sports Injuries: Prevention, Management and Risk Factors. Nova Science Publishers, Hauppauge, NY. USA. ISBN 978-1-63463-305-5.
- Brooks, G.A.; Fahey, T.D. & White, T.P. (1996). Exercise Physiology: Human Bioenergetics and Its Applications. Mayfield Publishing Co. ISBN 0-07-255642-0.
- Kennedy, Robert and Ross, Don (1988). Muscleblasting! Brief and Brutal Shock Training. Sterling Publishing Co., Inc. ISBN 0-8069-6758-7.
- Hutchins, Ken. Super Slow: The ULTIMATE Exercise Protocol. Casselberry FL: Super Slow Systems, 1989, 1992. ISBN 0-9633199-0-6.
- Tsatsouline, Pavel (2001). Relax into stretch: instant flexibility through mastering muscle tension. Dragon Door Publications. ISBN 978-0-938045-28-1.
- Kennedy, Robert and Ross, Don (1988). Muscleblasting! Brief and Brutal Shock Training. Sterling Publishing Co., Inc. ISBN 0-8069-6758-7.
- Rippetoe, Mark (2007). Starting Strength: Basic Barbell Training, p.8. The Aasgaard Company. p. 320. ISBN 0-9768054-2-1.

3

Effects of Exercise

Exercise has many benefits, but it also has effects. Excess of exercise can cause exercise induced nausea, exercise hypertension, exercise intolerance and muscle fatigue. Exercise should be properly done, initially under the assistance of an instructor to avoid any injury. Excess of exercise can never be good; overtraining can cause suppressed immune function.

Neurobiological Effects of Physical Exercise

The neurobiological effects of physical exercise are numerous and involve a wide range of interrelated effects on brain structure, brain function, and cognition. A large body of research in humans has demonstrated that consistent aerobic exercise (e.g., 30 minutes every day) induces persistent improvements in certain cognitive functions, healthy alterations in gene expression in the brain, and beneficial forms of neuroplasticity and behavioral plasticity; some of these long-term effects include: increased neuron growth, increased neurological activity (e.g., c-Fos and BDNF signaling), improved stress coping, enhanced cognitive control of behavior, improved declarative, spatial, and working memory, and structural and functional improvements in brain structures and pathways associated with cognitive control and memory. The effects of exercise on cognition have important implications for improving academic performance in children and college students, improving adult productivity, preserving cognitive function in old age, preventing or treating certain neurological disorders, and improving overall quality of life.

People who regularly perform aerobic exercise (e.g., running, jogging, brisk walking, swimming, and cycling) have greater scores on neuropsychological function and performance tests that measure certain cognitive functions, such as attentional control, inhibitory control, cognitive flexibility, working memory updating and capacity, declarative memory, spatial memory, and information processing speed. Aerobic exercise is also a potent antidepressant and euphoriant; as a result, consistent exercise produces general improvements in mood and self-esteem.

Regular aerobic exercise improves symptoms associated with a variety of central nervous system disorders and may be used as an adjunct therapy for these disorders. There is clear evidence of exercise treatment efficacy for major depressive disorder and attention deficit hyperactivity disorder. A large body of preclinical evidence and emerging clinical evidence supports the use of exercise therapy for treating and preventing the development of drug addictions. Reviews of clinical evidence also support the use of exercise as an adjunct therapy for certain neurodegenerative disorders, particularly Alzheimer's disease and Parkinson's disease. Regular exercise is also associated with a lower risk of developing neurodegenerative disorders. Regular exercise has also been proposed as an adjunct therapy for brain cancers.

Long-term Effects

Neuroplasticity

Neuroplasticity is the process by which neurons adapt to a disturbance over time, and most often occurs in response to repeated exposure to stimuli. Aerobic exercise increases the production of neurotrophic factors (e.g., BDNF, IGF-1, VEGF, and GDNF) which mediate improvements in cognitive functions and various forms of memory by promoting blood vessel formation in the brain, adult neurogenesis, and other forms of neuroplasticity. Consistent aerobic exercise over a period of several months induces clinically significant improvements in executive functions and increased gray matter volume in multiple brain regions, particularly those which give rise to executive functions. The brain structures that show the greatest improvements in gray matter volume in response to aerobic exercise are the prefrontal cortex, caudate nucleus, and hippocampus; less significant increases in gray matter volume occur in the anterior cingulate cortex, parietal cortex, cerebellum, and nucleus accumbens. The prefrontal cortex, caudate nucleus, and anterior cingulate cortex are among the most significant brain structures in the dopamine and norepinephrine systems that give rise to cognitive control. Exercise-induced neurogenesis (i.e., the increases in gray matter volume) in the hippocampus is associated with measurable improvements in spatial memory. Higher physical fitness scores, as measured by VO_2 max, are associated with better executive function, faster information processing speed, and greater gray matter volume of the hippocampus, caudate nucleus, and nucleus accumbens. Long-term aerobic exercise is also associated with persistent beneficial epigenetic changes that result in improved stress coping, improved cognitive function, and increased neuronal activity (c-Fos and BDNF signaling).

BDNF Signaling

One of the most significant effects of exercise on the brain is the increased synthesis and expression of BDNF, a neuropeptide hormone, in the brain and periphery, resulting in increased signaling through its tyrosine kinase receptor, tropomyosin receptor kinase B (TrkB). Since BDNF is capable of crossing the blood–brain barrier, higher peripheral BDNF synthesis also increases BDNF signaling in the brain. Exercise-induced increases in brain BDNF signaling are associated with beneficial epigenetic changes, improved cognitive function, improved mood, and improved memory. Furthermore, research has provided a great deal of support for the role of BDNF in hippocampal neurogenesis, synaptic plasticity, and neural repair. Engaging in moderate-high intensity aerobic exercise such as running, swimming, and cycling increases BDNF biosynthesis through myokine signaling, resulting in up to a threefold increase in blood plasma and brain BDNF levels; exercise intensity is positively correlated with the magnitude of increased BDNF biosynthesis and expression. A meta-analysis of studies involving the effect of exercise on BDNF levels found that consistent exercise modestly increases resting BDNF levels as well.

IGF-1 Signaling

IGF-1 is a peptide that mediates some of the effects of growth hormone and acts through the IGF-1 receptor to control tissue growth and remodeling. In the brain, IGF-1 functions as a neurotrophic factor that, like BDNF, plays a significant role in cognition, neurogenesis, and neuronal survival. Physical activity is associated with increased levels of IGF-1 in blood serum, which is known to contribute to neuroplasticity in the brain due to its capacity to cross the blood–brain barrier and blood–cerebrospinal fluid barrier; consequently, one review noted that IGF-1 is a key mediator of exercise-induced adult neurogenesis, while a second review characterized it as a factor which links "body fitness" with "brain fitness". The amount of IGF-1 released into blood plasma during exercise is positively correlated with exercise intensity and duration.

VEGF Signaling

VEGF is a neurotrophic and angiogenic (i.e., blood vessel growth promoting) signaling protein that binds to two receptor tyrosine kinases, VEGFR1 and VEGFR2, which are expressed in neurons and glial cells in the brain. Hypoxia, or inadequate cellular oxygen supply, strongly upregulates VEGF expression and VEGF exerts a neuroprotective effect in hypoxic neurons. Like BDNF and IGF-1, aerobic exercise has been shown to increase VEGF biosynthesis in peripheral tissue which subsequently crosses the blood–brain barrier and promotes neurogenesis and blood vessel formation the central nervous system. Exercise-induced increases in VEGF signaling have been shown to improve cerebral blood volume and contribute to exercise-induced neurogenesis in the hippocampus.

GDNF Signaling

Structural Growth

Reviews of neuroimaging studies indicate that consistent aerobic exercise increases gray matter volume in brain regions associated with memory processing, cognitive control, motor function, and reward; the most prominent gains in gray matter volume are seen in the prefrontal cortex, caudate nucleus, and hippocampus, which support cognitive control and memory processing, among other cognitive functions. Moreover, the left and right halves of the prefrontal cortex, the hippocampus, and the cingulate cortex appear to become more functionally interconnected in response to consistent aerobic exercise. Three reviews indicate that marked improvements in prefrontal and hippocampal gray matter volume occur in healthy adults that regularly engage in medium intensity exercise for several months. Other regions of the brain that demonstrate moderate or less significant gains in gray matter volume during neuroimaging include the anterior cingulate cortex, parietal cortex, cerebellum, and nucleus accumbens.

Regular exercise has been shown to counter the shrinking of the hippocampus and memory impairment that naturally occurs in late adulthood. Sedentary adults over age 55 show a 1–2% decline in hippocampal volume annually. A neuroimaging study with a sample of 120 adults revealed that participating in regular aerobic exercise increased the volume of the left hippocampus by 2.12% and the right hippocampus by 1.97% over a one-year period. Subjects in the low intensity stretching group who had higher fitness levels at baseline showed less hippocampal volume loss, providing evidence for exercise being protective against age-related cognitive decline. In general, individuals that exercise more over a given period have greater hippocampal volumes and better memory function. Aerobic exercise has also been shown to induce growth in the white matter tracts in the anterior corpus callosum, which normally shrink with age.

The various functions of the brain structures that show exercise-induced increases in gray matter volume include:

- Prefrontal and anterior cingulate cortices – required for the cognitive control of behavior, particularly: working memory, attentional control, decision-making, cognitive flexibility, social cognition, and inhibitory control of behavior; implicated in attention deficit hyperactivity disorder (ADHD) and addiction
- Nucleus accumbens – responsible for incentive salience ("wanting" or desire, the form of motivation associated with reward) and positive reinforcement; implicated in addiction
- Hippocampus – responsible for storage and consolidation of declarative memory and spatial memory; implicated in depression
- Cerebellum – responsible for motor coordination and motor learning
- Caudate nucleus – responsible for stimulus-response learning and inhibitory control; implicated in Parkinson's disease, Huntington's disease and ADHD
- Parietal cortex – responsible for sensory perception, working memory, and attention

Cognitive Control and Memory

Concordant with the functional roles of the brain structures that exhibit increased gray matter volumes, exercise has been shown to improve numerous aspects of cognitive control and memory function. In particular, consistent aerobic exercise has been shown to improve attentional control, information processing speed, cognitive flexibility (e.g., task switching), inhibitory control, working memory updating and capacity, declarative memory, and spatial memory. In adults, the effect sizes of improvements in cognitive function are largest for indices of executive functions and small to moderate for aspects of memory and information processing speed. Individuals who have a sedentary lifestyle tend to have impaired cognitive control relative to other more physically active non-exercisers. A reciprocal relationship between exercise and cognitive control has also been noted: improvements in control processes, such as attentional control and inhibitory control, increase an individual's tendency to exercise. A systematic review of studies conducted on children suggests that some of the exercise-induced improvements in executive function are apparent after single bouts of exercise, while other aspects (e.g., attentional control) only improve following consistent exercise on a regular basis.

Short-term Effects

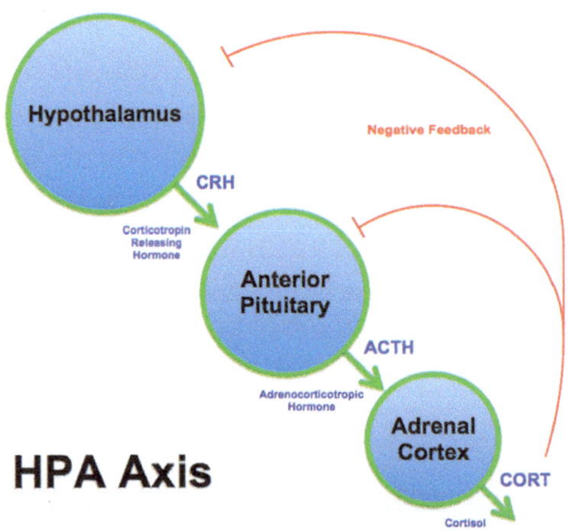

Diagram of the hypothalamic–pituitary–adrenal axis

Psychological Stress and Cortisol

The "stress hormone", cortisol, is a glucocorticoid that binds to glucocorticoid receptors. Psychological stress induces the release of cortisol from the adrenal gland by activating the hypothalamic–pituitary–adrenal axis (HPA axis). Short-term increases in cortisol levels are associated with adaptive cognitive improvements, such as enhanced inhibitory control; however, excessively high exposure or prolonged exposure to high levels of cortisol causes impairments in cognitive control and has neurotoxic effects in the human brain. For example, chronic psychological stress decreases BDNF expression which has detrimental effects on hippocampal volume and can lead to depression.

As a physical stressor, aerobic exercise stimulates cortisol secretion in an intensity-dependent manner; however, it does not result in long-term increases in cortisol production since this exercise-induced effect on cortisol is a response to transient negative energy balance. Individuals who have recently exercised exhibit improvements in stress coping behaviors. Aerobic exercise increases physical fitness and lowers neuroendocrine (i.e., HPA axis) reactivity and therefore reduces the biological response to psychological stress in humans (e.g., reduced cortisol release and attenuated heart rate response). Exercise also reverses stress-induced decreases in BDNF expression and signaling in the brain, thereby acting as a buffer against stress-related diseases like depression. Physical exercise also releases neurotransmitters like endorphins, which ease the negative feelings that come with depression.

Euphoria

Continuous exercise can produce short-term euphoria, an affective state associated with feelings of profound contentment, elation, and well-being, which is colloquially known as a "runner's high" in distance running or a "rower's high" in rowing. Current medical reviews indicate that several endogenous euphoriants are responsible for producing exercise-related euphoria, specifically phenethylamine (a stimulant), β-endorphin (an opioid), and anandamide (a cannabinoid).

Neurotransmitters, Neuromodulators, and Neuropeptides

β-Phenylethylamine

β-Phenylethylamine, commonly referred to as phenethylamine, is a potent human trace amine and neuromodulator which functions as endogenous amphetamine. Thirty minutes of moderate to high intensity physical exercise has been shown to induce an enormous increase in urinary β-phenylacetic acid, the primary metabolite of phenethylamine. Two reviews noted a study where the mean 24 hour urinary β-phenylacetic acid concentration following just 30 minutes of intense exercise rose 77% above its base level; the reviews suggest that phenethylamine synthesis sharply increases during physical exercise during which it is rapidly metabolized due to its short half-life of roughly 30 seconds. In a resting state, phenethylamine is synthesized in catecholamine neurons from L-phenylalanine by aromatic amino acid decarboxylase at approximately the same rate at which dopamine is produced.

In light of this observation, the original paper and both reviews suggest that phenethylamine plays a prominent role in mediating the mood-enhancing euphoric effects of a runner's high, as both phenethylamine and amphetamine are potent euphoriants.

β-Endorphin

β-Endorphins (contracted from "endogenous morphine") are endogenous opioid neuropeptides that bind to μ-opioid receptors, in turn producing euphoria and pain relief. A meta-analytic review found that exercise significantly increases the secretion of β-endorphins and that this secretion is correlated with improved mood states. β-endorphins have also been found to improve sleep. Moderate intensity exercise produces the greatest increase in β-endorphin synthesis, while higher and lower intensity forms of exercise are associated with smaller increases in β-endorphin synthesis.

A review on β-endorphins and exercise noted that an individual's mood improves for the remainder of the day following physical exercise and that one's mood is positively correlated with overall daily physical activity level. Exercise-induced improvements in mood occur in sedentary individuals, recreational exercisers, and marathoner runners, but recreational athletes and marathon runners experience more pronounced mood-lifting effects from exercising.

Anandamide

Anandamide is an endogenous cannabinoid neurotransmitter that binds to cannabinoid receptors. It has been shown that aerobic exercise causes an increase in plasma anandamide levels, where the magnitude of this increase is highest at moderate exercise intensity (i.e., exercising at ~70–80% maximum heart rate). Increases in plasma anandamide levels are associated with psychoactive effects because anandamide is able to cross the blood–brain barrier and act within the central nervous system. Thus, because anandamide is a euphoriant and aerobic exercise is associated with euphoric effects, it has been proposed that anandamide partly mediates the short-term mood-lifting effects of exercise (e.g., the euphoria of a runner's high) via exercise-induced increases in its synthesis.

In mice it was demonstrated that certain features of a runner's high depend on cannabinoid receptors. Pharmacological or genetic disruption of cannabinoid signaling via cannabinoid receptors prevents the analgesic and anxiety-reducing effects of running.

Monoamine Neurotransmitters

Glutamate

Glutamate, one of the most common neurochemicals in the brain, is an excitatory neurotransmitter involved in many aspects of brain function, including learning and memory. Exercise normalizes the cotransmission of glutamate and dopamine in the nucleus accumbens. A review of the effects of exercise on neurocardiac function in preclinical models noted that exercise-induced neuroplasticity of the rostral ventrolateral medulla (RVLM) has an inhibitory effect on glutamatergic neurotransmission, in turn reducing sympathetic activity; the review hypothesized that this neuroplasticity in the RVLM is a mechanism by which regular exercise prevents inactivity-related cardiovascular disease.

Effects in Children

Sibley and Etnier (2003) performed a meta-analysis that looked at the relationship between physical activity and cognitive performance in children. They reported a beneficial relationship in the categories of perceptual skills, intelligence quotient, achievement, verbal tests, mathematic tests, developmental level/academic readiness and other, with the exception of memory, that was found to be unrelated to physical activity. The correlation was strongest for the age ranges of 4–7 and 11–13 years. On the other hand, Chaddock and colleagues (2011) found results that contrasted Sibley and Etnier's meta-analysis. In their study, the hypothesis was that lower-fit children would perform poorly in executive control of memory and have smaller hippocampal volumes compared to higher-fit children. Instead of physical activity being unrelated to memory in children between 4 and 18 years of age, it may be that preadolescents of higher fitness have larger hippocampal volumes, than preadolescents of lower fitness. According to a previous study done by Chaddock and colleagues (Chaddock *et al.* 2010), a larger hippocampal volume would result in better executive control of memory. They concluded that hippocampal volume was positively associated with performance on relational memory tasks. Their findings are the first to indicate that aerobic fitness may relate to the structure and function of the preadolescent human brain. In Best's (2010) meta-analysis of the effect of activity on children's executive function, there are two distinct experimental designs used to assess aerobic exercise on cognition. The first is chronic exercise, in which children are randomly assigned to a schedule of aerobic exercise over several weeks and later assessed at the end. The second is acute exercise, which examines the immediate changes in cognitive functioning after each session. The results of both suggest that aerobic exercise may briefly aid children's executive function and also influence more lasting improvements to executive function. Other studies have suggested that exercise is unrelated to academic performance, perhaps due to the parameters used to determine exactly what academic achievement is. This area of study has been a focus for education boards that make decisions on whether physical education should be implemented in the school curriculum, how much time should be dedicated to physical education, and its impact on other academic subjects.

Animal studies have also shown that exercise can impact brain development early on in life. Mice that had access to running wheels and other such exercise equipment had better neuronal growth in the neural systems involved in learning and memory. Neuroimaging of the human brain has yielded similar results, where exercise leads to changes in brain structure and function. Some investigations have linked low levels of aerobic fitness in children with impaired executive function in older adults, but there is mounting evidence it may also be associated with a lack of selective attention, response inhibition, and interference control.

Effects on Central Nervous System Disorders

Addiction

Clinical and preclinical evidence indicate that consistent aerobic exercise, especially endurance exercise (e.g., marathon running), actually prevents the development of certain drug addictions and is an effective adjunct treatment for drug addiction, psychostimulant addiction in particular. Consistent aerobic exercise magnitude-dependently (i.e., by duration and intensity) reduces drug addiction risk, which appears to occur through the reversal of drug induced addiction-related neuroplasticity. One review noted that exercise may prevent the development of drug addiction by altering ΔFosB or c-Fos immunoreactivity in the striatum or other parts of the reward system. Moreover, aerobic exercise decreases psychostimulant self-administration, reduces the reinstatement (i.e., relapse) of drug-seeking, and induces opposite effects on striatal dopamine receptor

D_2 (DRD2) signaling (increased DRD2 density) to those induced by pathological stimulant use (decreased DRD2 density). Consequently, consistent aerobic exercise may lead to better treatment outcomes when used as an adjunct treatment for drug addiction. As of July 2015, more clinical research is still needed to understand the mechanisms and confirm the efficacy of exercise in drug addiction treatment and prevention.

Summary of addiction-related plasticity

Form of neuroplasticity or behavioral plasticity	Type of reinforcer						Sources
	Opiates	Psycho stimulants	High fat or sugar food	Sexual intercourse	Physical exercise (aerobic)	Environmental enrichment	
ΔFosB expression in nucleus accumbens D1-type MSNs	↑	↑	↑	↑	↑	↑	
Behavioral plasticity							
Escalation of intake	Yes	Yes	Yes				
Psychostimulant cross-sensitization	Yes	Not applicable	Yes	Yes	Attenuated	Attenuated	
Psychostimulant self-administration	↑	↑	↓		↓	↓	
Psychostimulant conditioned place preference	↑	↑	↓	↑	↓	↑	
Reinstatement of drug-seeking behavior	↑	↑			↓	↓	
Neurochemical plasticity							
CREB phosphorylation in the nucleus accumbens	↓	↓	↓		↓	↓	
Sensitized dopamine response in the nucleus accumbens	No	Yes	No	Yes			
Altered striatal dopamine signaling	↓DRD2, ↑DRD3	↑DRD1, ↓DRD2, ↑DRD3	↑DRD1, ↓DRD2, ↑DRD3		↑DRD2	↑DRD2	
Altered striatal opioid signaling	↑μ-opioid receptors	↑μ-opioid receptors ↑κ-opioid receptors	↑μ-opioid receptors	↑μ-opioid receptors	No change	No change	

Changes in striatal opioid peptides	↑dynorphin	↑dynorphin	↓enkephalin		↑dynorphin	↑dynorphin	
Mesocorticolimbic synaptic plasticity							
Number of dendrites in the nucleus accumbens	↓	↑		↑			
Dendritic spine density in the nucleus accumbens	↓	↑		↑			

Attention Deficit Hyperactivity Disorder

Regular physical exercise, particularly aerobic exercise, is an effective add-on treatment for ADHD in children and adults, particularly when combined with stimulant medication (i.e., amphetamine or methylphenidate), although the best intensity and type of aerobic exercise for improving symptoms are not currently known. In particular, the long-term effects of regular aerobic exercise in ADHD individuals include better behavior and motor abilities, improved executive functions (including attention, inhibitory control, and planning, among other cognitive domains), faster information processing speed, and better memory. Parent-teacher ratings of behavioral and socio-emotional outcomes in response to regular aerobic exercise include: better overall function, reduced ADHD symptoms, better self-esteem, reduced levels of anxiety and depression, fewer somatic complaints, better academic and classroom behavior, and improved social behavior. Exercising while on stimulant medication augments the effect of stimulant medication on executive function. It is believed that these short-term effects of exercise are mediated by an increased abundance of synaptic dopamine and norepinephrine in the brain.

Major Depressive Disorder

A number of medical reviews have indicated that exercise has a marked and persistent antidepressant effect in humans, an effect believed to be mediated through enhanced BDNF signaling in the brain. Several systematic reviews have analyzed the potential for physical exercise in the treatment of depressive disorders. The 2013 Cochrane Collaboration review on physical exercise for depression noted that, based upon limited evidence, it is more effective than a control intervention and comparable to psychological or antidepressant drug therapies. Three subsequent 2014 systematic reviews that included the Cochrane review in their analysis concluded with similar findings: one indicated that that physical exercise is effective as an adjunct treatment (i.e., treatments that are used together) with antidepressant medication; the other two indicated that physical exercise has marked antidepressant effects and recommended the inclusion of physical activity as an adjunct treatment for mild–moderate depression and mental illness in general. One systematic review noted that yoga may be effective in alleviating symptoms of prenatal depression. Another review asserted that evidence from clinical trials supports the efficacy of physical exercise as a treatment for depression over a 2–4 month period.

A 2015 review of clinical evidence and medical guideline for the treatment of depression with exercise noted that the available evidence on the effectiveness of exercise therapy for depression suffers from some limitations; nonetheless, it stated that there is clear evidence of efficacy for reducing symptoms of depression. The review also noted that patient characteristics, the type of depressive disorder, and the nature of the exercise program all affect the antidepressant properties of exercise therapy. A July 2016 meta-analysis concluded that physical exercise improves overall quality of life in individuals with depression relative to controls.

Neurodegenerative Disorders

Alzheimer's Disease

Alzheimer's Disease is a cortical neurodegenerative disorder and the most prevalent form of dementia, representing approximately 65% of all cases of dementia; it is characterized by impaired cognitive function, behavioral abnormalities, and a reduced capacity to perform basic activities of daily life. Two meta-analytic systematic reviews of randomized controlled trials with durations of 3–12 months have examined the effects of physical exercise on the aforementioned characteristics of Alzheimer's disease. The reviews found beneficial effects of physical exercise on cognitive function, the rate of cognitive decline, and the ability to perform activities of daily living in individuals with Alzheimer's disease. One review suggested that, based upon transgenic mouse models, the cognitive effects of exercise on Alzheimer's disease may result from a reduction in the quantity of amyloid plaque.

The Caerphilly Prospective study followed 2,375 male subjects over 30 years and examined the association between healthy lifestyles and dementia, among other factors. Analyses of the Caerphilly study data have found that exercise is associated with a lower incidence of dementia and a reduction in cognitive impairment. A subsequent systematic review of longitudinal studies also found higher levels of physical activity to be associated with a reduction in the risk of dementia and cognitive decline; this review further asserted that increased physical activity appears to be causally related with these reduced risks.

Parkinson's Disease

Parkinson's disease (PD) is a movement disorder that produces symptoms such as bradykinesia, rigidity, shaking, and impaired gait.

A review by Kramer and colleagues (2006) found that some neurotransmitter systems are affected by exercise in a positive way. A few studies reported seeing an improvement in brain health and cognitive function due to exercise. One particular study by Kramer and colleagues (1999) found that aerobic training improved executive control processes supported by frontal and prefrontal regions of the brain. These regions are responsible for the cognitive deficits in PD patients, however there was speculation that the difference in the neurochemical environment in the frontal lobes of PD patients may inhibit the benefit of aerobic exercise. Nocera and colleagues (2010) performed a case study based on this literature where they gave participants with early-to mid-staged PD, and the control group cognitive/language assessments with exercise regimens. Individuals performed 20 minutes of aerobic exercise three times a week for 8 weeks on a stationary exercise cycle. It was found that aerobic exercise improved several measures of cognitive function, providing evidence that such exercise regimens may be beneficial to patients with PD.

Fatigue (Medical)

Fatigue (also called exhaustion, tiredness, languidness, languor, lassitude, and listlessness) is a subjective feeling of tiredness which is distinct from weakness, and has a gradual onset. Unlike weakness, fatigue can be alleviated by periods of rest. Fatigue can have physical or mental causes. Physical fatigue is the transient inability of a muscle to maintain optimal physical performance, and is made more severe by intense physical exercise. Mental fatigue is a transient decrease in maximal cognitive performance resulting from prolonged periods of cognitive activity. It can manifest as somnolence, lethargy, or directed attention fatigue.

Medically, fatigue is a non-specific symptom, which means that it has many possible causes. Fatigue is considered a symptom, rather than a sign because it is a subjective feeling reported by the patient, rather than an objective one that can be observed by others. Fatigue and 'feelings of fatigue' are often confused.

Classification

Physical fatigue, or muscle fatigue, is the temporary physical inability of a muscle to perform optimally. The onset of muscle fatigue during physical activity is gradual, and depends upon an individual's level of physical fitness, and also upon other factors, such as sleep deprivation and overall health. It can be reversed by rest. Physical fatigue can be caused by a lack of energy in the muscle, by a decrease of the efficiency of the neuromuscular junction or by a reduction of the drive originating from the central nervous system. The central component of fatigue is triggered by an increase of the level of serotonin in the central nervous system. During motor activity, serotonin released in synapses that contact motoneurons promotes muscle contraction. During high level of motor activity, the amount of serotonin released increases and a spillover occurs. Serotonin binds to extrasynaptic receptors located on the axon initial segment of motoneurons with the result that nerve impulse initiation and thereby muscle contraction are inhibited.

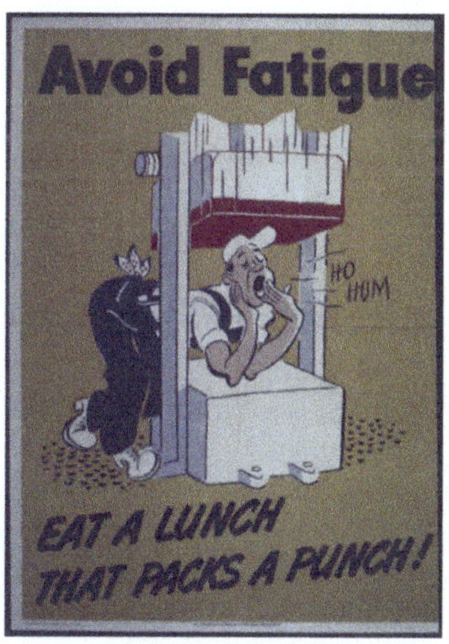
Avoid Fatigue
HO HUM
EAT A LUNCH
THAT PACKS A PUNCH!

Physical fatigue

Muscle strength testing can be used to determine the presence of a neuromuscular disease, but cannot determine its etiology. Additional testing, such as electromyography, can provide diagnostic information, but information gained from muscle strength testing alone is not enough to diagnose most neuromuscular disorders.

People with multiple sclerosis experience a form of overwhelming lassitude or tiredness that can occur at any time of the day, for any duration, and that does not necessarily recur in a recognizable pattern for any given patient, referred to as "neurological fatigue".

Mental Fatigue

Mental fatigue is a temporary inability to maintain optimal cognitive performance. The onset of mental fatigue during any cognitive activity is gradual, and depends upon an individual's cognitive ability, and also upon other factors, such as sleep deprivation and overall health. Mental fatigue has also been shown to decrease physical performance. It can manifest as somnolence, lethargy, or directed attention fatigue. Decreased attention is known as ego depletion and occurs when the limited 'self-regulatory capacity' is depleted. It may also be described as a more or less decreased level of consciousness. In any case, this can be dangerous when performing tasks that require constant concentration, such as operating large vehicles. For instance, a person who is sufficiently somnolent may experience microsleep. However, objective cognitive testing can be used to differentiate the neurocognitive deficits of brain disease from those attributable to tiredness.

The perception of mental fatigue is believed to be modulated by the brain's reticular activating system (RAS).

Comparison With Sleepiness

Fatigue is generally considered a more long-term condition than sleepiness (somnolence). Although sleepiness can be a symptom of medical issues, it usually results from lack of restful sleep, or a lack of stimulation. Chronic fatigue, on the other hand, is a symptom of a greater medical problem in most cases. It manifests in mental or physical weariness and inability to complete tasks at normal performance. Both are often used interchangeably and even categorized under the description of 'being tired.'

Causes

Fatigue is a normal result of working, mental stress, overstimulation and understimulation, jet lag or active recreation, depression, and also boredom, disease and lack of sleep. It may also have chemical causes, such as poisoning or mineral or vitamin deficiencies. Chronic blood loss frequently results in fatigue, as do other conditions that cause anemia. Fatigue is different from drowsiness, where a patient feels that sleep is required. Fatigue is a normal response to physical exertion or stress, but can also be a sign of a physical disorder.

Temporary fatigue is likely to be a minor illness like the common cold as one part of the sickness behavior response that happens when the immune system fights an infection.

Chronic Fatigue

Prolonged fatigue is a self-reported, persistent (constant) fatigue lasting at least one month. *Chronic fatigue* is a self-reported fatigue lasting at least six consecutive months. Chronic fatigue may be either persistent or relapsing. Chronic fatigue is a symptom of many diseases and conditions. Some major categories of diseases that feature fatigue include:

- Autoimmune diseases such as celiac disease, lupus, multiple sclerosis, myasthenia gravis, Sjögren's syndrome, and spondyloarthropathy
- Blood disorders such as anemia and hemochromatosis
- Cancer, in which case it is called cancer fatigue
- Chronic fatigue syndrome (CFS)
- Drug abuse including alcohol abuse
- Depression and other mental disorders that feature depressed mood
- Eating disorders, which can produce fatigue due to inadequate nutrition
- Endocrine diseases like diabetes mellitus and hypothyroidism
- Fibromyalgia
- Gulf War syndrome
- Heart disease
- HIV
- Inborn errors of metabolism such as fructose malabsorption.
- Infectious diseases such as infectious mononucleosis.
- Irritable bowel syndrome
- Leukemia or lymphoma
- Liver failure
- Lyme disease
- Neurological disorders such as narcolepsy, Parkinson's disease and post-concussion syndrome
- Physical trauma and other pain-causing conditions, such as arthritis
- Sleep deprivation or sleep disorders
- Spring fever
- Stroke
- Uremia, which is caused by kidney disease

Fatigue may also be a side effect of certain medications (e.g., lithium salts, ciprofloxacin); beta blockers, which can induce exercise intolerance; and many cancer treatments, particularly chemotherapy and radiotherapy.

Diagnosis

One study concluded about 50% of people who have fatigue receive a diagnosis that could explain the fatigue after a year with the condition. In those people who have a possible diagnosis, musculoskeletal (19.4%) and psychological problems (16.5%) are the most common. Definitive physical conditions were only found in 8.2% of cases.

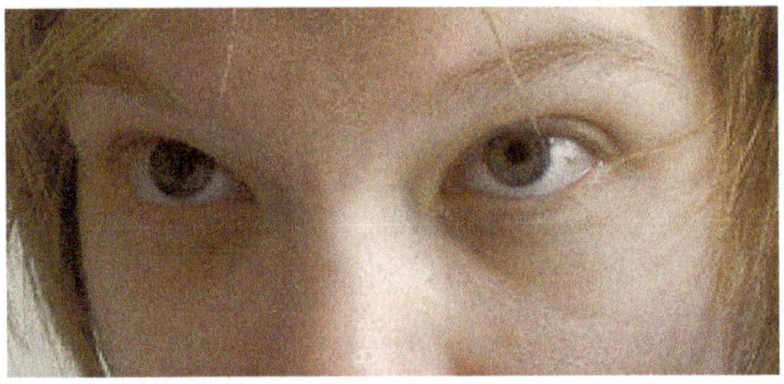

Minor dark circles, in addition to a hint of eye bags, a combination is suggestive of sleep deprivation.

If a person with fatigue decides to seek medical advice, the overall goal is to identify and rule out any treatable conditions. This is done by considering the person's medical history, any other symptoms that are present, and evaluating of the qualities of the fatigue itself. The affected person may be able to identify patterns to the fatigue, such as being more tired at certain times of day, whether fatigue increases throughout the day, and whether fatigue is reduced after taking a nap.

Because disrupted sleep is a significant contributor to fatigue, a diagnostic evaluation considers the quality of sleep, the emotional state of the person, sleep pattern, and stress level. The amount of sleep, the hours that are set aside for sleep, and the number of times that a person awakens during the night are important. A sleep study may be ordered to rule out a sleep disorder.

Depression and other psychological conditions can produce fatigue, so people who report fatigue are routinely screened for these conditions, along with drug abuse, poor diet, and lack of physical exercise, which paradoxically increases fatigue.

Basic medical tests may be performed to rule out common causes of fatigue. These include blood tests to check for infection or anaemia, a urinalysis to look for signs of liver disease or diabetes mellitus, and other tests to check for kidney and liver function, such as a comprehensive metabolic panel. Other tests may be chosen depending on the patient's social history, such as an HIV test or pregnancy test.

Muscle Fatigue

Muscle fatigue is the decline in ability of a muscle to generate force. It can be a result of vigorous exercise but abnormal fatigue may be caused by barriers to or interference with the different stages of muscle contraction. There are two main causes of muscle fatigue: the limitations of a nerve's ability to generate a sustained signal (neural fatigue) and the reduced ability of the muscle fiber to contract (metabolic fatigue).

Muscle Contraction

Muscle cells work by detecting a flow of electrical impulses from the brain which signals them to contract through the release of calcium by the sarcoplasmic reticulum. Fatigue (reduced ability to generate force) may occur due to the nerve, or within the muscle cells themselves.

Nervous Fatigue

Nerves are responsible for controlling the contraction of muscles, determining the number, sequence and force of muscular contraction. Most movements require a force far below what a muscle could potentially generate, and barring pathological nervous fatigue, is seldom an issue. But in extremely powerful contractions that are close to the upper limit of a muscle's ability to generate force, nervous fatigue (enervation), in which the nerve signal weakens, can be a limiting factor in untrained individuals.

In novice strength trainers, the muscle's ability to generate force is most strongly limited by nerve's ability to sustain a high-frequency signal. After a period of maximum contraction, the nerve's signal reduces in frequency and the force generated by the contraction diminishes. There is no sensation of pain or discomfort, the muscle appears to simply 'stop listening' and gradually cease to move, often going backwards. As there is insufficient stress on the muscles and tendons, there will often be no delayed onset muscle soreness following the workout.

Part of the process of strength training is increasing the nerve's ability to generate sustained, high frequency signals which allow a muscle to contract with its greatest force. It is this neural training that causes several weeks worth of rapid gains in strength, which level off once the nerve is generating maximum contractions and the muscle reaches its physiological limit. Past this point, training effects increase muscular strength through myofibrilar or sarcoplasmic hypertrophy and metabolic fatigue becomes the factor limiting contractile force.

Metabolic Fatigue

Though not universally used, 'metabolic fatigue' is a common term for the reduction in contractile force due to the direct or indirect effects of two main factors:

1. Shortage of fuel (substrates) within the muscle fiber

2. Accumulation of substances (metabolites) within the muscle fiber, which interfere either with the release of calcium (Ca^{2+}) or with the ability of calcium to stimulate muscle contraction.

Substrates

Substrates within the muscle generally serve to power muscular contractions. They include molecules such as adenosine triphosphate (ATP), glycogen and creatine phosphate. ATP binds to the myosin head and causes the 'ratchetting' that results in contraction according to the sliding filament model. Creatine phosphate stores energy so ATP can be rapidly regenerated within the muscle cells from adenosine diphosphate (ADP) and inorganic phosphate ions, allowing for sustained powerful contractions that last between 5–7 seconds. Glycogen is the intramuscular storage form of glucose, used to generate energy quickly once intramuscular creatine stores are exhausted, producing lactic acid as a metabolic byproduct.

Substrate shortage is one of the causes of metabolic fatigue. Substrates are depleted during exercise, resulting in a lack of intracellular energy sources to fuel contractions. In essence, the muscle stops contracting because it lacks the energy to do so.

Metabolites

Metabolites are the substances (generally waste products) produced as a result of muscular contraction. They include chloride, potassium, lactic acid, ADP, magnesium (Mg^{2+}), reactive oxygen species, and inorganic phosphate. Accumulation of metabolites can directly or indirectly produce metabolic fatigue within muscle fibers through interference with the release of calcium (Ca^{2+}) from the sarcoplasmic reticulum or reduction of the sensitivity of contractile molecules actin and myosin to calcium.

Chloride

Intracellular chloride partially inhibits the contraction of muscles. Namely, it prevents muscles from contracting due to "false alarms", small stimuli which may cause them to contract (akin to myoclonus). This natural brake helps muscles respond solely to the conscious control or spinal reflexes but also has the effect of reducing the force of conscious contractions.

Potassium

High concentrations of potassium (K^+) also causes the muscle cells to decrease in efficiency, causing cramping and fatigue. Potassium builds up in the t-tubule system and around the muscle fiber as a result of action potentials. The shift in K^+ changes the membrane potential around the muscle fiber. The change in membrane potential causes a decrease in the release of calcium (Ca^{2+}) from the sarcoplasmic reticulum.

Lactic Acid

It was once believed that lactic acid build-up was the cause of muscle fatigue. The assumption was lactic acid had a "pickling" effect on muscles, inhibiting their ability to contract. The impact of lactic acid on performance is now uncertain, it may assist or hinder muscle fatigue.

Produced as a by-product of fermentation, lactic acid can increase intracellular acidity of muscles. This can lower the sensitivity of contractile apparatus to Ca^{2+} but also has the effect of increasing cytoplasmic Ca^{2+} concentration through an inhibition of the chemical pump that actively transports calcium out of the cell. This counters inhibiting effects of potassium on muscular action potentials. Lactic acid also has a negating effect on the chloride ions in the muscles, reducing their inhibition of contraction and leaving potassium ions as the only restricting influence on muscle contractions, though the effects of potassium are much less than if there were no lactic acid to remove the chloride ions. Ultimately, it is uncertain if lactic acid reduces fatigue through increased intracellular calcium or increases fatigue through reduced sensitivity of contractile proteins to Ca^{2+}.

Lactic acid is now used as a measure of endurance training effectiveness and VO2 max.

Pathology

Muscle weakness may be due to problems with the nerve supply, neuromuscular disease (such as myasthenia gravis) or problems with muscle itself. The latter category includes polymyositis and other muscle disorders

Molecular Mechanisms

Muscle fatigue may be due to precise molecular changes that occur *in vivo* with sustained exercise. It has been found that the ryanodine receptor present in skeletal muscle undergoes a conformational change during exercise, resulting in "leaky" channels that are deficient in calcium release. These "leaky" channels may be a contributor to muscle fatigue and decreased exercise capacity.

Effect on Performance

Fatigue has been found to play a big role in limiting performance in just about every individual in every sport. In research studies, participants were found to show reduced voluntary force production in fatigued muscles (measured with concentric, eccentric, and isometric contractions), vertical jump heights, other field tests of lower body power, reduced throwing velocities, reduced kicking power and velocity, less accuracy in throwing and shooting activities, endurance capacity, anaerobic capacity, anaerobic power, mental concentration, and many other performance parameters when sport specific skills are examined.

Electromyography

Electromyography is a research technique that allows researchers to look at muscle recruitment in various conditions, by quantifying electrical signals sent to muscle fibers through motor neurons. In general, fatigue protocols have shown increases in EMG data over the course of a fatiguing protocol, but reduced recruitment of muscle fibers in tests of power in fatigued individuals. In most studies, this increase in recruitment during exercise correlated with a decrease in performance (as would be expected in a fatiguing individual).

Median power frequency is often used as a way to track fatigue using EMG. Using the median power frequency, raw EMG data is filtered to reduce noise and then relevant time windows are Fourier Transformed. In the case of fatigue in a 30-second isometric contraction, the first window may be the first second, the second window might be at second 15, and the third window could be the last second of contraction (at second 30). Each window of data is analyzed and the median power frequency is found. Generally, the median power frequency decreases over time, demonstrating fatigue. Some reasons why fatigue is found are due to action potentials of motor units having a similar pattern of repolarization, fast motor units activating and then quickly deactivating while slower motor units remain, and conduction velocities of the nervous system decreasing over time.

Dehydration

Dehydration refers to a deficit of total body water, with an accompanying disruption of metabolic processes. Dehydration is also a cause for hypernatremia. The term *dehydration* is distinct from hypovolemia (loss of blood volume, particularly plasma).

Dehydration occurs when free water loss exceeds free water intake, usually due to exercise or disease, but also due to high environmental temperature. Mild dehydration can be also be caused by immersion diuresis and this may increase risk of decompression sickness in divers. Most people can tolerate a three to four percent decrease in total body water without difficulty or adverse health effects. A five to eight percent decrease can cause fatigue and dizziness. Loss of over ten percent of total body water can cause physical and mental deterioration, accompanied by severe thirst. Death occurs at a loss of between fifteen and twenty-five percent of the body water. Mild dehydration is characterized by thirst and general discomfort and is usually resolved with oral rehydration.

Definition

Dehydration occurs when water intake is insufficient to replace free water lost due to normal physiologic processes (*e.g.* breathing or urination) and other causes (*e.g.* diarrhea or vomiting). Hypovolemia is a related condition specifically meaning a decrease in volume of blood plasma— not of total body water. Both (total body water and plasma volume) are regulated through independent mechanisms in humans and should not be conflated. Some authors have reported three types of dehydration based on serum sodium levels: hypotonic or hyponatremic (referring to this as primarily a loss of electrolytes, sodium in particular), hypertonic or hypernatremic (referring to this as primarily a loss of water), and isotonic or isonatremic (referring to this as equal loss of water and electrolytes). Indeed, in humans, it has been commonly thought that the most commonly seen type of dehydration (by far) is isotonic (isonatraemic) dehydration. This usage is incorrect and the terms *isotonic, isonatremic,* and *eunatremic dehydration* actually all refer to hypovolemia and should therefore be abandoned in favor of the latter. *Hyponatremic* dehydration cannot exist because by definition depletion of total body water can only lead to hypernatremia so this term actually refers to coexistence of two separate disorders - hyponatremia and hypovolemia and again the term dehydration must be avoided. A classic example of hyponatremia coexisting with hypovolemia is Addison's disease where cortisol deficiency leads to ADH excess and hyponatremia but mineralocorticoid deficiency simultaneously leads to sodium loss and hypovolemia. The latter subjects are not dehydrated, on the contrary they are over-hydrated (from free water retention due to ADH excess).

Dehydration is thus a term that has been very loosely used to either mean *true* dehydration or as a proxy for hypovolemia and only the former is the proper use of this term. This is important because total body water is not controlled via sodium regulation, only intravascular volume is so controlled and this distinction is important to guide therapy. Dehydration can be life-threatening when severe and lead to seizures or respiratory arrest, and also carries the risk of osmotic cerebral edema if rehydration is overtly rapid.

Signs and Symptoms

Patients who lose enough extracellular fluid (ECF) volume develop skin tenting (loss of skin elasticity), flat neck veins, and orthostatic or frank tachycardia and dizziness or fainting when standing up due to orthostatic hypotension, are often said to be dehydrated or *dry*. This is incorrect since these findings are *not* signs of dehydration and indicate ECF depletion, or hypovolemia for short.

The hallmarks of dehydration include thirst and neurological changes such as headaches, general discomfort, loss of appetite, decreased urine volume (unless polyuria is the cause of dehydration), confusion, unexplained tiredness, purple fingernails and even seizures. The symptoms of dehydration become increasingly severe with greater total body water loss. In people over age 50, the body's thirst sensation diminishes and continues diminishing with age. Many senior citizens suffer symptoms of dehydration. Dehydration contributes to morbidity in the elderly especially during conditions that promote insensible free water losses such as hot weather. A Cochrane review on this subject defined water-loss dehydration as *people with serum osmolality of 295 mOsm/kg or more* and found that the main symptoms in the elderly were expressing fatigue, missing drinks between meals and bioelectrical impedance analysis. However, this Cochrane review was also plagued by the same lack of clarity regarding the distinction between dehydration and hypovolemia seen in the literature, but confusion was avoided to a large extent by their use of hypertonicity to define dehydration. It must be pointed out that dehydration and hypovolemia may occur simultaneously in the same person at the same time and thus explains the lack of clarity in the literature regarding the symptoms and signs associated with these two conditions - however, their distinction is essential to guide therapy.

Cause

Risk factors for dehydration include but are not limited to: exerting oneself in hot and humid weather, habitation at high altitudes, endurance athletes, elderly adults, infants and children and people living with chronic illnesses.

In the elderly, blunted response to thirst and/or inadequate ability to access free water in the face of excess free water losses (especially hyperglycemia related) seem to be the main causes of dehydration. Excess free water or hypotonic water can leave the body in two ways - *sensible* loss such as osmotic diuresis, sweating, vomiting and diarrhea, and *insensible* water loss, occurring mainly through the skin and respiratory tract. In humans, dehydration can be caused by a wide range of diseases and states that impair water homeostasis in the body. These occur through the following main mechanisms:

Water/Hypotonic Fluid Loss (With Decreased Thirst and/or Impaired Access to Free Water)

- Insensible respiratory losses
- Fluid loss with a sodium plus potassium concentration less than that in the plasma, such as urinary losses in hyperglycemia (osmotic diuresis)
- Transient hypernatremia can occur when water shifts intracellularly caused by activities, such as severe exercise, and on cessation of activities the sodium returns to normal within 5 to 15 minutes

Sodium Excess

- Hypertonic sodium intake without appropriate water intake leads to hypernatremia, as the sodium load is excreted in water, leading to free water loss. This is the mechanism of free water loss when hypertonic saline is given in SIADH.

Prevention

For routine activities, thirst is normally an adequate guide to maintain proper hydration. With exercise, exposure to hot environments, or a decreased thirst response, additional water may be required.

In resting, thermoneutral individuals, whole-body insensible water loss is widely accepted to occur at about .03L/h and approximately 50% of this passes through the skin. The remaining 50% of normal insensible water loss occurs through the lungs as water vapor. Additional losses throughout the day occur through the kidneys as urine (some of which is obligatory water excretion that gets rid of solutes) and some water, in the absence of diarrhea, is also lost through the feces.

In warm or humid weather or during heavy exertion, however, the water loss can increase markedly, because humans have a large and widely variable capacity for the active secretion of sweat. For example, whole-body sweat losses in men can exceed 2 L/h during competitive sport, with rates of 3–4 L/h observed during short-duration, high-intensity exercise in the heat. When such large amounts of water are being lost through perspiration, electrolytes, especially sodium, are also being lost.

In most athletes exercising and sweating for 4–5 hours with a sweat sodium concentration of less than 50 mmol/L, the total sodium lost is less than 10% of total body stores (total stores are approximately 2,500 mmol, or 58 g for a 70-kg person). These losses appear to be well tolerated by most people. On the other hand, the inclusion of some sodium in fluid replacement drinks has some theoretical benefits and the addition of sodium poses little or no risk, so long as these fluids are hypotonic (since the mainstay of dehydration prevention is the replacement of free water losses).

Treatment

The treatment for minor dehydration, often considered the most effective, is drinking water and stopping fluid loss. Plain water restores only the volume of the blood plasma, inhibiting the thirst mechanism before solute levels can be replenished. Solid foods can contribute to fluid loss from vomiting and diarrhea. Urine concentration and frequency will customarily return to normal as dehydration resolves.

In more severe cases, correction of a dehydrated state is accomplished by the replenishment of necessary water and electrolytes (through oral rehydration therapy or fluid replacement by intravenous therapy). As oral rehydration is less painful, less invasive, less expensive, and easier to provide, it is the treatment of choice for mild dehydration. Solutions used for intravenous rehydration must be isotonic or hypotonic. Pure water injected into the veins will cause the breakdown (lysis) of red blood cells (erythrocytes).

When fresh water is unavailable (e.g. at sea or in a desert), seawater and ethanol will worsen the condition. Urine contains a similar solute concentration to seawater, and numerous guides advise against its consumption in survival situations.

For severe cases of dehydration where fainting, unconsciousness, or other severely inhibiting symptom is present (the patient is incapable of standing or thinking clearly), emergency attention is required. Fluids containing a proper balance of replacement electrolytes are given orally or intravenously with continuing assessment of electrolyte status; complete resolution is the norm in all but the most extreme cases.

Some research indicates that artificial hydration to alleviate symptoms of dry mouth and thirst in the dying patient may be futile.

Exercise Intolerance

Exercise intolerance is a condition of inability or decreased ability to perform physical exercise at the expected level or duration of someone with a specific physical condition. It also includes experiences of unusually severe post-exercise pain, fatigue, nausea, vomiting or other negative effects. Exercise intolerance is not a disease or syndrome in and of itself, but a primary symptom of chronic diastolic heart failure.

Since there are many possible specific reasons why exercise could be inhibited, this is a rather slippery term. For instance, the patient may experience unusual breathlessness (dyspnea), muscle pain (myalgia), tachypnoea (abnormally rapid breathing), tachycardia (having a heart rate that exceeds the normal range) or increasing muscle weakness while exercising, or may, after exercise, experience severe headache, nausea, dizziness, occasional muscle cramps or extreme fatigue.

In most cases, the specific reason that exercise is not tolerated is of considerable significance when trying to isolate the cause down to a specific disease. Dysfunctions involving the pulmonary, cardiovascular or neuromuscular systems have been frequently found to be associated with exercise intolerance, with behavioural causes also playing a part in it.

Causes

Cardiorespiratory Disorders

1. Cystic fibrosis; CF can cause skeletal muscle atrophy however more commonly it can cause exercise intolerance. The exercise intolerance is associated with reduced pulmonary function that is the origin of CF.
2. Bronchiectasis;
3. Spinal muscular atrophy; symptoms include exercise intolerance, cognitive impairment and fatigue.

Chronic Fatigue Syndrome

- Orthostatic intolerance (OI) occurs in CFS. OI includes exercise intolerance as one of the main symptoms. It also includes fatigue, nausea, headaches, cognitive problems and visual disturbances as other less major symptoms.

Post-concussion Syndrome

- Exercise intolerance is present in those with PCS however their intolerance to exercise may reduce over time.

- Individuals with postconcussion syndrome may also experience a level of exercise intolerance, however there is little known comparatively about exercise intolerance in PCS patients.

Rhabdomyolysis

Heart Conditions

1. Cardiac arrhythmia;
2. Aortic valve insufficiency;
3. Pulmonary artery hypertension; PAH has the following symptoms; dyspnea and fatigue, these systems consequently contribute to exercise intolerance.
4. Asymptomatic atrial septal defects; In the heart the right ventricular (RV) can have a volume overload which ultimately produces a pressure overload in the RV resulting in exercise intolerance as the RV is no longer able to control high pressure associated with exercise.
5. Chronic heart failure

Mutations

1. Mitochondrial complex 111; Currently it is suggested that there are 27 different mutations identified in cytochrome *b* (mitochondrial complex III is one of those mutations). This mutation can often lead to skeletal muscle weakness and as a result exercise intolerance.
2. a complex of Coenzyme Q10;
3. several proteins;
4. Skeletal muscle respiratory chain defect; This can result in serve exercise intolerance which is manifested by the following symptoms of Skeletal muscle respiratory chain defect; muscle fatigue and lactic acidosis.

- Exercise tolerance reflects the combined capacity of components in the oxygen cascade to supply adequate oxygen for ATP resynthesis. In individuals with diseases such as cancer, certain therapies can affect one or more components of this cascade and therefore reduce the body's ability to utilise or deliver oxygen, leading to exercise intolerance.

Cytochrome b Mutations

Cytochrome b mutations can frequently cause isolated exercise intolerance and myopathy and in some cases multisystem disorders. The mitochondrial respiratory chain complex III catalyses electron transfer to cytochrome c. Complex III is embedded in the inner membrane of the mitochondria and consists of 11 subunits. Cytochrome b is encoded by the mitochondrial DNA which differs from all other subunits which are encoded in the nucleus. Cytochrome b plays a major part in the correct fabricating and function of complex III.

This mutation occurred in an 18-year-old man who had experienced exercise intolerance for most of his adolescence. Symptoms included extreme fatigue, nausea, a decline in physical activity ability and myalgia.

Intracranial Hypertension - Individuals with elevated levels of cerebrospinal fluid can experience increased head pain, throbbing, pulsatile tinnitus, nausea and vomiting, faintness and weakness and even loss of consciousness after exercise or exertion.

Treatment

Exercise is key for many heart and back patients, and a variety of specific exercise techniques are available for both groups. Some exercise specialists are trained in modifications specific to these patients.

In individuals with heart failure and normal EF (ejection fraction), including aortic distensibility, blood pressure, LV diastolic compliance and skeletal muscle function, aerobic exercise has the potential to improve exercise tolerance. A variety of pharmacological interventions such as verapamil, enalapril, angiotensin receptor antagonism, and aldosterone antagonism could potentially improve exercise tolerance in these individuals as well.

Research on individuals suffering from Chronic obstructive pulmonary disease (COPD), has found a number of effective therapies in relation to exercise intolerance. These include:

1. Oxygen Supplementation
    - Reduces carotid body drive and slows respiration at a given level of exercise.
2. Treatment with bronchodilators
    - Clinically useful improvements in expiratory airflow, allows fuller exhalation in a given period of time, reduces dynamic hyperinflation, and prolongs exercise tolerance.
3. Heliox (79% Helium, 21% oxygen)
    - Heliox has a lower density than air.
    - Breathing heliox lowers expiratory airflow resistance, decreases dynamic hyperinflation, and prolongs exercise tolerance.
4. High intensity rehabilitative exercise training
    - Increasing the fitness of muscles decreases the amount of lactic acid released at any given level of exercise.
    - Since lactic acid stimulates respiration, after rehabilitative training exercising, ventilation is lower, respiration is slowed, and dynamic hyperinflation is reduced.

A combination of these therapies (Combined therapies), have shown the potential to improve exercise tolerance as well.

Hazards

Certain conditions in particular exist where exercise, particularly rehabilitation, may be contraindicated, including:

- Decompensated heart failure
- Recent myocardial infarction
- Hypertrophic cardiomyopathy or cardiomyopathy from recent myocarditis
- Active or suspected myocarditis or pericarditis
- Low left ventricular ejection fraction
- Severe aortic stenosis
- Unstable ischemia
- Unstable arrythmia
- Irregular or resting pulse greater than 100 bpm
- Resting systolic blood pressure >200 mm Hg or resting diastolic blood pressure >110 mm Hg
- Severe pulmonary hypertension
- Severe chronic fatigue syndrome
- Suspected or known dissecting aneurysm
- Recent systemic or pulmonary embolus
- Pneumothorax and haemoptysis
- thrombophlebitis

Other conditions may also preclude exercising under certain conditions. Passive physiotherapy can in some instances be an alternative for some patients unable to safely self-power.

Exercise-induced Bronchoconstriction

Exercise-induced asthma, or E.I.A., occurs when the airways narrow as a result of exercise. The preferred term for this condition is exercise-induced bronchoconstriction (EIB); exercise does not cause asthma, but is frequently an asthma trigger.

Signs and Symptoms

It might be expected that people with E.I.B. would present with shortness of breath, and/or an elevated respiratory rate and wheezing, consistent with an asthma attack. However, many will present with decreased stamina, or difficulty in recovering from exertion compared to team members, or paroxysmal coughing from an irritable airway. Similarly, examination may reveal wheezing and prolonged expiratory phase, or may be quite normal. Consequently, a potential for under-diagnosis exists. Measurement of airflow, such as peak expiratory flow rates, which can be done inexpensively on the track or sideline, may prove helpful.

Cause

While the potential triggering events for E.I.B. are well recognized, the underlying pathogenesis is poorly understood. It usually occurs after at least several minutes of vigorous, "aerobic" activity, which demands that normal nasal breathing be supplemented by mouth breathing. The resultant inhalation of air that has not been warmed and humidified by the nasal passages seems to generate increased blood flow to the linings of the bronchial tree, resulting in edema. Constriction of these small airways then follows, worsening the degree of obstruction to airflow. There is increasing evidence that the smooth muscle that lines the airways becomes progressively more sensitive to changes that occur as a result of injury to the airways from dehydration. The chemical mediators that provoke the muscle spasm appear to arise from mast cells.

Diagnosis

Exercise-induced bronchoconstriction can be difficult to diagnose clinically given the lack of specific symptoms and frequent misinterpretation as manifestations of vigorous exercise. There are many mimics that present with similar symptoms, such as vocal cord dysfunction, cardiac arrhythmias, cardiomyopathies, and gastroesophageal reflux disease. It is also important to distinguish those who have asthma with exercise worsening, and who consequently will have abnormal testing at rest, from true exercise-induced bronchoconstriction, where there will be normal baseline results. Because of the wide differential diagnosis of exertional respiratory complaints, the diagnosis of exercise-induced bronchoconstriction based on history and self-reported symptoms alone has been shown to be inaccurate and will result in an incorrect diagnosis more than 50% of the time.

Spirometry

Objective testing should begin with spirometry at rest. In true exercise-induced bronchoconstriction, the results should be within normal limits. Should resting values be abnormal, then asthma, or some other chronic lung condition, is present. There is, of course, no reason why asthma and exercise-induced bronchoconstriction should not co-exist but the distinction is important because without successful treatment of underlying asthma, treatment of an exercise component will likely be unsuccessful. If baseline testing is normal, some form of exercise or pharmacologic stress will be required, either on the sideline or practice venue, or in the laboratory.

Exercise Testing

Treadmill or ergometer-based testing in lung function laboratories are effective methods for diagnosing exercise-induced bronchoconstriction, but may result in false negatives if the exercise stimulus is not intense enough.

Field-exercise Challenge

Field-exercise challenge tests that involve the athlete performing the sport in which they are normally involved and assessing FEV_1 after exercise are helpful if abnormal but have been shown to be less sensitive than eucapnic voluntary hyperventilation.

Eucapnic Voluntary Hyperventilation Challenge

The International Olympic Committee recommends the eucapnic voluntary hyperventilation (EVH) challenge as the test to document exercise-induced asthma in Olympic athletes. In the EVH challenge, the patient voluntarily, without exercising, rapidly breathes dry air enriched with 5% CO_2 for six minutes. The presence of the enriched CO_2 compensates for the CO_2 losses in the expired air, not matched by metabolic production, that occurs during hyperventilation, and so maintains CO_2 levels at normal.

Pharmacological Challenge Tests

Pharmacological challenge tests, such as the methacholine challenge test, have a lower sensitivity for detection of exercise-induced bronchoconstriction in athletes and are also not a recommended first-line approach in the evaluation of exercise-induced asthma.

Mannitol inhalation has been recently approved for use in the United States.

It should be noted, however, that a relatively recent review of the literature has concluded that there is currently insufficient available evidence to conclude that either mannitol inhalation or eucapnic voluntary hyperventilation are suitable alternatives to exercise challenge testing to detect exercise-induced bronchoconstriction and that additional research is required.

Treatment

Lifestyle

The best treatment is avoidance of conditions predisposing to attacks, when possible. In athletes who wish to continue their sport or do so in adverse conditions, preventive measures include altered training techniques and medications.

Some take advantage of the refractory period by precipitating an attack by "warming up," and then timing competition such that it occurs during the refractory period. Step-wise training works in a similar fashion. Warm up occurs in stages of increasing intensity, using the refractory period generated by each stage to reach a full workload.

Medication

The treatment of EIB has been extensively studied in asthmatic subjects over the last 30 years, but not so in EIB. Thus, it is not known whether athletes with EIB or 'sports asthma' respond similarly to subjects with classical allergic or nonallergic asthma. However, there is no evidence supporting different treatment for EIB in asthmatic athletes and nonathletes.

The most common medication used is a beta agonist taken about 20 minutes before exercise. Some physicians prescribe inhaled anti-inflammatory mists such as corticosteroids or leukotriene antagonists, and mast cell stabilizers have also proven effective. A randomized crossover study compared oral montelukast with inhaled salmeterol, both given two hours before exercise. Both drugs had similar benefit but montelukast lasted 24 hours.

Three randomized double-blind cross-over trials have examined the effect of vitamin C on EIB. Pooling the results of the three vitamin C trials indicates an average 48% reduction in the FEV1 decline caused by exericise (Figure). The systematic review concluded that "given the safety and low cost of vitamin C, and the positive findings for vitamin C administration in the three EIB studies, it seems reasonable for physically active people to test vitamin C when they have respiratory symptoms such as cough associated with exercise." It should be acknowledged that the total number of subjects involved in all three trials was only 40.

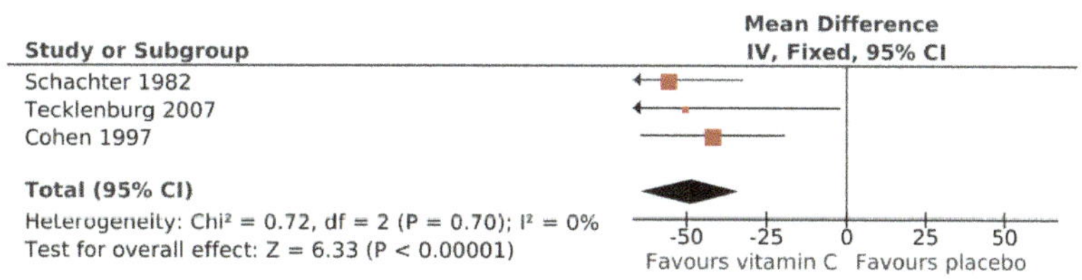

Figure: This forest plot shows the effect of vitamin C (0.5–2 g/day) on post-exercise decline in FEV1 in three studies with asthmatic participants. Constructed from data in Fig. 4 of Hemilä (2013). The three horizontal lines indicate the three studies, and the diamond shape at the bottom indicates the pooled effect of vitamin C: decrease in the post-exercise decline in FEV1 by 48% (95%CI: 33 to 64%).

In May 2013, the American Thoracic Society issued the first treatment guidelines for EIB.

Prognosis

As evidenced by many professional athletes who have overcome EIB using some combination of accepted treatments, the prognosis is usually very good. Olympic swimmers Tom Dolan, Amy Van Dyken, and Nancy Hogshead, Olympic track star Jackie Joyner-Kersee, baseball Hall of Famer Catfish Hunter, and American football player Jerome Bettis are among the many who have done so. Tour de France winner Chris Froome admitted to suffer from the condition after being spotted using a nasal inhaler during race. Other sportspeople with EIB include racing cyclist Simon Yates, distance runner Paula Radcliffe and cross-country skier Marit Bjørgen. Research by sports scientist John Dickinson found that 70 percent of UK-based members of the British swimming team had some form of asthma, as did a third of Team Sky cyclists, compared to a national asthma rate of eight to ten percent, whilst a study by the United States Olympic Committee in 2000 found that half of cross-country skiers had EIB.

School children are also one of the major groups impacted by EIB as exercise programs and sports activities form a big part of most schools. Proactive schools usually set special EIB friendly guidelines for students with EIB so that they can be included in mainstream student exercise programs.

Exercise Hypertension

Exercise hypertension is an excessive rise in blood pressure during exercise. Many of those with exercise hypertension have spikes in systolic pressure to 250 mmHg or greater.

A rise in systolic blood pressure to over 200 mmHg when exercising at 100 W is pathological and a rise in pressure over 220 mmHg needs to be controlled by the appropriate drugs.

Similarly, in healthy individuals the response of the diastolic pressure to 'dynamic' exercise (e.g. walking, running or jogging) of moderate intensity is to remain constant or to fall slightly (due to the improved blood flow), but in some individuals a rise of 10 mmHg or greater is found.

Recent work at Johns Hopkins involving a group of athletes aged 55 to 75 with mild hypertension has found a correlation of those with exercise hypertension to a reduced ability of the major blood vessels to change in size in response to increased blood flow (probably due to impaired function of the endothelial cells in the vessel walls). This is to be differentiated from stiffness of the blood-vessel walls, which was not found to be correlated with the effect.

Exercise-induced Nausea

Exercise-induced nausea is a feeling of sickness or vomiting which can occur shortly after exercise has stopped as well as during exercise itself. It may be a symptom of either over-exertion during exercise, or from too abruptly ending an exercise session. People engaged in high-intensity exercise such as aerobics and bicycling have reported suffering from exercise-induced nausea. A study of 20 volunteers conducted at Nagoya University, Japan associated a higher degree of exercise-induced nausea after eating.

Lack of hydration during exercise is a well known cause of headache and nausea during exercise. Exercising at a heavy rate causes blood flow to be taken away from the stomach, causing nausea.

Another possible cause of exercise induced nausea is overhydration. Drinking too much water before, during, and/or after extreme exercise (such as a marathon) can cause nausea, diarrhea, confusion, and muscle tremors. Excessive water consumption reduces or dilutes electrolyte levels in the body causing hyponatremia.

Exercise-associated Hyponatremia

Exercise-associated hyponatremia, or EAH, is a fluid-electrolyte disorder caused by a decrease in sodium levels (hyponatremia) during or up to 24 hours after prolonged physical activity. This disorder can develop when marathon runners or endurance event athletes drink more fluid, usually water or sports drinks, than their kidneys can excrete. This excess water can severely dilute the level of sodium in the blood needed for organs, especially the brain, to function properly.

The incidence of EAH in athletes has increased in recent years, especially in the United States, as marathon races and endurance events have become more popular. A recent study showed 13% of the Boston 2002 marathon runners experienced EAH; most cases were mild. Eight deaths from EAH have been documented since 1985.

Mechanism

Sodium is an important electrolyte needed for maintaining blood pressure. Sodium is mainly found in the body fluids that surround the cells and is necessary for nerves, muscles, and other body tissues to function properly.

Many factors may contribute to the development of EAH. Under normal conditions, sodium and water levels are regulated by the renal and hormonal systems. The decrease in sodium levels can occur due to a defect in the renal and hormonal systems, an overwhelming increase in water consumption and excessive loss of sodium through sweating. When the sodium levels outside of the cells decrease, water moves into the cells. The cells begin to increase in size. When several cells in one area begin to increase in size, swelling occurs in the affected area. Swelling is commonly observed in hands, legs, and feet.

Sodium is also important in regulating the amount of water that passes through the blood-brain barrier. Decreased sodium blood levels result in increased permeability of water across the blood-brain barrier. This increased influx of water causes brain swelling which leads to severe neurological symptoms.

Symptoms

Symptoms may be absent or mild for the early onset of EAH and can include impaired exercise performance, nausea, vomiting, headache, bloating, and swelling of hands, legs, and feet. As water retention increases, weight gain may also occur. More severe symptoms include pulmonary edema and hyponatremic encephalopathy. Symptoms of hyponatremic encephalopathy are associated with an altered level of consciousness and can include sullenness, sleepiness, withdrawing from social interaction, photophobia, and seizures. In some reported cases, death has occurred.

Diagnosis

EAH is categorized by having a blood serum or plasma sodium level below normal, which is less than 135 mmol/l. Asymptomatic EAH is not normally detected unless the athlete has had a sodium blood serum or plasma test. Hyponatremic encephalopathy may be detect using brain imaging studies and pulmonary edema may be confirmed by x-ray.

Causes and Prevention

The primary causes of EAH include excessive fluid retention during exercise with a significant sodium deficit and excessive fluid intake leading to an increase in total body water resulting in a reduction in blood sodium levels.

Athlete-specific risk factors are being of female gender, use of non-steroidal anti-inflammatory drugs or NSAIDs, slow running, excessive fluid ingestion, low body weight, and event inexperience. Event-specific risk factors are high availability of drinking fluids, duration of exercise exceeds 4 hours, unusually hot environmental conditions, and extreme cold temperature.

Prevention of EAH focuses on reducing fluid consumption to avoid fluid retention before, during, and after exercise.

The Role of Thirst

In a published statement of the Third International Exercise-Associated Hyponatremia Consensus Development Conference, researchers concluded that drinking in accordance with the sensation of thirst is sufficient for preventing both dehydration and hyponatremia. This advice is contradicted by the American College of Sports Medicine, which has previously recommended athletes drink "as much as tolerable. In October of 2015, ACSM President W. Larry Kenney stated that "[T]he clear and important health message should be that thirst alone is not the best indicator of dehydration or the body's fluid needs."

In a letter to the editors of The Journal of Wilderness and Environmental Medicine, Brad L. Bennett, PhD claimed "perpetuation of the myth that one needs to drink beyond the dictates of thirst can be deadly." Similarly, authors of the Statement of the Third International Exercise-Associated Hyponatremia Consensus Development Conference claim this advice has "facilitated inadvertent overdrinking and pathological dilutional EAH."

Critics of the ACSM's view have questioned their motives, pointing out that Gatorade is one of the organizations "platinum sponsors."

Treatment and Prognosis

Treatments are focused on the underlying cause of hyponatremia and include

- fluid restriction
- 0.9% saline and hypertonic saline intravenously
- 100 ml of 3% saline hourly

When EAH is treated early, complete recovery is expected.

In addition to the above treatments, athletes experiencing EAH encephalopathy may also receive high-flow oxygen and a rapid infusion of 100 ml of 3% NaCl to reduce brain edema.

Recent Research

As the incidence of EAH has increased in recent years, current research has focused on the prevalence of EAH in marathon runners and endurance athletes. One study found 26% of the athletes competing in the Triple Iron ultra-triathlon developed EAH. A similar study measured the prevalence of EAH in open-water ultra-endurance swimmers and found 8% of males and 36% of females developed EAH.

Current research has also focused on the determining the most effective treatment for EAH. The data from one study suggests that immediate administration of 100 ml intravenous bolus of 3% hypertonic saline was more effective at normalizing blood sodium levels than oral administration for asymptomatic EAH.

Hives

Hives also known as urticaria, is a kind of skin rash with red, raised, itchy bumps. They may also burn or sting. Often the patches of rash move around. Typically they last a few days and do not leave any long lasting skin changes. Fewer than 5% of cases last for more than six weeks. The condition frequently recurs.

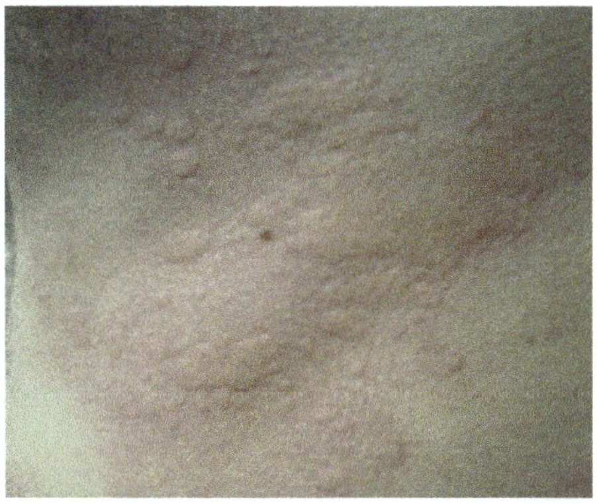

Hives on the left chest wall. Notice that they are slightly raised.

Hives frequently occur following an infection or as a result of an allergic reaction such as to medication, insect bites, or food. Psychological stress, cold temperature, or vibration may also be a trigger. In half of cases the cause remains unknown. Risk factors include having conditions such as hay fever or asthma. Diagnosis is typically based on the appearance. Patch testing may be useful to determine the allergy.

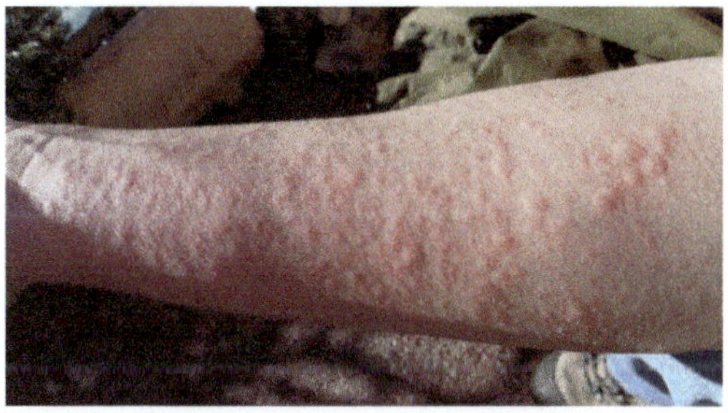

After contact with a conifer

Prevention is by avoiding whatever it is that causes the condition. Treatment is typically with antihistamines such as diphenhydramine and ranitidine. In severe cases, corticosteroids or leukotriene inhibitors may also be used. Keeping the environmental temperature cool is also useful. For cases that last more than six weeks immunosuppressants such as ciclosporin may be used.

About 20% of people are affected. Cases of short duration occur equally in males and females while cases of long duration are more common in females. Cases of short duration are more common among children while cases of long duration are more common among those who are middle aged. Hives have been described at least since the time of Hippocrates. The term urticaria is from the Latin *urtica* meaning “nettle”.

Welts (raised areas surrounded by a red base) from urticaria can appear anywhere on the surface of the skin. Whether the trigger is allergic or not, a complex release of inflammatory mediators, including histamine from cutaneous mast cells, results in fluid leakage from superficial blood vessels. Welts may be pinpoint in size, or several inches in diameter.

Angioedema is a related condition (also from allergic and nonallergic causes), though fluid leakage is from much deeper blood vessels in the subcutaneous or submucosal layers. Individual hives that are painful, last more than 24 hours, or leave a bruise as they heal are more likely to be a more serious condition called urticarial vasculitis. Hives caused by stroking the skin (often linear in appearance) are due to a benign condition called dermatographic urticaria.

Cause

Urticaria can also be classified by the purported causative agent. Many different substances in the environment may cause urticaria, including medications, food and physical agents. In perhaps more than 50% of people with chronic urticaria of unknown cause, it is due to an autoimmune reaction.

Medications

Drugs that have caused allergic reactions evidenced as urticaria include codeine, dextroamphetamine, aspirin, ibuprofen, penicillin, clotrimazole, trichazole, sulfonamides, anticonvulsants, cefaclor, piracetam, vaccines, and antidiabetic drugs. The antidiabetic sulphonylurea glimepiride, in particular, has been documented to induce allergic reactions manifesting as urticaria. Drug-induced urticaria has been known to have an effect on severe cardiorespiratory failure.

Food

The most common food allergies in adults are shellfish and nuts. The most common food allergies in children are shellfish, nuts, eggs, wheat, and soy. One study showed Balsam of Peru, which is in many processed foods, to be the most common cause of immediate contact urticaria. A less common cause is exposure to certain bacteria, such as *Streptococcus* species or possibly *Helicobacter pylori*.

Infection or Environmental Agent

Urticaria including chronic spontaneous urticaria can be a complication and symptom of a parasitic infection, such as blastocystosis and strongyloidiasis among others.

The rash that develops from poison ivy, poison oak, and poison sumac contact is commonly mistaken for urticaria. This rash is caused by contact with urushiol and results in a form of contact dermatitis called urushiol-induced contact dermatitis. Urushiol is spread by contact, but can be washed off with a strong grease- or oil-dissolving detergent and cool water and rubbing ointments.

Dermatographic Urticaria

Dermatographic urticaria (also known as dermatographism or "skin writing") is marked by the appearance of weals or welts on the skin as a result of scratching or firm stroking of the skin. Seen in 4–5% of the population, it is one of the most common types of urticaria, in which the skin becomes raised and inflamed when stroked, scratched, rubbed, and sometimes even slapped.

The skin reaction usually becomes evident soon after the scratching, and disappears within 30 minutes. Dermatographism is the most common form of a subset of chronic hives, acknowledged as "physical hives".

It stands in contrast to the linear reddening that does not itch seen in healthy people who are scratched. In most cases, the cause is unknown, although it may be preceded by a viral infection, antibiotic therapy, or emotional upset. Dermographism is diagnosed by taking a tongue blade and drawing it over the skin of the arm or back. The hives should develop within a few minutes. Unless the skin is highly sensitive and reacts continually, treatment is not needed. Taking antihistamines can reduce the response in cases that are annoying to the patient.

Pressure or Delayed Pressure

This type of urticaria can occur right away, precisely after a pressure stimulus or as a deferred response to sustained pressure being enforced to the skin. In the deferred form, the hives only appear after about six hours from the initial application of pressure to the skin. Under normal circumstances, these hives are not the same as those witnessed with most urticariae. Instead, the protrusion in the affected areas is typically more spread out. The hives may last from eight hours to three days. The source of the pressure on the skin can happen from tight fitted clothing, belts, clothing with tough straps, walking, leaning against an object, standing, sitting on a hard surface, etc. The areas of the body most commonly affected are the hands, feet, trunk, abdomen, buttocks, legs and face. Although this appears to be very similar to dermatographism, the cardinal difference is that the swelled skin areas do not become visible quickly and tend to last much longer. This form of the skin disease is, however, rare.

Cholinergic or Stress

Cholinergic urticaria (CU) is one of the physical urticaria which is provoked during sweating events such as exercise, bathing, staying in a heated environment, or emotional stress. The hives produced are typically smaller than classic hives and are generally shorter-lasting.

Multiple subtypes have been elucidated, each of which require distinct treatment.

Cold-induced

The cold type of urticaria is caused by exposure of the skin to extreme cold, damp and windy conditions; it occurs in two forms. The rare form is hereditary and becomes evident as hives all over the body 9 to 18 hours after cold exposure. The common form of cold urticaria demonstrates itself with the rapid onset of hives on the face, neck, or hands after exposure to cold. Cold urticaria is common and lasts for an average of five to six years. The population most affected is young adults, between 18 and 25 years old. Many people with the condition also suffer from dermographism and cholinergic urticaria.

Severe reactions can be seen with exposure to cold water; swimming in cold water is the most common cause of a severe reaction. This can cause a massive discharge of histamine, resulting in low blood pressure, fainting, shock and even loss of life. Cold urticaria is diagnosed by dabbing an ice cube against the skin of the forearm for 1 to 5 minutes. A distinct hive should develop if a patient suffers cold urticaria. This is different from the normal redness that can be seen in people without cold urticaria. Patients with cold urticaria need to learn to protect themselves from a hasty drop in body temperature. Regular antihistamines are not generally efficacious. One particular antihistamine, cyproheptadine (Periactin), has been found to be useful. The tricyclic antidepressant doxepin has also been found to be an effective blocking agent of histamine discharge. Finally, a medication named ketotifen, which keeps mast cells from discharging histamine, has also been employed with widespread success.

Solar Urticaria

This form of the disease occurs on areas of the skin exposed to the sun; the condition becomes evident within minutes of exposure.

Water-induced

This type of urticaria is also termed rare, and occurs upon contact with water. The response is not temperature-dependent and the skin appears similar to cholinergic form of the disease. The appearance of hives is within one to 15 minutes of contact with the water, and can last from 10 minutes to two hours. This kind of hives do not seem to be stimulated by histamine discharge like the other physical hives. Most researchers believe this condition is actually skin sensitivity to additives in the water, such as chlorine. Water urticaria is diagnosed by dabbing tap water and distilled water to the skin and observing the gradual response. Aquagenic urticaria is treated with capsaicin (Zostrix) administered to the chafed skin. This is the same treatment used for shingles. Antihistamines are of questionable benefit in this instance, since histamine is not the causative factor.

Chizzola maculae is a very specific skin lesion due to fluoride exposure. The size of a coin, these lesions may resemble small blue bruises or be wholly pink. Doctors George Waldbott and V. A. Cecilioni named the lesions after a town in Italy, where they were common in young women and children. According to Waldbott, chizzola maculae are early symptoms of fluoride intoxication.

Exercise

The condition was first distinguished in 1980. People with exercise urticaria (EU) experience hives, itchiness, shortness of breath and low blood pressure five to 30 minutes after beginning exercise. These symptoms can progress to shock and even sudden death. Jogging is the most common exercise to cause EU, but it is not induced by a hot shower, fever, or with fretfulness. This differentiates EU from cholinergic urticaria.

EU sometimes occurs only when someone exercises within 30 minutes of eating particular foods, such as wheat or shellfish. For these individuals, exercising alone or eating the injuring food without exercising produces no symptoms. EU can be diagnosed by having the patient exercise and then observing the symptoms. This method must be used with caution and only with the appropriate resuscitative measures at hand. EU can be differentiated from cholinergic urticaria by the hot water immersion test. In this test, the patient is immersed in water at 43 °C (109.4 °F). Someone with EU will not develop hives, while a person with cholinergic urticaria will develop the characteristic small hives, especially on the neck and chest.

The immediate symptoms of this uncanny type are treated with antihistamines, epinephrine and airway support. Taking antihistamines prior to exercise may be effective. Ketotifen is acknowledged to stabilise mast cells and prevent histamine release, and has been effective in treating this hives disorder. Avoiding exercise or foods that cause the mentioned symptoms is very important. In particular circumstances, tolerance can be brought on by regular exercise, but this must be under medical supervision.

Pathophysiology

The skin lesions of urticarial disease are caused by an inflammatory reaction in the skin, causing leakage of capillaries in the dermis, and resulting in an edema which persists until the interstitial fluid is absorbed into the surrounding cells.

Urticaria is caused by the release of histamine and other mediators of inflammation (cytokines) from cells in the skin. This process can be the result of an allergic or nonallergic reaction, differing in the eliciting mechanism of histamine release.

Allergic Urticaria

Histamine and other proinflammatory substances are released from mast cells in the skin and tissues in response to the binding of allergen-bound IgE antibodies to high-affinity cell surface receptors. Basophils and other inflammatory cells are also seen to release histamine and other mediators, and are thought to play an important role, especially in chronic urticarial diseases.

Autoimmune Urticaria

Over half of all cases of chronic idiopathic urticaria are the result of an autoimmune trigger. Roughly 50% of patients with chronic urticaria spontaneously develop autoantibodies directed at the receptor FcεRI located on skin mast cells. Chronic stimulation of this receptor leads to chronic hives. Patients often have other autoimmune conditions, such as autoimmune thyroiditis, celiac disease, type 1 diabetes, rheumatoid arthritis, Sjögren's syndrome or systemic lupus erythematosus.

Infections

Hive-like rashes commonly accompany viral illnesses, such as the common cold. They usually appear three to five days after the cold has started, and may even appear a few days after the cold has resolved.

Nonallergic Urticaria

Mechanisms other than allergen-antibody interactions are known to cause histamine release from mast cells. Many drugs, for example morphine, can induce direct histamine release not involving any immunoglobulin molecule. Also, a diverse group of signaling substances, called neuropeptides, have been found to be involved in emotionally induced urticaria. Dominantly inherited cutaneous and neurocutaneous porphyrias (porphyria cutanea tarda, hereditary coproporphyria, variegate porphyria and erythropoietic protoporphyria) have been associated with solar urticaria. The occurrence of drug-induced solar urticaria may be associated with porphyrias. This may be caused by IgG binding, not IgE.

Dietary Histamine Poisoning

This is termed scombroid food poisoning. Ingestion of free histamine released by bacterial decay in fish flesh may result in a rapid-onset, allergic-type symptom complex which includes urticaria. However, the urticaria produced by scombroid is reported not to include wheals.

Stress and Chronic Idiopathic Urticaria

Chronic idiopathic urticaria has been anecdotally linked to stress since the 1940s. A large body of evidence demonstrates an association between this condition and both poor emotional well-being and reduced health-related quality of life. A link between stress and this condition has also been shown. A recent study has demonstrated an association between stressful life events (e.g. bereavement, divorce, etc.) and chronic idiopathic urticaria and also an association between post-traumatic stress and chronic idiopathic urticaria.

Diagnosis

The cause of chronic urticaria can rarely be determined. In some cases regular extensive allergy testing over a long period of time is requested in hopes of getting new insight. No evidence shows regular allergy testing results in identification of a problem or relief for people with chronic urticaria. Regular allergy testing for people with chronic urticaria is not recommended.

Acute Versus Chronic

- Acute urticaria is defined as the presence of evanescent wheals which completely resolve within six weeks. Acute urticaria becomes evident a few minutes after the person has been exposed to an allergen. The outbreak may last several weeks, but usually the hives are gone in six weeks. Typically, the hives are a reaction to food, but in about half the cases, the trigger is unknown. Common foods may be the cause, as well as bee or wasp stings, or skin contact with certain fragrances. Acute viral infection is another common cause of acute urticaria (viral exanthem). Less common causes of hives include friction, pressure, temperature extremes, exercise, and sunlight.
- Chronic urticaria (ordinary urticaria) is defined as the presence of evanescent wheals which persist for greater than six weeks. Some of the more severe chronic cases have lasted more than 20 years. A survey indicated chronic urticaria lasted a year or more in more than 50% of sufferers and 20 years or more in 20% of them.

Acute and chronic urticaria are visually indistinguishable.

Related Conditions

Angioedema

Angioedema is similar to urticaria, but in angioedema, the swelling occurs in a lower layer of the dermis than in urticaria, as well as in the subcutis. This swelling can occur around the mouth, eyes, in the throat, in the abdomen, or in other locations. Urticaria and angioedema sometimes occur together in response to an allergen, and is a concern in severe cases, as angioedema of the throat can be fatal.

Vibratory Angioedema

This very rare form of angioedema develops in response to contact with vibration. In vibratory angioedema, symptoms develop within two to five minutes after contact with a vibrating object, and abate after about an hour. Patients with this disorder do not suffer from dermographism or pressure urticaria. Vibratory angioedema is diagnosed by holding a vibrating device such as a laboratory vortex machine against the forearm for four minutes. Speedy swelling of the whole forearm extending into the upper arm is also noted later. The principal treatment is avoidance of vibratory stimulants. Antihistamines have also been proven helpful.

Management

The mainstay of therapy for both acute and chronic urticaria is patient education, avoiding triggers and using antihistamines.

Chronic urticaria can be difficult to treat and lead to significant disability. Unlike the acute form, 50-80% of people with chronic urticaria have no identifiable triggers. Fortunately, 50% of people with chronic urticaria will experience remission within 1 year. Overall, treatment is geared towards symptomatic management. Individuals with chronic urticaria may need other medications in addition to antihistamines to control symptoms. Patients who experience urticaria with angioedema require emergency treatment as this is a life-threatening condition.

Treatment guidelines for the management of chronic urticaria have been published by professional allergy and dermatology groups. According to the 2014 American practice parameters, treatment involves a step wise approach. Step 1 consists of second generation, H1 receptor blocking antihistamines. Systemic glucocorticoids can also be used for episodes of severe disease but should not be used for long term due to their long list of side effects. Step 2 consists of increasing the dose of the current antihistamine, adding other antihistamines, or adding a leukotriene receptor antagonist such as montelukast. Step 3 consists of adding or replacing the current treatment with hydroxyzine or doxepin. If the individual doesn't respond to steps 1-3 then they are considered to have refractory symptoms. At this point, anti-inflammatory medications (dapsone, sulfasalazine), immunosuppressants (cyclosporin, sirolimus) or other medications like omalizumab can be used. These options are explained in more detail below.

Antihistamines

Antihistamines that block the histamine H1 receptors are the first line of therapy. First generation antihistamines such as diphenhydramine (Benadryl) or hydroxyzine (Atarax) block both central and peripheral H1 receptors and can be very sedating. Second generation antihistamines such as loratadine (Claritin), cetirizine (Zyrtec), or desloratadine (Clarinex) selectively antagonize only the peripheral H1 receptors and are therefore less sedating, less anticholinergic, and generally preferred over the first generation antihistamines. To obtain the maximal benefit, it is important to take the antihistamines daily instead of only during acute exacerbations.

Patients who don't respond to the maximum dose of H1 antihistamines may benefit from the addition of H2 antihistamines. However, not all combinations have proven beneficial. Studies have shown improvement with the combination of hydroxyzine and cimetidine but not with the combination of cetirizine and cimetidine.

Systemic Steroids

Oral glucocorticoids are effective in controlling symptoms of chronic urticaria however they have an extensive list of adverse effects such as adrenal suppression, weight gain, osteoporosis, hyperglycemia, etc. Therefore, their use should be limited to a couple of weeks. In addition, one study found that systemic glucocorticoids combined with antihistamines did not hasten the time to symptom control compared with antihistamines alone.

Leukotriene-receptor Antagonists

Leukotrienes are released from mast cells along with histamine. The medications, montelukast and zafirlukast block leukotriene receptors and can be used as add on treatment or in isolation for patients with CU. It is important to note that these medications may be more beneficial for patients with NSAID induced CU.

Other

Other options for refractory symptoms of chronic urticaria include anti-inflammatory medications, omalizumab, and immunosuppressants. Potential anti-inflammatory agents include dapsone, sulfasalazine, and hydroxychloroquine. Dapsone is a sulfone antimicrobial agent and is thought to suppress prostaglandin and leukotriene activity. It is helpful in therapy-refractory cases and is contraindicated in patients with G6PD deficiency. Sulfasalazine, a 5-ASA derivative, is thought to alter adenosine release and inhibit IgE mediated mast cell degranulation, Sulfasalazine is a good option for people with anemia who cannot take dapsone. Hydroxychloroquine is an antimalarial agent that suppresses T lymphocytes. It has a low cost however it takes longer than dapsone or sulfasalazine to work.

Omalizumab was approved by the FDA in 2014 for patients 12 years old and above with chronic urticaria. It is a monoclonal antibody directed against IgE. Significant improvement in pruritus and quality of life was observed in a phase III, multicenter, randomized control trial.

Immunosuppressants used for CU include cyclosporine, tacrolimus, sirolimus, and mycophenolate. Calcineurin inhibitors, such as cyclosporine and tacrolimus, inhibit cell responsiveness to mast cell products and inhibit T cell activity. They are preferred by some experts to treat severe symptoms. Sirolimus and mycophenolate have less evidence for their use in the treatment of chronic urticaria but reports have shown them to be efficacious. Immunosuppressants are generally reserved as the last line of therapy for severe cases due to their potential for serious adverse effects.

Tennis Elbow

Tennis elbow or lateral epicondylitis is a condition in which the outer part of the elbow becomes sore and tender. The forearm muscles and tendons become damaged from overuse — repeating the same strenuous motions again and again. This leads to pain and tenderness on the outside of the elbow.

Any activity, including playing tennis, which involves the repetitive use of the extensor muscles of the forearm can cause acute or chronic tendonitis of the tendinous insertion of these muscles at the lateral epicondyle of the elbow. The condition is common in carpenters and laborers who swing a hammer or other tool with the forearm,continuing activity after onset of the condition and avoiding mandatory rest may lead to permanent onset of pain and only treatable via surgery. Dr. F. Runge (a German physician) is usually credited for the first description of the condition in 1873; he called it "writer's cramp" (*Schreibekrampfes*). Later, it was called "washer women's elbow". As it also occurred in tennis, it soon was called "tennis elbow" after British surgeon Henry Morris published an article in *The Lancet* describing "the lawn tennis arm," 1883. The term "tennis elbow" first appeared in an 1883 paper by H.P. Major as "lawn-tennis elbow".

Signs and Symptoms

- Pain on the outer part of the elbow (lateral epicondyle)
- Point tenderness over the lateral epicondyle—a prominent part of the bone on the outside of the elbow
- Pain from gripping and movements of the wrist, especially wrist extension and lifting movements
- Pain from activities that use the muscles that extend the wrist (e.g. pouring a container of liquid, lifting with the palm down, sweeping, especially where wrist movement is required)

Symptoms associated with tennis elbow include, but are not limited to: radiating pain from the outside of the elbow to the forearm and wrist, pain during extension of wrist, weakness of the forearm, a painful grip while shaking hands or torquing a doorknob, and not being able to hold relatively heavy items in the hand. The pain is similar to the condition known as *golfer's elbow*, but the latter occurs at the medial side of the elbow.

Causes

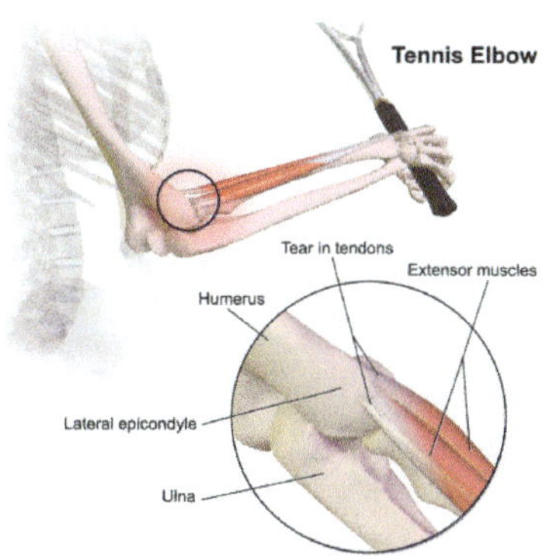

Tennis elbow

Tennis elbow is a type of repetitive strain injury, resulting from tendon overuse and failed healing of the tendon. In addition, the extensor carpi radialis brevis muscle plays a key role.

Early experiments suggested that tennis elbow was primarily caused by overexertion. However, studies show that trauma such as direct blows to the epicondyle, a sudden forceful pull, or forceful extension cause more than half of these injuries. It has also been known that incorrectly playing tennis may cause early stages of tennis elbow as shock is received when mishitting the ball.

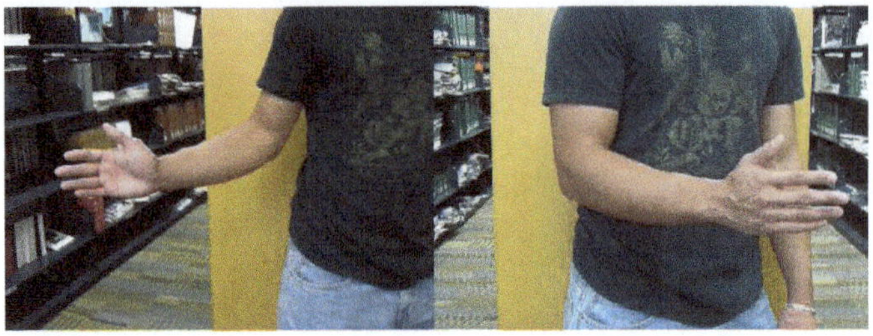

Example of repetitive movement that may cause tennis elbow

Cyriax proposes one explanation of how tennis elbow may come about. The hypothesis states that there are microscopic and macroscopic tears between the common extensor tendon and the periosteum of the lateral humeral epicondyle. An operation conducted in this study showed that 28 out of 39 patients showed tearing at the tendon cuff. Kaplan stated that the radial nerve was significantly involved in tennis elbow. He noted the constriction of the radial nerve by adhesions to the capsule of the radiohumeral joint and the short extensor muscle of the wrist. He found evidence that many differed in how they contracted tennis elbow. Disorders such as calcification of the rotator cuff, bicipital tendinitis, or carpal tunnel syndrome may increase chances of tennis elbow.

Pathophysiology

Histological findings include granulation tissue, microrupture, degenerative changes, and there is no traditional inflammation. As a consequence, "lateral elbow tendinopathy or tendinosis" is used instead of "lateral epicondylitis".

Examination of tennis elbow tissue reveals noninflammatory tissue, and therefore, the term "angio-fibroblastic tendinosis" is used.

Longitudinal sonogram of the lateral elbow displays thickening and heterogeneity of the common extensor tendon that is consistent with tendinosis, as the ultrasound reveals calcifications, intrasubstance tears, and marked irregularity of the lateral epicondyle. Although the term "epicondylitis" is frequently used to describe this disorder, most histopathologic findings of studies have displayed no evidence of an acute, or a chronic inflammatory process. Histologic studies have demonstrated that this condition is the result of tendon degeneration, which causes normal tissue to be replaced by a disorganized arrangement of collagen. Therefore, the disorder is more appropriately referred to as "tendinosis" or "tendinopathy" rather than "tendinitis."

Colour Doppler ultrasound reveals structural tendon changes, with vascularity and hypo-echoic areas that correspond to the areas of pain in the extensor origin.

The pathophysiology of lateral epicondylitis is degenerative. Non-inflammatory, chronic degenerative changes of the origin of the extensor carpi radialis brevis (ECRB) muscle are identified in surgical pathology specimens. It is unclear if the pathology is affected by prior injection of corticosteroid.

Tennis players generally believe tennis elbow is caused by the repetitive nature of hitting thousands of tennis balls, which leads to tiny tears in the forearm tendon attachment at the elbow.

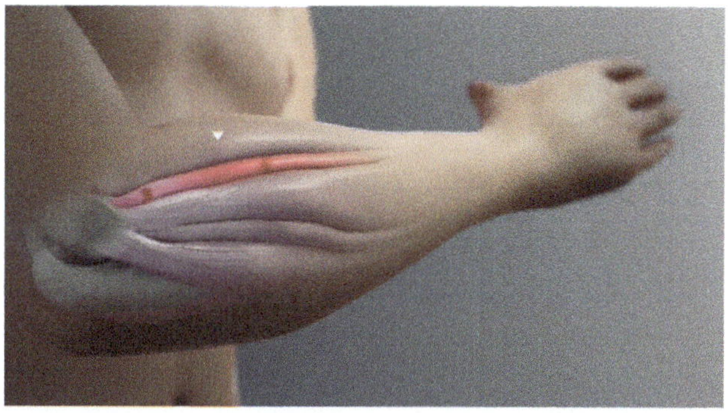

A 3D medical animation still shot illustrating the medical condition known as Tennis Elbow

The extensor digiti minimi also has a small origin site medial to the elbow that this condition can affect. The muscle involves the extension of the little finger and some extension of the wrist allowing for adaption to "snap" or flick the wrist—usually associated with a racquet swing. Most often, the extensor muscles become painful due to tendon breakdown from over-extension. Improper form or movement allows for power in a swing to rotate through and around the wrist—creating a moment on that joint instead of the elbow joint or rotator cuff. This moment causes pressure to build impact forces to act on the tendon causing irritation and inflammation.

The following speculative rationale is offered by proponents of an overuse theory of etiology: The extensor carpi radialis brevis has a small origin and does transmit large forces through its tendon during repetitive grasping. It has also been implicated as being vulnerable during shear stress during all movements of the forearm.

While it is commonly stated that lateral epicondylitis is caused by repetitive microtrauma/overuse, this is a speculative etiological theory with limited scientific support that is likely overstated. Other speculative risk factors for lateral epicondylitis include taking up tennis later in life, unaccustomed strenuous activity, decreased mental chronometry and speed and repetitive eccentric contraction of muscle (controlled lengthening of a muscle group).

Prevention

Another factor of tennis elbow injury is experience and ability. The proportion of players who reported a history of tennis elbow had an increased number of playing years. As for ability, poor technique increases the chance for injury much like any sport. Therefore, an individual must learn proper technique for all aspects of their sport. The competitive level of the athlete also affects the incidence of tennis elbow. Class A and B players had a significantly higher rate of tennis elbow occurrence compared to class C and novice players. However, an opposite, but not statistically significant, trend is observed for the recurrence of previous cases, with an increasingly higher rate as ability level decreases.

Other ways to prevent tennis elbow:

- Decrease the amount of playing time if already injured or feeling pain in outside part of the elbow.

- Stay in overall good physical shape.
- Strengthen the muscles of the forearm: (pronator quadratus, pronator teres, and supinator muscle)—the upper arm: (biceps, triceps)—and the shoulder (deltoid muscle) and upper back (trapezius). Increased muscular strength increases stability of joints such as the elbow.
- Like other sports, use equipment appropriate to your ability, body size, and muscular strength.
- Avoid any repetitive lifting or pulling of heavy objects (especially over your head)

Vibration dampeners (otherwise known as "gummies") are not believed to be a reliable preventative measure. Rather, proper weight distribution in the racket is thought to be a more viable option in negating shock.

Diagnosis

To diagnose tennis elbow, the physician performs a battery of tests in which he places pressure on the affected area while asking the patient to move the elbow, wrist, and fingers. X-rays can confirm and distinguish possibilities of existing causes of pain that are unrelated to tennis elbow, such as fracture or arthritis. Medical ultrasonography and magnetic resonance imaging (MRI) are other valuable tools for diagnosis but are frequently avoided due to the high cost. MRI screening can confirm excess fluid and swelling in the affected region in the elbow, such as the connecting point between the forearm bone and the extensor carpi radialis brevis.

Diagnosis is made by clinical signs and symptoms that are discrete and characteristic. With the elbow fully extended, the patient feels points of tenderness over the affected point on the elbow—which is the origin of the extensor carpi radialis brevis muscle from the lateral epicondyle (extensor carpi radialis brevis origin). There is also pain with passive wrist flexion and resistive wrist extension (Cozen's test). Resisted middle finger extension might indicate the involvement of Extensor Digitorum also. These tests shall be used to measure the prognosis of the condition.

Depending upon severity and quantity of multiple tendon injuries that have built up, the extensor carpi radialis brevis may not be fully healed by conservative treatment. Nirschl defines four stages of lateral epicondylitis, showing the introduction of permanent damage beginning at Stage 2.

1. Inflammatory changes that are reversible
2. Nonreversible pathologic changes to origin of the extensor carpi radialis brevis muscle
3. Rupture of ECRB muscle origin
4. Secondary changes such as fibrosis or calcification.

Treatment

Evidence for the treatment of lateral epicondylitis before 2010 was poor. There were clinical trials addressing many proposed treatments, but the trials were of poor quality.

A 2009 study looked at using eccentric exercise with a rubber bar in addition to standard treatment: the trial was stopped after 8 weeks because the improvement using the bar for therapy was so significant. Based on small sample size and a follow-up only 7 weeks from commencement of treatment, the study shows short-term improvements. This along with other studies allowed doctors to conclude that approximately 80-95% of all tennis elbow cases can be treated without surgery. However, long-term results have not yet been determined.

In some cases, severity of tennis elbow symptoms mend without any treatment, within six to 24 months. Tennis elbow left untreated can lead to chronic pain that degrades quality of daily living.

Physical

There are several recommendations regarding prevention, treatment, and avoidance of recurrence that are largely speculative including stretches and progressive strengthening exercises to prevent re-irritation of the tendon and other exercise measures.

One way to help treat minor cases of tennis elbow is to simply relax the affected arm. The rest will allow the stress and tightness within the forearm to slowly relax and eventually have the arm in working condition once again in a day or two, depending on the case.

Evidence from the Tyler study suggests that eccentric exercise using a rubber bar is highly effective at eliminating pain and increasing strength. The exercise involves grasping a rubber bar, twisting it, then slowly untwisting it.

Moderate evidence exists demonstrating that joint manipulation directed at the elbow and wrist and spinal manipulation directed at the cervical and thoracic spinal regions results in clinical changes to pain and function. There is also moderate evidence for short-term and mid-term effectiveness of cervical and thoracic spine manipulation as an add-on therapy to concentric and eccentric stretching plus mobilisation of wrist and forearm. Although not yet conclusive, the short-term analgesic effect of manipulation techniques may allow more vigorous stretching and strengthening exercises, resulting in a better and faster recovery process of the affected tendon in lateral epicondylitis.

Low level laser therapy, administered at specific doses and wavelengths directly to the lateral elbow tendon insertions, offers short-term pain relief and less disability in tennis elbow, both alone and in conjunction with an exercise regimen. Of late, dry needling has been gaining popularity in various types of tendinopathies and pain of muscular origin. Even in lateral epicondylitis, dry needling is widely employed by many physical therapists across the world. It is believed that dry needling would cause a tiny local injury in order to bring about various desirable growth factors in the vicinity. Dry needling is also aimed at eliciting local twitch response (LTR) in the extensor muscles, as in some cases of tennis elbow the extensor muscles of the forearm would harbor trigger points, which itself could be a major source of pain.

Orthotic Devices

Orthosis is a device externally used on the limb to improve the function or reduce the pain. Orthotics are useful therapeutic interventions for initial therapy of tennis elbow. There are two main types of orthoses prescribed for this problem: counterforce elbow orthoses and wrist extension orthoses.

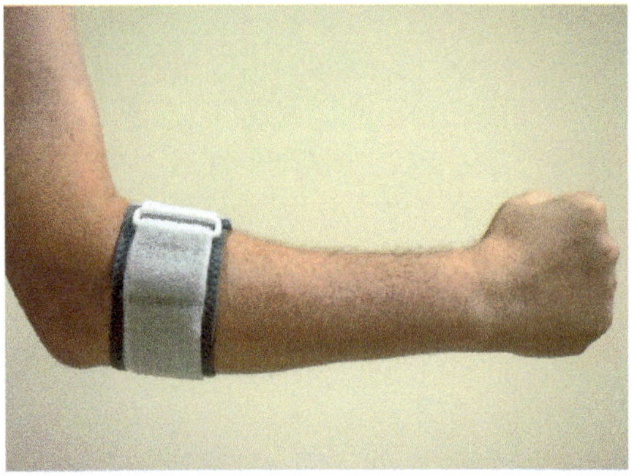

Counterforce orthosis reduces the elongation within the musculotendinious fibers

Counterforce orthosis has a circumferential structure surrounding the arm. This orthosis usually has a strap which applies a binding force over the origin of the wrist extensors. The applied force by orthosis reduces the elongation within the musculotendinious fibers. Wrist extensor orthosis maintains the wrist in the slight extension. This position reduces the overloading strain at the lesion area.

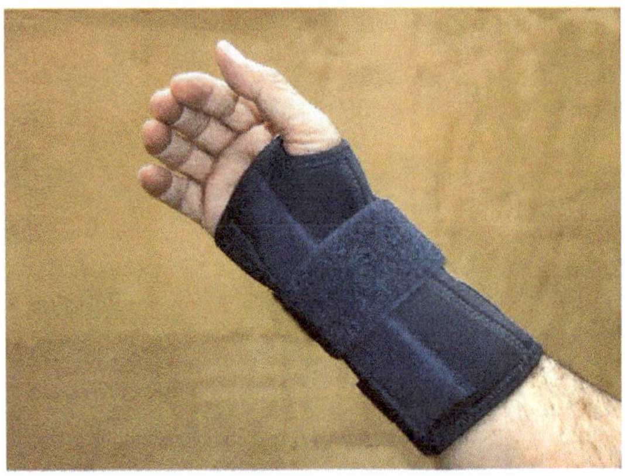

Wrist extensor orthosis reduces the overloading strain at the lesion area

Studies indicated both type of orthoses improve the hand function and reduce the pain in people with tennis elbow.

Medication

Although anti-inflammatories are a commonly prescribed treatment for tennis elbow, the evidence for their effect is usually anecdotal with only limited studies showing a benefit. A systematic review found that topical non-steroidal anti-inflammatory drugs (NSAIDs) may improve pain in the short term (up to 4 weeks) but was unable to draw firm conclusions due to methodological issues. Evidence for oral NSAIDs is mixed.

Evidence is poor for an improvement from injections of any type, be it corticosteroids, botulinum toxin, prolotherapy or other substances. Corticosteroid injection may be effective in the short term however are of little benefit after a year, compared to a wait-and-see approach. A recent randomized control trial comparing the effect of corticosteroid injection, physiotherapy, or a combination of corticosteroid injection and physiotherapy found that patients treated with corticosteroid injection versus placebo had lower complete recovery or improvement at 1 year (Relative risk 0.86). Patients that received corticosteroid injection also had a higher recurrence rate at 1 year versus placebo (54% versus 12%, relative risk 0.23). Complications from repeated steroid injections include skin problems such as hypopigmentation and fat atrophy leading to indentation of the skin around the injection site. Botulinum toxin type A to paralyze the forearm extensor muscles in those with chronic tennis elbow that has not improved with conservative measures may be reasonable.

Surgery

In recalcitrant cases, surgery may be an option. Surgical methods include:

- Lengthening, release, debridement, or repair of the origin of the extrinsic extensor muscles of the hand at the lateral epicondyle
- Rotation of the anconeus muscle
- Denervation of the lateral epicondyle
- Decompression of the posterior interosseous nerve

Surgical techniques for lateral epicondylitis can be done by open surgery, percutaneous surgery or arthroscopic surgery, with no evidence that any particular type is better or worse than another.

Prognosis

Response to initial therapy is common, but so is relapse (25% to 50%) and/or prolonged, moderate discomfort (40%).

Epidemiology

In tennis players, about 39.7% have reported current or previous problems with their elbow. Less than one quarter (24%) of these athletes under the age of 50 reported that the tennis elbow symptoms were "severe" and "disabling," while 42% were over the age of 50. More women (36%) than men (24%) considered their symptoms severe and disabling. Tennis elbow is more prevalent in individuals over 40, where there is about a four-fold increase among men and two-fold increase among women. Tennis elbow equally affects both sexes and, although men have a marginally higher overall prevalence rate as compared to women, this is not consistent within each age group, nor is it a statistically significant difference.

Playing time is a factor in tennis elbow occurrences. However, increased incidence with increased playing time is statistically significant only for respondents under 40. Individuals over 40 who played over two hours had a two-fold increase in chance of injury. Those under 40 had a 3.5 times increase compared to those who played less than two hours per day.

Tendinosis

Tendinosis, sometimes called chronic tendinitis, chronic tendinopathy, or chronic tendon injury, is damage to a tendon at a cellular level (the suffix "osis" implies a pathology of chronic degeneration without inflammation). It is thought to be caused by microtears in the connective tissue in and around the tendon, leading to an increase in tendon repair cells. This may lead to reduced tensile strength, thus increasing the chance of tendon rupture. Tendinosis is often misdiagnosed as tendinitis because of the limited understanding of tendinopathies by the medical community. Classic characteristics of "tendinosis" include degenerative changes in the collagenous matrix, hypercellularity, hypervascularity, and a lack of inflammatory cells which has challenged the original misnomer "tendinitis".

Causes

Tendinosis of the common extensor tendon of the elbow ("tennis elbow") is a common cause of elbow pain for adults.

The general opinion is that tennis elbow tendinosis is due to tendon overuse, and failed healing of the tendon. In addition, the extensor carpi radialis brevis muscle plays a key role.

Tendinosis of the tensor fasciae lateralis where it arises from the anterior part of the outer lip of the iliac crest; from the outer surface of the anterior superior iliac spine, and part of the outer border of the notch below it, between the gluteus medius and sartorius; and from the deep surface of the fascia lata. Pain in the hip area is a common symptom which is often misdiagnosed as hip pain.

Diagnosis

Symptoms can vary from an ache or pain and stiffness to the local area of the tendon, or a burning that surrounds the whole joint around the affected tendon. With this condition, the pain is usually worse during and after activity, and the tendon and joint area can become stiffer the following day as swelling impinges on the movement of the tendon. Many patients report stressful situations in their life in correlation with the beginnings of pain, which may contribute to the symptoms.

Swelling in a region of micro damage or partial tear may be detected visually or by touch.

Medical Imaging

Ultrasound imaging can be used to evaluate tissue strain, as well as other mechanical properties.

Ultrasound-based techniques are becoming more popular because of its affordability, safety, and speed. Ultrasound can be used for imaging tissues, and the sound waves can also provide information about the mechanical state of the tissue.

Increased water content and disorganized collagen matrix in tendon lesions may be detected by ultrasonography or magnetic resonance imaging.

Pathophysiology

Histological findings include granulation tissue, microrupture, degenerative changes, and there is no traditional inflammation. As a consequence, "lateral elbow tendinopathy or tendinosis" is used instead of "lateral epicondylitis".

Examination of tennis elbow tissue reveals noninflammatory tissue, so the term "angiofibroblastic tendinosis" is used.

Cultures from tendinopathic tendons contain an increased production of type III collagen.

Longitudinal sonogram of the lateral elbow displays thickening and heterogeneity of the common extensor tendon that is consistent with tendinosis, as the ultrasound reveals calcifications, intrasubstance tears, and marked irregularity of the lateral epicondyle. Although the term "epicondylitis" is frequently used to describe this disorder, most histopathologic findings of studies have displayed no evidence of an acute, or a chronic inflammatory process. Histologic studies have demonstrated that this condition is the result of tendon degeneration, which causes normal tissue to be replaced by a disorganized arrangement of collagen. Therefore, the disorder is more appropriately referred to as "tendinosis" or "tendinopathy" rather than "tendinitis."

Colour Doppler ultrasound reveals structural tendon changes, with vascularity and hypo-echoic areas that correspond to the areas of pain in the extensor origin.

Load-induced non-rupture tendinopathy in humans is associated with an increase in the ratio of collagen III:I proteins, a shift from large to small diameter collagen fibrils, buckling of the collagen fascicles in the tendon extracellular matrix, and buckling of the tenocyte cells and their nuclei.

Treatment

An injured tendon is very slow to heal. Partial tears heal by the rapid production of disorganized type-III collagen which is weaker than normal tendon. Recurrence of injury in the damaged region of the tendon is common.

Rehabilitation, rest, and gradual return to the activity in which tendinosis was experienced is a common therapy. There is evidence to suggest that tendinosis is not an inflammatory disorder; anti-inflammatory drugs are not an effective treatment; and inflammation is not the cause of this type of tendon dysfunction. There is a variety of treatment options but more research is necessary to determine their effectiveness. Initial recovery is usually within 2 to 3 months, and full recovery usually within 3 to 6 months. About 80% of patients will fully recover within 12 months. If the conservative therapy doesn't work, then surgery can be an option. This surgery consists of the excision of abnormal tissue. Time required to recover from surgery is about 4 to 6 months. Studies with a rat model of fatigue-damaged tendons suggested that delaying exercise until after the initial inflammatory stage of repair could promote remodelling more rapidly.

Research

Both eccentric loading and extracorporeal shockwave therapy are currently being researched as possible treatments for tendinosis. One study found both modalities to be equally effective in treating tendinosis of the Achilles tendon and more effective than a 'wait and see' approach. Other treatments for which research is on-going includes vitamin E, vitamin B6, nitric oxide, Platlet Rich Plasma (PRP), and stem cell injections.

Vitamin E

Vitamin E has been found to increase the activity of fibroblasts, leading to increased collagen fibrils and synthesis, which seems to speed up the regeneration and increase the regenerative capacity of tendons.

Nitric Oxide

Nitric oxide (NO) also appears to play a role in tendon healing and inhibition of its synthesis impairs tendon healing. The use of a nitric oxide delivery system (glyceryl trinitrate patches) applied over the area of maximal tenderness was tested in three clinical trials for the treatment of tendinopathies and was found to significantly reduce pain and increase range of motion and strength.

Soft Tissue Mobilization

Augmented Soft Tissue Mobilization (ASTM) is a form of manual therapy that has been shown in studies on rats to speed the healing of tendons by increasing fibroblast activity. One case study showed ASTM resulting in full recovery in the case of an athlete suffering from chronic ankle pain and fibrosis, after an unsuccessful course of surgery and conventional physical therapy.

Eccentric Loading

A promising line of therapy involves eccentric loading exercises involving lengthening muscular contractions.

Inflatable Brace

The use of an inflatable brace (AirHeel) was shown to be as effective as eccentric loading in the treatment of chronic Achilles tendinopathy. Both modalities produced significant reduction in pain scores, but their combination was no more effective than either treatment alone.

Shock-wave Therapy

Shock-wave therapy (SWT) may be effective in treating calcific tendinosis in both humans and rats. In rat subjects, SWT increased levels of healing hormones and proteins leading to increased cell proliferation and tissue regeneration in tendons. Another study found no evidence that SWT was useful in treating chronic pain in the Achilles tendon.

Tendon Bioengineering

The future of non-surgical care for tendinosis is likely bioengineering. Ligament reconstruction is possible using mesenchymal stem cells and a silk scaffold. These same stem cells were capable of seeding repair of damaged animal tendons. Autologous tenocyte implantation is currently being tested for tendinosis. There is a large randomized, double-blind, placebo controlled trial being conducted in the Netherlands to test the safety and efficacy of tenocyte therapy. Results from the trial are expected by April 2013.

Autologous Tenocyte Injection

A study investigated autologous tenocyte injection for the treatment of severe, chronic resistant lateral epicondylitis. A needle biopsy was used on the patellar tendon, and the extracted tendon cells were expanded by in vitro culture. The autologous tenocytes were sorted and purified by real-time polymerase chain reaction, and amplified by flow cytometry. The tenocytes were then injected into the injured tendinopathy site, which was the origin of the extensor carpi radialis brevis tendon, under the guidance of an ultrasound. After the autologous tenocyte injection treatment, patients with chronic lateral epicondylitis showed improved clinical function and structural repair at the origin of the common extensor tendon.

Nonbulbar Dermal Sheath Cells

RepliCel has planned a Phase 1/2 Achilles tendinosis clinical trial using fibroblasts that are isolated from the nonbulbar dermal sheath cells of a hair follicle, and is recruiting in Q1 2015. The tendon treatment will be tested in approximately 28 subjects. Nonbulbar dermal sheath cells are used because they produce more type I collagen than fibroblasts that are derived from adipose tissue. Type I collagen is the primary collagen in tendons. Nonbulbar dermal sheath cells will be replicated, and then reintroduced into the wounded tendons with ultrasound. After the injections, subjects will be assessed for pain, safety, and function, as well as changes in interstitial tears, tendon thickness, echotexture, and neovascularity.

Injections of microRNA

Scientists found that mir-29a, a single microRNA, through its interaction with a protein, interleukin 33, plays a key role in regulating the production of collagens in tendon disease. Loss of miR29a from human tendons results in an increase in collagen type-3 production, which is a key feature of tendon disease. The replacement of miR-29a in the damaged tendon cells in the laboratory restores collagen production to pre injury levels. A trial will put injections of microRNA – small molecules that help regulate gene expression – into the tendon to decrease the production of type 3 collagen and switch to type-1.

Allogenic Adipose-derived Mesenchymal Stem Cells

As of November 2013, researchers at the Seoul National University Hospital will be looking to recruit participants into a clinical trial to evaluate the efficacy of allogenic adipose-derived mesenchymal stem cells (ALLO-ASC) for the treatment of a lateral epicondylitis tendon injury where the duration of the symptoms is over six months. Adipose-derived mesenchymal stem cells will be administrated to the patients with lateral epicondylitis (tennis elbow) by an ultrasonographic-guided injection.

Elastography Ultrasound

Researchers have tried to analyze tissue strain and mechanical properties using elastography, which is an acoustical imaging technique that measures strain distributions in tissues that result from stress or compression of the tissue. Strain is inversely related to stiffness, so under a given amount of stress, tissue that displays less strain is assumed to be stiffer than tissue that exhibits more strain. Elastography is therefore an indirect method to estimate tissue stiffness.

One limitation of elastography is that it is inherently linear when ultrasound wave velocity and the material properties do not change during the strain measurement. This is a problem in soft tissues like tendons, as they are nonlinear in stiffness, and can undergo large deformations in activity. Elastography measures strain, and to more completely described the mechanical behavior, more data, like stiffness or stress would be required.

Acoustoelastography Ultrasound

Acoustoelastic theory is based on the principle that the acoustic properties of a material are altered as the material is loaded and deformed. The properties can be measured as a change in amplitude and wave velocity.

With the use of A-mode ultrasound, researchers have derived an acoustic relationship between reflected wave amplitude, and strain-dependent stiffness and stress in a deformed material.

As tendon tension increases, the intensity of reflected ultrasonic echoes increases. The increased intensity results in a brighter B-mode ultrasound image.

Acoustoelastography is an ultrasound technique that relates ultrasonic wave amplitude changes to the mechanical properties of a tendon.

It is an ultrasound-based model that can be used evaluate tendon function. Gradual deformations of a tendon can produce cine loops, where changes in echo intensity can be observed. By analyzing the echo intensity changes with Acoustoelastography, one can deduce the stiffness gradient, which is the rate of change of normalised stiffness as a function of strain.

EchoSoft ultrasound software from the Wisconsin Alumni Research Foundation and Echometrix applies the theory of acoustoelasticity to measure musculoskeletal (tendon and ligament) tissue. The software examines previously unused information found by ultrasound waves to quantify the extent of musculoskeletal injuries, or a patient's progress in a healing process.

Ultrasonic Percutaneous Tenotomy

Percutaneous ultrasonic tenotomy provided continued pain relief and functional improvement for recalcitrant tennis elbow at a 3-year follow-up.

Other Animals

Bowed tendon is a horseman's term for tendinitis (inflammation) and tendinosis (degeneration), most commonly seen in the superficial digital flexor tendon (SDFT) in the front leg.

Diagnosis

When the superficial digital flexor tendon of horses is damaged, there is a thickening of the tendon, giving it a bowed appearance when the leg is viewed from the side.

Medical Imaging

A study tested the repeatability and feasibility of using acoustoelastography for in vivo measurement of stiffness gradients in the superficial digital flexor tendons (SDFTs) of clinically normal horses. The results show that acoustoelastography is a repeatable and feasible technique for measuring stiffness gradients of superficial digital flexor tendons in clinically normal horses, and acoustoelastography has the potential to be used for comparing diseased and healthy tendon states.

A report describes the use of acoustoelastography to monitor the mechanical healing of an Achilles tendon laceration in a dog after suture repair. Serial acoustoelastography examinations of the tendon showed that mechanical properties improved throughout the recovery period. At 29 weeks, the mechanical properties of the repaired tendon were similar to that of the normal contralateral Achilles mechanism.

A study shows that acoustoelastography is a repeatable and feasible method for measuring stiffness gradients in equine superficial digital flexor tendons.

The acoustoelastic strain gauge is an ultrasound-based tissue evaluation technique that relates echo intensity changes that are observed during the stretching or relaxation tendons to the mechanical properties of the tissue. The method deduces stiffness gradient (the rate of change of normalized stiffness as a function of tissue strain) by evaluating the ultrasound dynamic images that are captured from tissue as it gradually deforms. Acoustoelastic strain gauge has been shown to accurately model stiffness and strain within tendons in vitro. To determine the repeatability and feasibility of in vivo ASG measurements of canine tendon function, stiffness gradients for the gastrocnemius tendons of dogs were recorded. Findings indicate that acoustoelastic strain gauge is a repeatable and feasible technique for measuring stiffness gradients in canine tendons.

Pathophysiology

Achilles tendons in rats were studied with acoustoelastography ultrasound. After a tendon injury, and during tendon healing, vascularity changes and cellular activity are vital to the formation of granular tissue in the tendon gap, and the subsequent development of neo-tendinous tissue that replaces damaged native tissue. Normal, intact tendon is composed mainly of type I collagen, and type III collagen increases after injury. Another study has recorded an association between collagen fibers and echogenicity tendon during Achilles tendon healing.

This report further indicates that a decrease in type I procollagen (and increase in type III collagen and periostin) correlates to reduced strength, echo intensity, and normalized stiffness. It shows that tissue normalized stiffness is linearly correlated to procollagen I, while echo intensity is seen to be nonlinearly correlated to type I procollagen. Furthermore, the increase in M1 macrophages, blood vessels, and proliferating cells that occur within two weeks of the injury are associated with a formation of granulation tissue. Ultimate stress, echo intensity, and normalized stiffness are all their lowest during these times. The results assert that the reduction in stress and normalized stiffness that is measured by ultrasonic and mechanical methods correlate well with the biological aspect of tendon healing.

Treatment

Mesenchymal stem cells, derived from a horse's bone marrow or fat, are currently being used for tendon repair in horses.

Confusion Between Tendonitis Versus Tendinosis

Tendonitis is a very common, but misleading term. Corticosteroids are drugs that reduce inflammation. They are typically injected along with a small amount of a numbing drug called lidocaine.

By definition, anything that ends in "itis" means "inflammation of." Research shows that tendons are weaker following corticosteroid injections. Tendinitis is still a very common diagnosis, though research increasingly documents that what is thought to be tendinitis is usually tendinosis.

Patellofemoral Pain Syndrome

Patellofemoral pain syndrome (PFPS) is a syndrome characterized by knee pain ranging from severe to mild discomfort seemingly originating from the contact of the posterior surface of the patella (back of the kneecap) with the femur (thigh bone).

The population most at risk from PFPS are runners, cyclists, basketball players and other sports participants. Onset can be gradual or the result of a single incident and is often caused by a change in training regime that includes dramatic increases in training time, distance or intensity, it can be compounded by worn or the wrong type of footwear. Symptoms include discomfort while sitting with bent knees or descending stairs and generalised knee pain. Treatment involves resting and physical therapy that includes stretching and strengthening exercises for the legs.

Definition

There is no universally accepted definition. Selected definitions include:

- "anterior knee pain involving the patella and retinaculum that excludes other intraarticular and peri-patellar pathology"

Runner's Knee

PFPS is one of a handful of conditions sometimes referred to as runner's knee; the other conditions being Chondromalacia patellae, Iliotibial band syndrome, and Plica syndrome.

Patellofemoral Pain Syndrome Vs. Chondromalacia Patellae

Chondromalacia patellae is a term sometimes treated synonymously with PFPS. However, there is general consensus that PFPS is a term that applies only to individuals without cartilage damage, thereby distinguishing it from chondromalacia patellae, a condition characterized by softening of the patellar articular cartilage. Despite this academic distinction, the diagnosis of PFPS is typically made clinically, based only on the history and physical examination rather than on the results of any medical imaging. Therefore, it is unknown whether most persons with a diagnosis of PFPS have cartilage damage or not, making the difference between PFPS and chondromalacia theoretical rather than practical. It is thought that only some individuals with anterior knee pain will have true chondromalacia patellae.

Signs and Symptoms

The onset of the condition is usually gradual, although some cases may appear suddenly following trauma.

- Knee pain - the most common symptom is diffuse peripatellar pain (vague pain around the kneecap) and localized retropatellar pain (pain focused behind the kneecap). Affected individuals typically have difficulty describing the location of the pain, and may place their hands over the anterior patella or describe a circle around the patella (the "circle sign"). Pain is usually initiated when load is put on the knee extensor mechanism, e.g. ascending or descending stairs or slopes, squatting, kneeling, cycling, running or prolonged sitting with flexed (bent) knees. The latter feature is sometimes termed the "movie sign" or "theatre sign" because individuals might experience pain while sitting to watch a film or similar activity. The pain is typically aching with occasional sharp pains.
- Crepitus (joint noises) may be present
- Giving-way of the knee may be reported

Causes

In most patients with PFPS an examination of their history will highlight a precipitating event that caused the injury. Changes in activity patterns such as excessive increases in running mileage, repetitions such as running up steps and the addition of strength exercises that affect the patellofemoral joint are commonly associated with symptom onset. Excessively worn or poorly fitted footwear often contribute. To prevent recurrence the causal behaviour should be identified and managed correctly.

The medical cause of PFPS is thought to be increased pressure on the patellofemoral joint. There are several theorized mechanisms relating to how this increased pressure occurs:

- Increased levels of physical activity
- Malalignment of the patella as it moves through the femoral groove
- Quadriceps muscle imbalance
- Tight anatomical structures, e.g. retinaculum or iliotibial band.

The cause of pain and dysfunction often results from either abnormal forces (e.g. increased pull of the lateral quadriceps retinaculum with acute or chronic lateral PF subluxation/dislocation) or prolonged repetitive compressive or shearing forces (running or jumping) on the PF joint. The result is synovial irritation and inflammation and subchondral bony changes in the distal femur or patella known as "bone bruises". Secondary causes of PF Syndrome are fractures, internal knee derangement, osteoarthritis of the knee and bony tumors in or around the knee.

Diagnosis

Differential Diagnosis

The diagnosis of patellofemoral pain syndrome is made by ruling out patellar tendinitis, prepatellar bursitis, plica syndrome, Sinding-Larsen and Johansson syndrome, and Osgood–Schlatter disease.

Examination

Patellofemoral grinding test.

Treatment

As patellofemoral pain syndrome is the most common cause of anterior knee pain in the outpatient, a variety of treatments for patellofemoral pain syndrome are implemented. Most patients with patellofemoral pain syndrome respond well to conservative therapy.

Exercises

There is consistent but very low quality evidence that exercise therapy for PFPS reduces pain, improves function and aids long-term recovery. However, there is insufficient evidence to compare the effectiveness of different types of exercises with each other, and exercises with other forms of treatment.

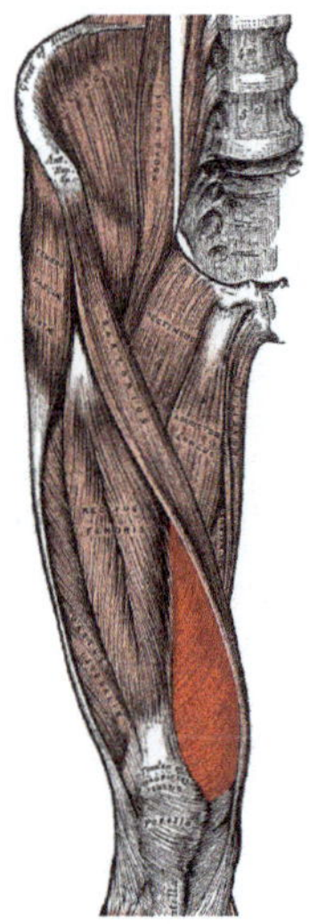

Exercise therapy is the recommended first line treatment of PFPS. Various exercises have been studied and recommended. Exercises are described according to 3 parameters:

- Type of muscle activity (concentric, eccentric or isotonic)
- Type of joint movement (dynamic, isometric or static)
- Reaction forces (closed or open kinetic chain)

Concentric muscle activity involves contraction (shortening) of the muscle(s). During eccentric activities muscles lengthen in an actively controlled manner. During isotonic activity the muscle tension remains the same.

Static/isometric exercises are those in which the position of the knee does not change, whereas dynamic exercises involves a change in the position of the knee. Isokinetic exercises are where the lower leg moves at a predetermined fixed speed, requiring an isokinetic dynamometer to control velocity.

Where the foot is held in contact with a fixed surface, the term closed kinetic chain is used, and open kinetic chain when the surface is not fixed.

The majority of exercise programs intended to treat PFPS are designed to strengthen the quadriceps muscles. Emphasis during exercise may be placed on coordinated contraction of the medial and lateral parts of the quadriceps as well as of the hip adductor, hip abductor and gluteal muscles. Many exercise programs include stretches designed to improve lower limb flexibility. Electromyographic biofeedback allows visualization of specific muscle contractions and may help individuals performing the exercises to target the intended muscles during the exercise. Electrostimulation may be used to apply external stimuli resulting in contraction of specific muscles and thus exercise.

A 2011 systematic review stated that evidence supports the use of quadriceps exercise for managing patellofemoral pain syndrome and that quadriceps strengthening is considered to be the "gold" standard treatment for patellofemoral pain syndrome. Quadriceps strengthening is commonly suggested because the quadriceps muscles help to stabilize the patella. Quadriceps weakness and quadriceps muscle imbalance may contribute to abnormal patellar tracking. If the strength of the vastus medialis muscle is inadequate, the usually larger and stronger vastus lateralis muscle will pull sideways (laterally) on the kneecap. Strengthening the vastus medialis to prevent or counter the lateral force of the vastus lateralis is one way of relieving PFPS. Moderate evidence supports the addition of hip abductor and external rotator strengthening, as well as exercises targeting hip flexion and hip extension. When executing these exercises, proper form is very important in order to ensure that the musculature is activated in such a way that will not lead to further injury. Inflexibility has often been cited as a source of patellofemoral pain syndrome. Stretching of the laterial knee has been suggested to help.

Medication

Non-steroidal anti-inflammatory drugs (NSAIDs) are widely used to treat PFPS, however there is only very limited evidence that they are effective. NSAIDs may reduce pain in the short term, overall however, after three months pain is not improved. There is no evidence that one type of NSAID is superior to another in PFPS, and therefore some authors have recommended that the NSAID with least side effects and which is cheapest should be used.

Glycosaminoglycan polysulfate (GAGPS) inhibits proteolytic enzymes and increases synthesis and degree of polymerization of hyaluronic acid in synovial fluid. There is contradictory evidence that it is effective in PFPS.

Medical Imaging

Magnetic resonance imaging rarely can give useful information for managing patellofemoral pain syndrome and treatment should focus on an appropriate rehabilitation program including correcting strength and flexibility concerns. In the uncommon cases where a patient has mechanical symptoms like a locked knee, knee effusion, or failure to improve following physical therapy, then an MRI may give more insight into diagnosis and treatment.

Rest

Patellofemoral pain syndrome may also result from overuse or overload of the PF joint. For this reason, knee activity should be reduced until the pain is resolved.

Ice

To reduce inflammation ice can be applied to the PF joint after an activity. The ice should be kept in place for 10 to 15 minutes.

Braces and Taping

There is no statistically or clinically significant difference in pain symptoms between taping and non-taping in individuals with PFPS.

Knee braces are ineffective in treating PFPS. The technique of McConnell taping involves pulling the patella medially with tape (medial glide). Findings from some studies suggest that there is limited benefit with patella taping or bracing when compared to quadriceps exercises alone.

Arch Support

Low arches can cause overpronation or the feet to roll inward too much increasing the Q angle and genu valgum. Poor lower extremity biomechanics may cause stress on the knees and ultimately patellofemoral pain syndrome. Stability or motion control shoes are designed for people with pronation issues. Arch supports and custom orthotics may also help to improve lower extremity biomechanics.

Surgery

The scientific consensus is that surgery should be avoided except in very severe cases in which conservative treatments fail. The majority of individuals with PFPS receive nonsurgical treatment.

Treatments Lacking Supportive Research

There is no evidence to support the use of acupuncture, low-level laser therapy, or chiropractic patellar mobilization to treat PFPS. Most studies touting the benefits of alternative therapies for PFPS were conducted with flawed experimental design, and therefore did not produce reliable results.

Epidemiology

Specific populations at high risk of primary Patellofemoral Syndrome include runners, bicyclists, basketball players, young athletes and females.

Repetitive Strain Injury

A repetitive strain injury (RSI) is an "injury to the musculoskeletal and nervous systems that may be caused by repetitive tasks, forceful exertions, vibrations, mechanical compression, or sustained or awkward positions." RSIs are also known as cumulative trauma disorders, repetitive stress injuries, repetitive motion injuries or disorders, musculoskeletal disorders, and occupational or sports overuse syndromes.

Definition

Repetitive strain injury (RSI) and associative trauma orders are umbrella terms used to refer to several discrete conditions that can be associated with repetitive tasks, forceful exertions, vibrations, mechanical compression, or sustained/awkward positions. Examples of conditions that may sometimes be attributed to such causes include edema, tendinosis (or less often tendinitis), carpal tunnel syndrome, cubital tunnel syndrome, De Quervain syndrome, thoracic outlet syndrome, intersection syndrome, golfer's elbow (medial epicondylitis), tennis elbow (lateral epicondylitis), trigger finger (so-called stenosing tenosynovitis), radial tunnel syndrome, and focal dystonia.

Since the 1970s there has been a worldwide increase in RSIs of the arms, hands, neck, and shoulder attributed to the widespread use of typewriters/computers in the workplace that require long periods of repetitive motions in a fixed posture.

Popular Terms

Specific sources of discomfort have been popularly referred to by terms such as Blackberry thumb, iPod finger, mouse arm disease, PlayStation thumb, Rubik's wrist or "cuber's thumb", stylus finger, raver's wrist, and Emacs pinky, among others.

Symptoms

Some examples of symptoms experienced by patients with RSI are aching, pulsing pain, tingling and extremity weakness, initially presenting with intermittent discomfort and then, with a higher degree of frequency.

Causes and Risk Factors

Workers in certain fields are at risk of repetitive strains. Most occupational injuries are musculoskeletal disorders, and many of these are caused by cumulative trauma rather than a single event. Miners and poultry workers, for example, must make repeated motions which can cause tendon, muscular, and skeletal injuries.

Diagnosis

RSIs are assessed using a number of objective clinical measures. These include effort-based tests such as grip and pinch strength, diagnostic tests such as Finkelstein's test for Dequervain's tendinitis, Phalen's Contortion, Tinel's Percussion for carpal tunnel syndrome, and nerve conduction velocity tests that show nerve compression in the wrist. Various imaging techniques can also be used to show nerve compression such as x-ray for the wrist, and MRI for the thoracic outlet and cervico-brachial areas.

Treatment

The most-often prescribed treatments for early-stage RSIs include analgesics, myofeedback, biofeedback, physical therapy, relaxation, and ultrasound therapy. Low-grade RSIs can sometimes resolve themselves if treatments begin shortly after the onset of symptoms. However, some RSIs may require more aggressive intervention including surgery and can persist for years.

The most-often prescribed treatments for early-stage RSIs include analgesics, myofeedback, biofeedback, physical therapy, relaxation, and ultrasound therapy. Low-grade RSIs can sometimes resolve themselves if treatments begin shortly after the onset of symptoms. However, some RSIs may require more aggressive intervention including surgery and can persist for years.

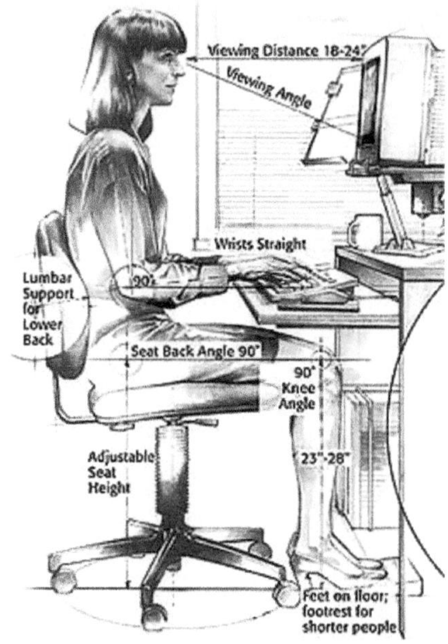

Ergonomics: the science of designing the job, equipment, and workplace

General exercise has been shown to decrease the risk of developing RSI. Doctors sometimes recommend that RSI sufferers engage in specific strengthening exercises, for example to improve sitting posture, reduce excessive kyphosis, and potentially thoracic outlet syndrome. Modifications of posture and arm use (human factors and ergonomics) are often recommended.

History

Although seemingly a modern phenomenon, RSIs have long been documented in the medical literature. In 1700, the Italian physician Bernardino Ramazzini first described RSI in more than 20 categories of industrial workers in Italy, including musicians and clerks. Carpal tunnel syndrome was first identified by the British surgeon James Paget in 1854.

Lee Jackson's 2006 work "A Dictionary of Victorian London", quotes a paragraph from the April 1875 issue of The Graphic describing "telegraphic paralysis".

The Swiss surgeon Fritz de Quervain first identified De Quervain's tendinitis in Swiss factory workers in 1895. The French neurologist Jules Tinel (1879–1952) developed his percussion test for compression of the median nerve in 1900. The American surgeon George Phalen improved the understanding of the aetiology of carpal tunnel syndrome with his clinical experience of several hundred patients during the 1950s and 1960s.

References

- Fleisher, Gary Robert; Ludwig, Stephen (2010). Textbook of Pediatric Emergency Medicine. Lippincott Williams & Wilkins. p. 811. ISBN 978-1-60547-159-4.

- Murray, Robert; Stofan, John (2001). "Ch. 8: Formulating carbohydrate-electrolyte drinks for optimal efficacy". In Maughan, Ron J.; Murray, Robert. Sports Drinks: Basic Science and Practical Aspects. CRC Press. pp. 197–224. ISBN 978-0-8493-7008-3.
- Douglas B. McKeag; James L. Moeller; American College of Sports Medicine (3 July 2007). ACSM's Primary Care Sports Medicine. Lippincott Williams & Wilkins. p. 167. ISBN 978-0-7817-7028-6. Retrieved 21 April 2012.
- Zuberbier, Torsten; Grattan, Clive; Maurer, Marcus (2010). Urticaria and Angioedema. Springer Science & Business Media. p. 38. ISBN 9783540790488.
- Griffiths, Christopher; Barker, Jonathan; Bleiker, Tanya; Chalmers, Robert; Creamer, Daniel (2016). Rook's Textbook of Dermatology, 4 Volume Set (9 ed.). John Wiley & Sons. p. Chapter 42.3. ISBN 9781118441176.
- James, William; Berger, Timothy; Elston, Dirk (2005). Andrews' Diseases of the Skin: Clinical Dermatology (10th ed.). Saunders. p. 150. ISBN 0-7216-2921-0.
- Rapini, Ronald P.; Bolognia, Jean L.; Jorizzo, Joseph L. (2007). Dermatology: 2-Volume Set. St. Louis: Mosby. p. 265. ISBN 1-4160-2999-0.
- Gerard A. Malanga, Scott F. Nadler (2006). Musculoskeletal physical examination : an evidence-based approach. Philadelphia, Penns.: Elsevier Mosby. pp. 302–304. ISBN 9781560535911.
- Arendt, edited by Stefano Zaffagnini, David Dejour, Elizabeth A. (2010). Patellofemoral pain, instability, and arthritis clinical presentation, imaging, and treatment. Berlin: Springer. p. 134. ISBN 9783642054242.
- Gardner, Amanda (17 February 2010). "For Olympians and weekend warriors, winter sports can trigger asthma". cnn.com. Retrieved 29 April 2016.
- "Reply to: Is drinking to thirst a prudent guideline to avoid hyponatremia? - Wilderness & Environmental Medicine". www.wemjournal.org. Retrieved 2016-01-13.

4

Benefits of Exercise

To maintain a physically fit body with a fit mind, it is very important to exercise. The benefits of exercising include physical strength, fighting depression, obesity and diabetes. The aspects elucidated in this chapter are of vital importance, and provide a better understanding of exercise. The topics discussed in the chapter are of great importance to broaden the existing knowledge on exercise physiology.

Agility

Agility or *nimbleness* is the ability to change the body's position efficiently, and requires the integration of isolated movement skills using a combination of balance, coordination, speed, reflexes, strength, and endurance. Agility is the ability to change the direction of the body in an efficient and effective manner and to achieve this requires a combination of

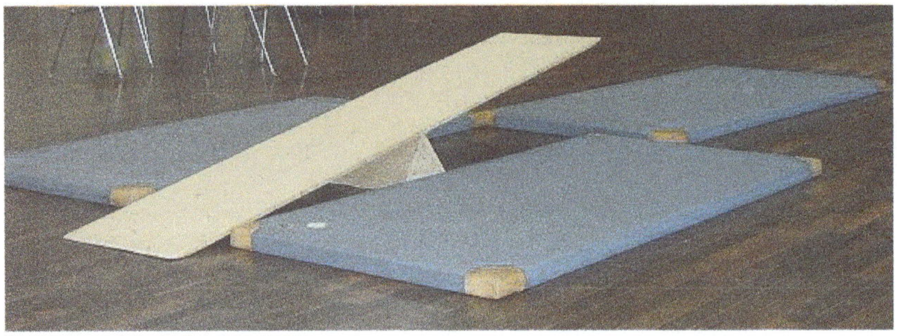

Material to exercise the balance agility for children

- balance – the ability to maintain equilibrium when stationary or moving (i.e. not to fall over) through the coordinated actions of our sensory functions (eyes, ears and the proprioceptive organs in our joints);
- static balance – the ability to retain the centre of mass above the base of support in a stationary position;
- dynamic balance – the ability to maintain balance with body movement;
- speed - the ability to move all or part of the body quickly;
- strength - the ability of a muscle or muscle group to overcome a resistance; and lastly,
- coordination – the ability to control the movement of the body in co-operation with the body's sensory functions (e.g., in catching a ball [ball, hand, and eye coordination]).

In sports, agility is often defined in terms of an individual sport, due to it being an integration of many components each used differently (specific to all of sorts of different sports). Sheppard and

Young (2006) defined agility as a "rapid whole body movement with change of velocity or direction in response to a stimulus".

Agility is also an important attribute in many role playing games, both computer games and pen-and-paper or tabletop games such as *Dungeons & Dragons*. Agility may affect the character's ability to evade an enemy's attack or land their own, move more quickly, navigate uneven terrain, or engage in stealthy activities such as lockpicking or pickpocketing.

Motor Coordination

Motor coordination is the combination of body movements created with the kinematic (such as spatial direction) and kinetic (force) parameters that result in intended actions. Motor coordination is achieved when subsequent parts of the same movement, or the movements of several limbs or body parts are combined in a manner that is well timed, smooth, and efficient with respect to the intended goal. This involves the integration of proprioceptive information detailing the position and movement of the musculoskeletal system with the neural processes in the brain and spinal cord which control, plan, and relay motor commands. The cerebellum plays a critical role in this neural control of movement and damage to this part of the brain or its connecting structures and pathways results in impairment of coordination, known as ataxia.

Properties

Nonexact Reproduction

Examples of motor coordination are the ease with which people can stand up, pour water into a glass, walk, and reach for a pen. These are created reliably, proficiently and repeatedly, but these movements rarely are reproduced exactly in their motor details, such as joint angles when pointing or standing up from sitting.

Combination

The complexity of motor coordination can be seen in the task of picking up a bottle of water and pouring it in a glass. This apparently simple task is actually a combination of complex tasks that are processed at different levels. The levels of processing include: (1) for the prehension movement to the bottle, the reach and hand configuration have to be coordinated, (2) when lifting the bottle, the load and the grip force applied by the fingers need to be coordinated to account for weight, fragility, and slippage of the glass, and (3) when pouring the water from the bottle to the glass, the actions of both arms, one holding the glass and the other that is pouring the water, need to be coordinated with each other. This coordination also involves all of the eye–hand coordination processes. The brain interprets actions as spatial-temporal patterns and when each hand performs a different action simultaneously, bimanual coordination is involved. Additional levels of organization are required depending on whether the person will drink from the glass, give it to someone else, or simply put it on a table.

Degree of Freedom Problem

The problem with understanding motor coordination arises from the biomechanical redundancy caused by the large number of musculoskeletal elements involved. These different elements create many degrees of freedom by which any action can be done because of the range of ways of arranging, turning, extending and combining the various muscles, joints, and limbs in a motor task. Several hypotheses have been developed in explanation of how the nervous system determines a particular solution from a large set of possible solutions that can accomplish the task or motor goals equally well.

Theories

Muscle Synergies

Nikolai Bernstein proposed the existence of muscle synergies as a neural strategy of simplifying the control of multiple degrees of freedom. A functional muscle synergy is defined as a pattern of co-activation of muscles recruited by a single neural command signal. One muscle can be part of multiple muscle synergies, and one synergy can activate multiple muscles. The current method of finding muscle synergies is to measure EMG (electromyography) signals from the muscles involved in a certain movement so that specific patterns of muscle activation can be identified. Statistical analyses are applied to the filtered EMG data to determine the number of muscle synergies that best represent the original EMG. Alternatively, coherence analysis of EMG data can be used to determine the coupling between muscles and the frequency of common input. A reduced number of control elements (muscle synergies) are combined to form a continuum of muscle activation for smooth motor control during various tasks. These synergies work together to produce movements such as walking or balance control. Directionality of a movement has an effect on how the motor task is performed (i.e. walking forward vs. walking backward, each uses different levels of contraction in different muscles). Researchers have measured EMG signals for perturbation applied in multiple directions in order to identify muscle synergies that are present for all directions.

Initially, it was thought that the muscle synergies eliminated the redundant control of a limited number of degrees of freedom by constraining the movements of certain joints or muscles (flexion and extension synergies). However, whether these muscle synergies are a neural strategy or whether they are the result of kinematic constraints has been debated. Recently the term of sensory synergy has been introduced supporting the assumption that synergies are the neural strategies to handle sensory and motor systems.

Uncontrolled Manifold Hypothesis

A more recent hypothesis propose that the central nervous system does not eliminate the redundant degrees of freedom, but instead it uses all of them to ensure flexible and stable performance of motor tasks. The central nervous system makes use of this abundance from the redundant systems instead of restricting them like previously hypothesized. Uncontrolled Manifold (UCM) Hypothesis provides a way to quantify the muscle synergy. This hypothesis defines "synergy" a little differently from that stated above; a synergy represents an organization of elemental variables (degrees of freedom) that stabilizes an important performance variable. Elemental variable is the smallest sensible variable that can be used to describe a system of interest at a selected level of analysis, and a performance variable refers to the potentially important variables produced by the system as a whole. For example, in multi-joint reaching task, the angles and the positions of certain joints are the elemental variables, and the performance variables are the endpoint coordinates of the hand.

This hypothesis proposes that the controller (the brain) acts in the space of elemental variables (i.e. the rotations shared by the shoulder, elbow, and wrist in arm movements) and selects in the space of manifolds (i.e. sets of angular values corresponding to a final position). This hypothesis acknowledges that variability is always present in human movements, and it categorizes it into two types: (1) bad variability and (2) good variability. Bad variability affects the important performance variable and causes large errors in the final result of a motor task, and a good variability keeps the performance task unchanged and maintains successful outcome. An interesting example of the good variability was observed in the tongue's movements, which are responsible for the speech production. The prescription of the stiffness' level to the tongue's body creates some variability (in terms of the acoustical parameters of speech, such as formants), which is, however, not significant for the quality of speech (at least, in the reasonable range of stiffness' levels). One of the possible explanations might be that the brain only works to decrease the bad variability that hinders the desired final result, and it does so by increasing the good variability in the redundant domain.

Types

Inter-limb

Inter-limb coordination concerns how movements are coordinated across limbs. J. A. Scott Kelso and colleagues have proposed that coordination can be modeled as coupled oscillators, a process that can be understood in the HKB (Haken, Kelso, and Bunz) model. The coordination of complex inter-limb tasks is highly reliant on the temporal coordination. An example of such temporal coordination can be observed in the free pointing movement of the eyes, hands, and arms to direct at the same motor target. These coordination signals are sent simultaneously to their effectors. In bimanual tasks (tasks involving two hands), it was found that the functional segments of the two hands are tightly synchronized. One of the postulated theories for this functionality is the existence of a higher, "coordinating schema" that calculates the time it needs to perform each individual task and coordinates it using a feedback mechanism. There are several areas of the brain that are found to contribute to temporal coordination of the limbs needed for bimanual tasks, and these areas include the premotor cortex(PMC), the parietal cortex, the mesial motor cortices, more specifically the supplementary motor area (SMA), the cingulate motor cortex (CMC), the primary motor cortex (M1), and the cerebellum.

Intra-limb

Intra-limb coordination involves the planning of trajectories in the Cartesian planes. This reduces computational load and the degrees of freedom for a given movement, and it constrains the limbs to act as one unit instead of sets of muscles and joints. This concept is similar to "muscle synergies" and "coordinative structures." An example of such concept is the Hogan and Flash minimum-jerk model, which predicts that the parameter that the nervous system controls is the spatial path of the hand, i.e. the end-effector (which implies that the movement is planned in the Cartesian coordinates). Other early studies showed that the end-effector follows a regularized kinematic pattern relating movement's curvature to speed and that the central nervous system is devoted to its coding. In contrast to this model, the joint-space model postulates that the motor system plans movements in joint coordinates. For this model, the controlled parameter is the position of each joint contributing to the movement. Control strategies for goal directed movement differ according to the task that the subject is assigned. This was proven by testing two different conditions: (1) subjects moved cursor in the hand to the target and (2) subjects move their free hand to the target. Each condition showed different trajectories: (1) straight path and (2) curved path.

Eye–hand

Eye–hand coordination concerns how eye movements are coordinated with and affect hand movements. Typical findings relate to the eye looking at an object before the hand starts moving towards that object.

Learning

Bernstein proposed that individuals learn coordination first by restricting the degrees of freedom that they use. By controlling only a limited set of degrees of freedom, this enables the learner to simplify the dynamics of the body parts involved and the range of movement options. Once the individual has gained some proficiency, these restrictions can be relaxed so allowing them to use the full potential of their body.

Physical Strength

Physical strength is the measure of an animal's exert of ability on physical objects. Increasing physical strength is the goal of strength training.

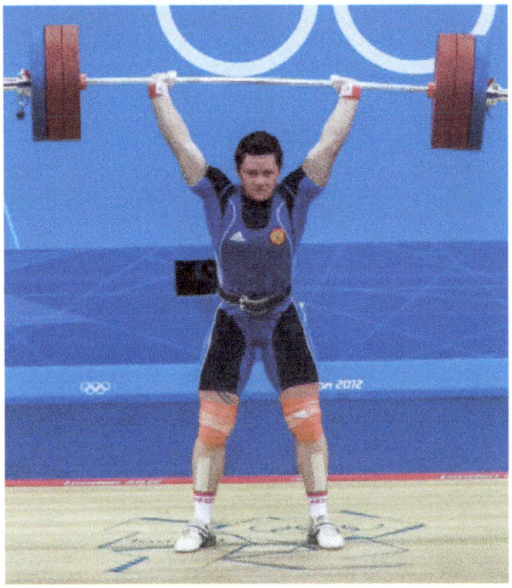

Natalia Zabolotnaya lifting 160 kilograms over her head

Overview

An individual's physical strength is determined by two factors; the cross-sectional area of muscle fibers recruited to generate force and the intensity of the recruitment. Individuals with a high proportion of type I slow twitch muscle fibers will be relatively weaker than a similar individual with a high proportion of type II fast twitch fibers, but would have a greater inherent capacity for physical endurance. The genetic inheritance of muscle fiber type sets the outermost boundaries of physical strength possible (barring the use of enhancing agents such as testosterone), though the unique position within this envelope is determined by training. Individual muscle fiber ratios can be determined through a muscle biopsy. Other considerations are the ability to recruit muscle fibers for a particular activity, joint angles, and the length of each limb. For a given cross-section, shorter limbs are able to lift more weight. The ability to gain muscle also varies person to person, based mainly upon genes dictating the amounts of hormones secreted, but also on sex, age, health of the person, and adequate nutrients in the diet. A one rep maximum is the test to determine maximum muscular strength.

Strength Capability

There are various ways to measure physical strength of a person or population. Strength capability analysis is usually done in the field of ergonomics where a particular task (e.g. lifting a load, pushing a cart, etc.) and/or a posture is evaluated and compared to the capabilities of the section of the population that the task is intended towards. The external reactive moments and forces on the joints are usually used in such cases. The strength capability of the joint is denoted by the amount of moment that the muscle force can create at the joint to counter the external moment.

Skeletal muscles produce reactive forces and moments at the joints. To avoid injury or fatigue, when person is performing a task, such as pushing or lifting a load, the external moments created at the joints due to the load at the hand and the weight of the body segments must be ideally less than the muscular moment strengths at the joint.

One of the first sagittal-plane models to predict strength was developed by Chaffin in 1969. Based on this model, the external moments at each joint must not exceed the muscle strength moments at that joint.

$$M_{j/L} < S_j$$

Where, S_j is the muscle strength moment at joint, j, and $M_{j/L}$ is the external moment at the joint, j, due to load, L and the body segments preceding the joint in the top-down analysis.

Top-down analysis is the method of calculating the reactive moments and forces at each joint starting at the hand, all the way till the ankle and foot. In a 6-segment model, the joints considered are elbow, shoulder, L5/S1 disc of the spine, hip, knee and ankle. It is common to ignore the wrist joint in manual calculations. Software intended for such calculation use the wrist joint also, dividing the lower arm into hand and forearm segments.

Prediction of Static Strength

Static strength prediction is the method of predicting the strength capabilities of a person or a population (based on anthropometry) for a particular task and/or posture (an isometric contraction). Manual calculations are usually performed using the top-down analysis on a six or seven-link model, based on available information about the case and then compared to standard guidelines, such as the one provided by the National Institute for Occupational Safety and Health, to predict capability.

Muscle Hypertrophy

Muscle hypertrophy involves an increase in size of skeletal muscle through a growth in size of its component cells. Two factors contribute to hypertrophy: sarcoplasmic hypertrophy, which focuses more on increased muscle glycogen storage; and myofibrillar hypertrophy, which focuses more on increased myofibril size.

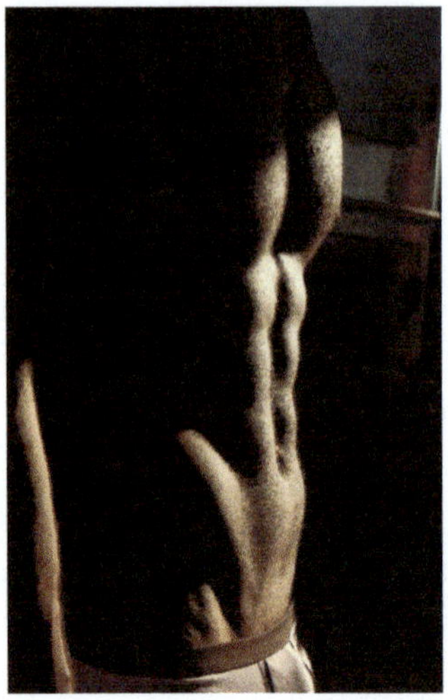

Athletes use a combination of strength training, diet, and supplementation to induce muscle hypertrophy.

Hypertrophy Stimulation

A range of stimuli can increase the volume of muscle cells. These changes occur as an adaptive response that serves to increase the ability to generate force or resist fatigue in anaerobic conditions.

Strength Training

Strength training typically produces a combination of the two different types of hypertrophy: contraction against 80 to 90% of the one-repetition maximum for 2–6 repetitions (reps) causes myofibrillated hypertrophy to dominate (as in powerlifters, Olympic lifters and strength athletes), whereas several repetitions (generally 8–12 for bodybuilding or 12 or more for muscular endurance) against a submaximal load facilitates mainly sarcoplasmic hypertrophy (professional bodybuilders and endurance athletes). The first measurable effect is an increase in the neural drive stimulating muscle contraction. Within just a few days, an untrained individual can achieve measurable strength gains resulting from "learning" to use the muscle. As the muscle continues to receive increased demands, the synthetic machinery is upregulated. Although all the steps are not yet clear, this upregulation appears to begin with the ubiquitous second messenger system (including phospholipases, protein kinase C, tyrosine kinase, and others). These, in turn, activate the family of immediate-early genes, including c-fos, c-jun and myc. These genes appear to dictate the contractile protein gene response.

Progressive overload is considered the most important principle behind hypertrophy, so increasing the weight, repetitions (reps), and sets will all have a positive impact on growth. Some experts create complex plans that manipulate weight, reps, and sets, increasing one while decreasing the others to keep the schedule varied and less repetitive.

Anaerobic Training

The best approach to specifically achieve muscle growth remains controversial (as opposed to focusing on gaining strength, power, or endurance); it was generally considered that consistent anaerobic strength training will produce hypertrophy over the long term, in addition to its effects on muscular strength and endurance. Muscular hypertrophy can be increased through strength training and other short-duration, high-intensity anaerobic exercises. Lower-intensity, longer-duration aerobic exercise generally does not result in very effective tissue hypertrophy; instead, endurance athletes enhance storage of fats and carbohydrates within the muscles, as well as neovascularization.

Factors Affecting Hypertrophy

Several biological factors such as age and nutrition can affect muscle hypertrophy. During puberty in males, hypertrophy occurs at an increased rate. Natural hypertrophy normally stops at full growth in the late teens. An adequate supply of amino acids is essential to produce muscle hypertrophy. As testosterone is one of the body's major growth hormones, on average, men find hypertrophy much easier to achieve than women. Taking additional testosterone, as in anabolic steroids, will increase results. It is also considered a performance-enhancing drug, the use of which can cause competitors to be suspended or banned from competitions. Testosterone is also a medically regulated substance in most countries, making it illegal to possess without a medical prescription. Anabolic steroid use can cause testicular atrophy, cardiac arrest, and gynecomastia.

Changes in Protein Synthesis and Muscle Cell Biology Associated with Stimuli

Protein Synthesis

The message filters down to alter the pattern of gene expression. The additional contractile proteins appear to be incorporated into existing myofibrils (the chains of sarcomeres within a muscle cell). There appears to be some limit to how large a myofibril can become: at some point, they split. These events appear to occur within each muscle fiber. That is, hypertrophy results primarily from the growth of each muscle cell, rather than an increase in the number of cells. Skeletal muscle cells are however unique in the body in that they can contain multiple nuclei, and the number of nuclei can increase.

Cortisol decreases amino acid uptake by muscle tissue, and inhibits protein synthesis. The short-term increase in protein synthesis that occurs subsequent to resistance training returns to normal after approximately 28 hours in adequately fed male youths. Another study determined that muscle protein synthesis was elevated even 72 hours following training.

A small study performed on young and elderly found that ingestion of 340 grams of lean beef (90 g protein) did not increase muscle protein synthesis any more than ingestion of 113 grams of lean beef (30 g protein). In both groups, muscle protein synthesis increased by 50%. The study concluded that more than 30 g protein in a single meal did not further enhance the stimulation of muscle protein synthesis in young and elderly. However, this study didn't check protein synthesis in relation to training; therefore conclusions from this research are controversial.

It is not uncommon for bodybuilders to advise a protein intake as high as 2–4 g per kilogram of bodyweight per day. However, scientific literature has suggested this is higher than necessary, as protein intakes greater than 1.8 g per kilogram of body weight showed to have no greater effect on muscle hypertrophy. A study carried out by American College of Sports Medicine (2002) put the recommended daily protein intake for athletes at 1.2–1.8 g per kilogram of body weight. Conversely, Di Pasquale (2008), citing recent studies, recommends a minimum protein intake of 2.2 g/kg "for anyone involved in competitive or intense recreational sports who wants to maximize lean body mass but does not wish to gain weight. However athletes involved in strength events (..) may need even more to maximize body composition and athletic performance. In those attempting to minimize body fat and thus maximize body composition, for example in sports with weight classes and in bodybuilding, it's possible that protein may well make up over 50% of their daily caloric intake."

Microtrauma

Microtrauma, which is tiny damage to the fibers, may play a significant role in muscle growth. When microtrauma occurs (from weight training or other strenuous activities), the body responds by overcompensating, replacing the damaged tissue and adding more, so that the risk of repeat damage is reduced. Damage to these fibers has been theorized as the possible cause for the symptoms of delayed onset muscle soreness (DOMS), and is why progressive overload is essential to continued improvement, as the body adapts and becomes more resistant to stress. However, work examining the time course of changes in muscle protein synthesis and their relationship to hypertrophy showed that damage was unrelated to hypertrophy. In fact, in that study the authors showed that it was not until the damage subsided that protein synthesis was directed to muscle growth.

Myofibrillar Vs. Sarcoplasmic Hypertrophy

In the bodybuilding and fitness community and even in some academic books skeletal muscle hypertrophy is described as being in one of two types: Sarcoplasmic or myofibrillar. According to this hypothesis, during sarcoplasmic hypertrophy, the volume of sarcoplasmic fluid in the muscle cell increases with no accompanying increase in muscular strength, whereas during myofibrillar hypertrophy, actin and myosin contractile proteins increase in number and add to muscular strength as well as a small increase in the size of the muscle. Sarcoplasmic hypertrophy is greater in the muscles of bodybuilders while myofibrillar hypertrophy is more dominant in Olympic weightlifters. These two forms of adaptations rarely occur completely independently of one another; one can experience a large increase in fluid with a slight increase in proteins, a large increase in proteins with a small increase in fluid, or a relatively balanced combination of the two.

In Sports

Examples of increased muscle hypertrophy are seen in various professional sports, mainly strength related sports such as boxing, bodybuilding, mixed martial arts, rugby, professional wrestling and various forms of gymnastics. These athletes train extensively in strength as well as cardiovascular and muscular endurance training.

References

- Strength, National; editors, Conditioning Association ; Thomas R. Baechle, Roger W. Earle, (2008). Essentials of strength training and conditioning (3rd ed.). Champaign, IL: Human Kinetics. ISBN 978-0736058032.
- Manchester KL (1970). "33 – Sites of Hormonal Regulation of Protein Metabolism". Mammalian Protein Metabolism. Academic Press, New York. p. 229. doi:10.1016/B978-0-12-510604-7.50011-6. ISBN 978-0-12-510604-7.
- Di Pasquale, Mauro G. (2008). "Utilization of Proteins in Energy Metabolism". In Ira Wolinsky, Judy A. Driskell. Sports Nutrition: Energy metabolism and exercise. CRC Press. p. 79. ISBN 978-0-8493-7950-5.
- Kraemer, William J.; Zatsiorsky, Vladimir M. (2006). Science and practice of strength training. Champaign, IL: Human Kinetics. p. 50. ISBN 0-7360-5628-9.

5

Scientific Study of Body Movements

To understand the effect that physical activity has at the cellular level and on the body as a whole is the main concern of sports science. Kinesiology on the other hand concentrates on the biomechanics and orthopedics of a body in motion. This chapter also discusses movement assessment and kinathropometry. Exercise physiology is an emerging field of study; the following chapter will not only provide an overview, it will also delve deep into the variegated topics related to it.

Sports Science

Sports science (also sport science) is a discipline that studies how the healthy human body works during exercise, and how sport and physical activity promote health from cellular to whole body perspectives. The study of sports science traditionally incorporates areas of physiology (exercise physiology), psychology (sport psychology), anatomy, biomechanics, biochemistry and biokinetics. Sports scientists and performance consultants are growing in demand and employment numbers, with the ever-increasing focus within the sporting world on achieving the best results possible. Through the study of science and sport, researchers have developed a greater understanding on how the human body reacts to exercise, training, different environments and many other stimuli.

Origins of Exercise Physiology

Sports Science can trace its origins to ancient Greece. The noted ancient Greek physician Galen (131–201) wrote 87 detailed essays about improving health (proper nutrition), aerobic fitness, and strengthening muscles. Assyrian Hunayn ibn Ishaq translated Galen's work, along with that of Hippocrates, into Arabic which led to the spread of Greek physiology throughout the Middle East and Europe. Between 776 BC to 393 AD, the ancient Greek physicians planned the training regimens and diets of the Olympic competitors.

New ideas upon the working and functioning of the human body emerged during the renaissance as anatomists and physicians challenged the previously known theories. These spread with the implementation of the printed word, the result of Gutenberg's printing press in the 15th century. Allied with this was a large increase in academia in general, universities were forming all around the world. Importantly these new scholars went beyond the simplistic notions of the early Greek physicians, and shed light upon the complexities of the circulatory, and digestive systems. Furthermore, by the middle of the 19th century early medical schools (such as the Harvard Medical School, formed 1782) began appearing in the United States, whose graduates went on to assume positions of importance in academia and allied medical research.

Medical journal publications increased significantly in number during this period. In 1898, three articles on physical activity appeared in the first volume of the *American Journal of Physiology*. Other articles and reviews subsequently appeared in prestigious journals. The German applied physiology publication, *Internationale Zeitschrift fur Physiologie einschliesslich Arbeitphysiologie* (1929–1940; now known as the European Journal of Applied Physiology and Occupational Physiology), became a significant journal in the field of research.

A number of key figures have made significant contributions to the discipline, including the following:

- Austin Flint, Jr., (1836–1915) One of the first American pioneer physicians, studied physiological responses to exercise in his influential medical textbooks.
- Edward Hitchcock, Jr., (1828–1911) Amherst College Professor of hygiene and physical education, devoted his academic career to the scientific study of physical exercise, training and the body. Coauthored 1860 text on exercise physiology.
- George Wells Fitz, M.D. (1860–1934) Created the first departmental major in Anatomy, Physiology, and Physical Training at Harvard University in 1891.
- August Krogh (1874–1949) Won the 1920 Nobel prize in physiology for discovering the mechanism that controlled capillary blood flow in resting or active muscle.
- Per-Olof Astrand (1922–2015) Professor at the Department of physiology, Karolinska Institute, Stockholm. Wrote seminal paper which evaluated the physical working capacity of men and women aged 4–33 years.

Study of Sports Science

Higher-education degrees in Sports Science or Human Physiology are also becoming increasingly popular with many universities now offering both undergraduate, postgraduate and distance learning degrees in the discipline. Opportunities for graduates in these fields employment as a Physical Education teacher, Dietician or Nutritionist, Performance Analyst, Sports coach, Sports therapist, Fitness centre manager, Sports administrator, Strength and Conditioning specialist or retail manager of a Sports store. Graduates may also be well positioned to undertake further training to become an accredited Physiotherapist, Exercise Physiologist, Research Scientist and Sports Medical Doctor.

There are many noted institutions in the United Kingdom which run courses in Sports Science. Some of the better known are University of Brighton, St Mary's University, Twickenham University of Kent – School of Sport & Exercise Sciences, Nottingham Trent University, Durham, University of Derby (fastest rising in the league tables at this time 2014 Guardian League table) Leeds, Loughborough, Exeter, Oxford Brookes University, Bath, Bangor, Birmingham, University of Chichester, Edinburgh, Liverpool John Moores, University of Portsmouth, Manchester Metropolitan University and Stirling.

In the United States, institutions offering related degrees include Jackson State University, University of Connecticut, University of Nebraska-Lincoln, Ohio State University, University of Florida, University of Missouri.

Kinesiology

Kinesiology is a scientific study of human or non-human body movement. Kinesiology addresses physiological, biomechanical, and psychological mechanisms of movement. Applications of kinesiology to human health (i.e. human Kinesiology) include biomechanics and orthopedics; strength and conditioning; sport psychology; methods of rehabilitation, such as physical and occupational therapy; and sport and exercise. Studies of human and animal motion include measures from motion tracking systems, electrophysiology of muscle and brain activity, various methods for monitoring physiological function, and other behavioral and cognitive research techniques.

Kinesiology as described above should not be confused with applied kinesiology, a controversial medical diagnostic method.

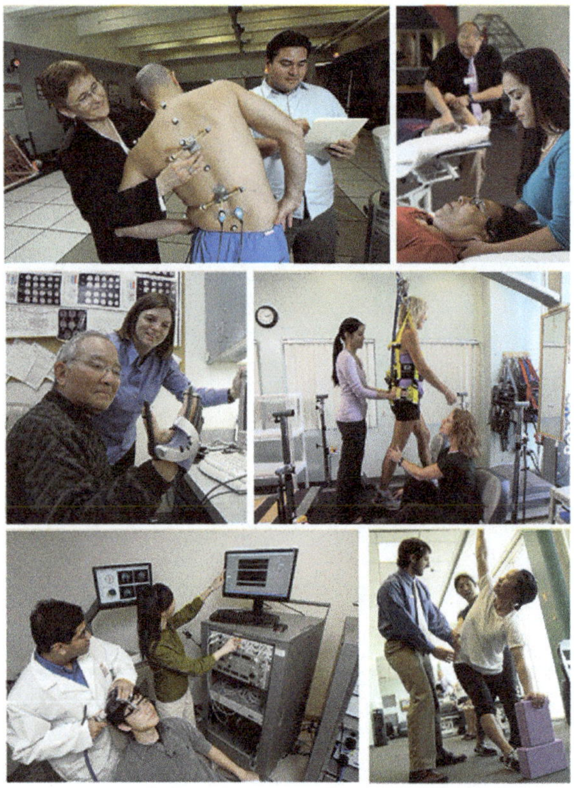

A series of images that represent research (left) and practice (right) in the field of kinesiology.

Basics

Kinesiology is the study of human and nonhuman animal-body movements, performance, and function by applying the sciences of biomechanics, anatomy, physiology, psychology, and neuroscience. Applications of kinesiology in human-health include physical education teacher, the rehabilitation professions, such as physical and occupational therapy, as well as applications in the sport and exercise industries. Kinesiology is a field of scientific study, and does not prepare individuals for clinical practice. A bachelor's degree in kinesiology can provide strong preparation for graduate study in biomedical research, as well as in professional programs, such as allied health and medicine.

Whereas the term "kinesiologist" is neither a licensed nor professional designation in the United States nor most countries (with the exception of Canada), individuals with training in this area can teach physical education, provide consulting services, conduct research and develop policies related to rehabilitation, human motor performance, ergonomics, and occupational health and safety. In North America, kinesiologists may study to earn a Bachelor of Science, Master of Science, or Doctorate of Philosophy degree in Kinesiology or a Bachelor of Kinesiology degree, while in Australia or New Zealand, they are often conferred an Applied Science (Human Movement) degree (or higher). Many doctoral level faculty in North American kinesiology programs received their doctoral training in related disciplines, such as neuroscience, mechanical engineering, psychology, and physiology.

The world's first kinesiology department was launched in 1967 at the University of Waterloo, Canada.

Principles

Adaptation Through Exercise

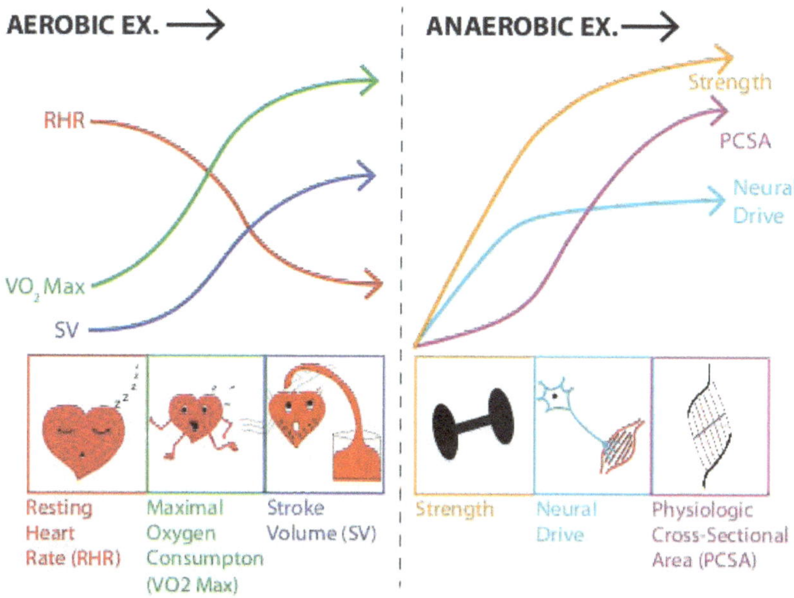

Summary of long-term adaptations to regular aerobic and anaerobic exercise. Aerobic exercise can cause several central cardiovascular adaptations, including an increase in stroke volume (SV) and maximal aerobic capacity (VO_2 max), as well as a decrease in resting heart rate (RHR). Long-term adaptations to resistance training, the most common form of anaerobic exercise, include muscular hypertrophy, an increase in the physiological cross-sectional area (PCSA) of muscle(s), and an increase in neural drive, both of which lead to increased muscular strength. Neural adaptations begin more quickly and plateau prior to the hypertrophic response.

Adaptation through exercise is a key principle of kinesiology that relates to improved fitness in athletes as well as health and wellness in clinical populations. Exercise is a simple and established intervention for many movement disorders and musculoskeletal conditions due to the neuroplasticity of the brain and the adaptability of the musculoskeletal system. Therapeutic exercise has been shown to improve neuromotor control and motor capabilities in both normal and pathological populations.

There are many different types of exercise interventions that can be applied in kinesiology to athletic, normal, and clinical populations. Aerobic exercise interventions help to improve cardiovascular endurance. Anaerobic strength training programs can increase muscular strength, power, and lean body mass. Decreased risk of falls and increased neuromuscular control can be attributed to balance intervention programs. Flexibility programs can increase functional range of motion and reduce the risk of injury.

As a whole, exercise programs can reduce symptoms of depression and risk of cardiovascular and metabolic diseases. Additionally, they can help to improve quality of life, sleeping habits, immune system function, and body composition.

The study of the physiological responses to physical exercise and their therapeutic applications is known as exercise physiology, which is an important area of research within kinesiology.

Neuroplasticity

Adaptive plasticity along with practice in three levels. In behavior level, performance (e.g., successful rate, accuracy) improved after practice. In cortical level, motor representation areas of the acting muscles enlarged; functional connectivity between primary motor cortex (M1) and supplementary motor area (SMA) is strengthened. In neuronal level, the number of dendrites and neurotransmitter increase with practice.

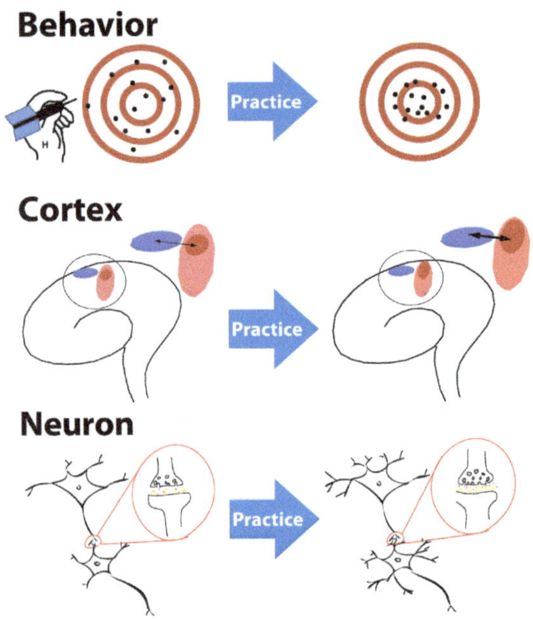

Neuroplasticity is also a key scientific principle used in kinesiology to describe how movement and changes in the brain are related. The human brain adapts and acquires new motor skills based on this principle, which includes both adaptive and maladaptive brain changes.

Adaptive Plasticity

Recent empirical evidence indicates the significant impact of physical activity on brain function; for example, greater amounts of physical activity are associated with enhanced cognitive function in older adults. The effects of physical activity can be distributed throughout the whole brain, such as higher gray matter density and white matter integrity after exercise training, and/or on specific brain areas, such as greater activation in prefrontal cortex and hippocampus. Neuroplasticity is also the underlying mechanism of skill acquisition. For example, after long-term training, pianists showed greater gray matter density in sensorimotor cortex and white matter integrity in the internal capsule compared to non-musicians.

Maladaptive Plasticity

Maladaptive plasticity is defined as neuroplasticity with negative effects or detrimental consequences in behavior. Movement abnormalities may occur among individuals with and without brain injuries due to abnormal remodeling in central nervous system. Learned non-use is an example commonly seen among patients with brain damage, such as stroke. Patients with stroke learned to suppress paretic limb movement after unsuccessful experience in paretic hand use; this may cause decreased neuronal activation at adjacent areas of the infarcted motor cortex.

There are many types of therapies that are designed to overcome maladaptive plasticity in clinic and research, such as constraint-induced movement therapy (CIMT), body weight support treadmill training (BWSTT) and virtual reality therapy. These interventions are shown to enhance motor function in paretic limbs and stimulate cortical reorganization in patients with brain damage.

Motor Redundancy

Motor redundancy is a widely used concept in kinesiology and motor control which states that, for any task the human body can perform, there are effectively an unlimited number of ways the nervous system could achieve that task. This redundancy appears at multiple levels in the chain of motor execution:

- Kinematic redundancy means that for a desired location of the endpoint (e.g. the hand or finger), there are many configurations of the joints that would produce the same endpoint location in space.
- Muscle redundancy means that the same net joint torque could be generated by many different relative contributions of individual muscles.
- Motor unit redundancy means that for the same net muscle force could be generated by many different relative contributions of motor units within that muscle.

The concept of motor redundancy is explored in numerous studies, usually with the goal of describing the relative contribution of a set of motor elements (e.g. muscles) in various human movements, and how these contributions can be predicted from a comprehensive theory. Two distinct (but not incompatible) theories have emerged for how the nervous system coordinates redundant elements: simplification and optimization. In the simplification theory, complex movements and muscle actions are constructed from simpler ones, often known as primitives or synergies, resulting in a simpler system for the brain to control. In the optimization theory, motor actions arise from the minimization of a control parameter, such as the energetic cost of movement or errors in movement performance.

Scope of Practice

In Canada, kinesiology is a professional designation as well as an area of study. In the province of Ontario the scope has been officially defined as, "the assessment of human movement and performance and its rehabilitation and management to maintain, rehabilitate or enhance movement and performance"

Kinesiologists work in a variety of roles as health professionals. They work as rehabilitation providers in hospitals, clinics and private settings working with populations needing care for musculoskeletal, cardiac and neurological conditions. They provide rehabilitation to persons injured at work and in vehicular accidents. Kinesiologists also work as functional assessment specialists, exercise therapists, ergonomists, return to work specialists, case managers and medical legal evaluators. They can be found in hospital, long term care, clinic, work, and community settings. Additionally, kinesiology is applied in areas of health and fitness for all levels of athletes, but more often found with training of elite athletes. All too often biomechanical analysis focuses on the kinetic energy or the working numbers in execution of technique. More emphasis should be placed on muscle and joints as they are involved in the action and the role they play in execution of the technique is critical.

Licensing and Regulation

Canada

In Canada, Kinesiology has been designated a regulated health profession in Ontario only. Kinesiology was granted the right to regulate in the province of Ontario in the summer of 2007 and similar proposals have been made for other Canadian provinces. The College of Kinesiologists of Ontario (http://www.coko.ca/) achieved proclamation on April 1, 2013, at which time the professional title "Kinesiologist" became protected by law. In Ontario only members of the college may call themselves a Registered Kinesiologist. Individuals who have earned degrees in kinesiology can work in research, the fitness industry, clinical settings, and in industrial environments.

Health Service

- Health Promotion

  Kinesiologists working in the health promotion industry work with individuals to enhance the health, fitness, and well-being of the individual. Kinesiologists can be found working in fitness facilities, personal training/corporate wellness facilities, and industry.

- Clinical/Rehabilitation

  Kinesiologists work with individuals with disabling conditions to assist in regaining their optimal physical function. They work with individuals in their home, fitness facilities, rehabilitation clinics, and at the worksite. They also work alongside physiotherapists and occupational therapists.

- Ergonomics

  Kinesiologists work in industry to assess suitability of design of workstations and provide suggestions for modifications and assistive devices.

- Health and Safety.

  Kinesiologists are involved in consulting with industry to identify hazards and provide recommendations and solutions to optimize the health and safety of workers.

- Disability Management/Case Coordination

  Kinesiologists recommend and provide a plan of action to return an injured individual to their optimal function in all aspects of life.

- Management/Research/Administration/Health and Safety

  Kinesiologists frequently fulfill roles in all above areas, perform research, and manage businesses.

- Health Education

  Kinesiologists working in health education teach people about behaviors that promote wellness. They develop and implement strategies to improve the health of individuals and communities. Community health workers collect data and discuss health concerns with members of specific populations or communities.

- Athletic Training

  Kinesiologists working in athletic training work in cooperation with physicians. Athletic trainers strive to prevent athletes from suffering injuries, diagnose them if they have suffered an injury and apply the appropriate treatment.

- Athletic Coaches and Scouts

  Kinesiologists who pursue a career as an athletic coach develop new talent and guide an athlete's progress in a specific sport. They teach amateur or professional athletes the skills they need to succeed at their sport. Many coaches are also involved in scouting. Scouts look for new players and evaluate their skills and likelihood for success at the college, amateur, or professional level.

- Physical Education Teacher

  Kinesiologists working as physical education teachers are responsible for teaching fitness, sports and health. They help students stay both mentally and physically fit by teaching them to make healthy choices.

Kinanthropometry

It is a scientific discipline that is concerned with the measurement of individuals in a variety of morphological perspectives, its application to movement and those factors which influence movement, including: components of body build, body measurements, proportions, composition, shape and maturation; motor abilities and cardiorespiratory capacities; physical activity including recreational activity as well as highly specialized sports performance. The predominant focus is upon obtaining detailed measurements upon the body composition of a given person.

Kinanthropometry is the interface between human anatomy and movement. It is the application of a series of measurements made on the body and from these we can use the data that we gather directly or perform calculations using the data to produce various indices and body composition predictions and to measure and describe physique.

Kinanthropometry is an unknown word for many people except those inside the field of sport science. Describing the etymology of the word kinanthropometry can help illustrate simply what you are going to talk about. However, if you have to say just a few sentences about the general scope of it, some problems will arise immediately. Is it a science? Why are its central definitions so ambiguous and various? For what really matter the kinanthropometric assessment. And so on.

Defining a particular aim for kinanthropometry is central for its full understanding. Ross et al. (1972) said "K is a scientific discipline that studies the body size, the proportionality, the performance of movement, the body composition and principal functions of the body. This so well cited definition is not completely exact as the last four words show. What are the kinanthropometric methods that truly tell us something about principal functions of the body? In principle an amount or distribution of fat mass or muscular mass could be correlated or show a level of causation with any disease. The morpho-physiological mechanisms involved in those explanations are big enigmas today. Few diseases are in practice diagnosed using anthropometric measures and body composition methods at any public health care system. The use of body composition outcomes for predicting health status due to their associations with a lot of physiological variables is valid. However, this purpose is not included within the kinanthropometric perspective because the absent of movement prediction's probability in those diagnoses. The countless uses of some of its fundamental methods have to be accepted but they should not change the theoretical core of the scientific discipline. On the other hand, this definition omits some important objectives of quantifying the body that are an indelible part of its frame; for example: the study of human shape using the method of the anthropometric somatotype of Carter and Heath (1990). Besides that, the performance of movement is why one studies the body size, proportionality, body composition, and human shape. It is confusing to write at the same level the performance of movement because then one never clearly portrays the purpose of the discipline, meaning that a descriptive knowledge of the body is the sole purpose while you are mixing the real scope in the statement.

Stewart (2010) defined kinanthropometry as "The academic discipline that involves the use of anthropometric measures in relation to other scientific parameters and/or thematic areas such as human movement, physiology or applied health sciences".

For Betancourt (2009), kinanthropometry is a scientific discipline of biomechanics that can be defined as: the set of theoretical assumptions that explain the relationships between the morpho-functional structure of healthy individuals and their biological potentiality of performing an efficient motion in an ontogenic moment.

Movement Assessment

Movement assessment is the practice of analysing movement performance during functional tasks to determine the kinematics of individual joints and their effect on the kinetic chain. Three-dimensional or two-dimensional analysis of the biomechanics involved in sporting tasks can assist in prevention of injury and enhancing athletic performance. Identification of abnormal movement mechanics provides physical therapists with the ability to prescribe more accurate corrective exercise programs to prevent injury and improve exercise rehabilitation and progression following injury and assist in determining readiness to return to sport.

Landing Error Scoring System (LESS)

The LESS is a valid and reliable tool for the biomechanical assessment of the jump landing technique. The LESS involves the scoring of 22 biomechanical criteria of the lower extremity and trunk, with the outcomes being associated with the risk of anterior cruciate ligament (ACL) and patellofemoral injury. LESS scoring is split into the following categories: excellent (0-3); good (4-5); moderate (6-7); and poor (>7). Identification of biomechanical abnormalities in landing technique, the effect of fatigue and differences between gender allow for more precise clinical exercise intervention to reduce the risk of injury.

Unsupported Single Leg Squat

The single leg squat is an exercise that was developed into a functional test by Liebenson to examine the biomechanics of the lower extremity, assess hip muscle dysfunction and provide an indication of mechanics during daily functional tasks. The test requires the person to stand on the limb being tested, with the non-weight bearing limb in about 45° of hip flexion and about 90° of knee flexion. The person's arms should be in 90° of shoulder flexion and full elbow extension. The athlete is required to squat down to at least 60° of knee flexion and return to the start position within 6 seconds.

Single Leg Hop for Distance

Single leg hop tests are commonly used to assess functional knee performance by assessing limb symmetry after an anterior cruciate ligament injury or following anterior cruciate ligament reconstruction. The hop tests mainly used are: the single leg hop for distance; crossover hop test; triple hop test; 6m timed hop test; square hop test and side-to-side hop test. The limb symmetry is assessed by means of the limb symmetry index (LSI). Normal values for return to play criteria following ACL reconstruction indicate that the injured limb should be greater than or equal to 90% of the uninjured limb.

6

Metabolism and its Mechanisms

The sum total of all the chemical processes that occur in the body and help sustain life is referred to as metabolism. Some of the mechanisms explained in this chapter are metabolic equivalent, basal metabolic rate and metabolic age. The aspects elucidated in this chapter are of vital importance, and provide a better understanding of exercise physiology.

Metabolism

Metabolism is the set of life-sustaining chemical trans-formations within the cells of living organisms. The three main purposes of metabolism are the conversion of food/fuel to energy to run cellular processes, the conversion of food/fuel to building blocks for proteins, lipids, nucleic acids, and some carbohydrates, and the elimination of nitrogenous wastes. These enzyme-catalyzed reactions allow organisms to grow and reproduce, maintain their structures, and respond to their environments. The word metabolism can also refer to the sum of all chemical reactions that occur in living organisms, including digestion and the transport of substances into and between different cells, in which case the set of reactions within the cells is called intermediary metabolism or intermediate metabolism.

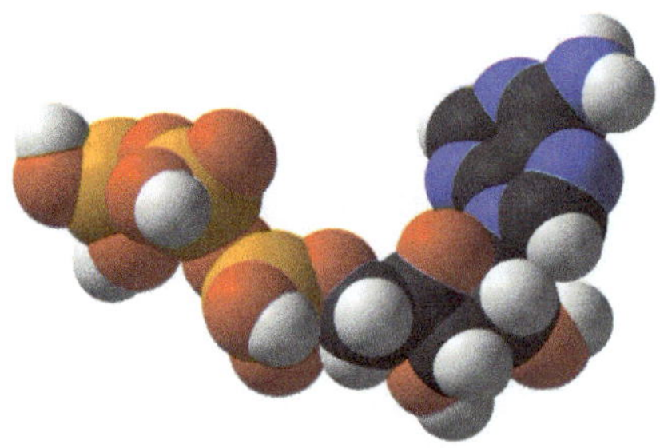

Structure of adenosine triphosphate (ATP), a central intermediate in energy metabolism

Metabolism is usually divided into two categories: catabolism, the *breaking down* of organic matter, for example, by cellular respiration, and anabolism, the *building up* of components of cells such as proteins and nucleic acids. Usually, breaking down releases energy and building up consumes energy.

The chemical reactions of metabolism are organized into metabolic pathways, in which one chemical is transformed through a series of steps into another chemical, by a sequence of enzymes. Enzymes are crucial to metabolism because they allow organisms to drive desirable reactions that require energy that will not occur by themselves, by coupling them to spontaneous reactions that release energy. Enzymes act as catalysts that allow the reactions to proceed more rapidly. Enzymes also allow the regulation of metabolic pathways in response to changes in the cell's environment or to signals from other cells.

The metabolic system of a particular organism determines which substances it will find nutritious and which poisonous. For example, some prokaryotes use hydrogen sulfide as a nutrient, yet this gas is poisonous to animals. The speed of metabolism, the metabolic rate, influences how much food an organism will require, and also affects how it is able to obtain that food.

A striking feature of metabolism is the similarity of the basic metabolic pathways and components between even vastly different species. For example, the set of carboxylic acids that are best known as the intermediates in the citric acid cycle are present in all known organisms, being found in species as diverse as the unicellular bacterium *Escherichia coli* and huge multicellular organisms like elephants. These striking similarities in metabolic pathways are likely due to their early appearance in evolutionary history, and their retention because of their efficacy.

Key Biochemicals

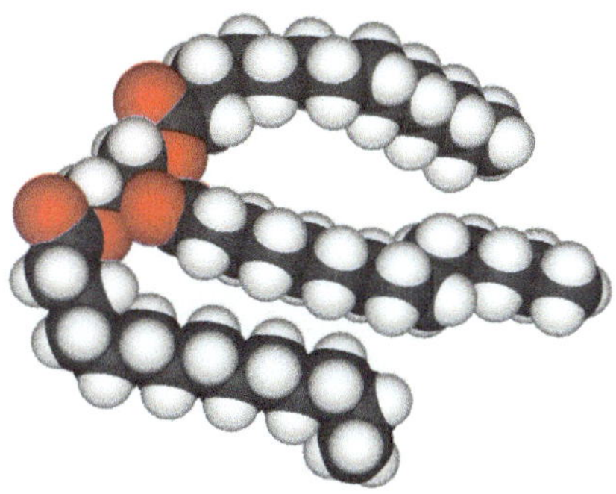

Structure of a triacylglycerol lipid

Most of the structures that make up animals, plants and microbes are made from three basic classes of molecule: amino acids, carbohydrates and lipids (often called fats). As these molecules are vital for life, metabolic reactions either focus on making these molecules during the construction of cells and tissues, or by breaking them down and using them as a source of energy, by their digestion. These biochemicals can be joined together to make polymers such as DNA and proteins, essential macromolecules of life.

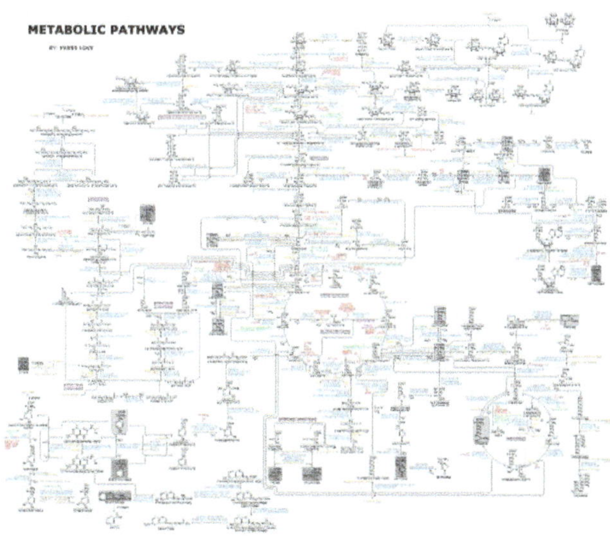

This is a diagram depicting a large set of human metabolic pathways.

Type of molecule	Name of monomer forms	Name of polymer forms	Examples of polymer forms
Amino acids	Amino acids	Proteins (made of polypeptides)	Fibrous proteins and globular proteins
Carbohydrates	Monosaccharides	Polysaccharides	Starch, glycogen and cellulose
Nucleic acids	Nucleotides	Polynucleotides	DNA and RNA

Amino Acids and Proteins

Proteins are made of amino acids arranged in a linear chain joined together by peptide bonds. Many proteins are enzymes that catalyze the chemical reactions in metabolism. Other proteins have structural or mechanical functions, such as those that form the cytoskeleton, a system of scaffolding that maintains the cell shape. Proteins are also important in cell signaling, immune responses, cell adhesion, active transport across membranes, and the cell cycle. Amino acids also contribute to cellular energy metabolism by providing a carbon source for entry into the citric acid cycle (tricarboxylic acid cycle), especially when a primary source of energy, such as glucose, is scarce, or when cells undergo metabolic stress.

Lipids

Lipids are the most diverse group of biochemicals. Their main structural uses are as part of biological membranes both internal and external, such as the cell membrane, or as a source of energy. Lipids are usually defined as hydrophobic or amphipathic biological molecules but will dissolve in organic solvents such as benzene or chloroform. The fats are a large group of compounds that contain fatty acids and glycerol; a glycerol molecule attached to three fatty acid esters is called a triacylglyceride. Several variations on this basic structure exist, including alternate backbones such as sphingosine in the sphingolipids, and hydrophilic groups such as phosphate as in phospholipids. Steroids such as cholesterol are another major class of lipids.

Carbohydrates

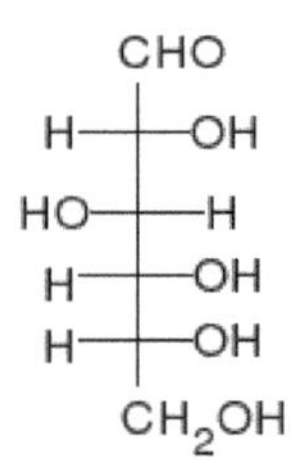

Glucose can exist in both a straight-chain and ring form.

Carbohydrates are aldehydes or ketones, with many hydroxyl groups attached, that can exist as straight chains or rings. Carbohydrates are the most abundant biological molecules, and fill numerous roles, such as the storage and transport of energy (starch, glycogen) and structural components (cellulose in plants, chitin in animals). The basic carbohydrate units are called monosaccharides and include galactose, fructose, and most importantly glucose. Monosaccharides can be linked together to form polysaccharides in almost limitless ways.

Nucleotides

The two nucleic acids, DNA and RNA, are polymers of nucleotides. Each nucleotide is composed of a phosphate attached to a ribose or deoxyribose sugar group which is attached to a nitrogenous base. Nucleic acids are critical for the storage and use of genetic information, and its interpretation through the processes of transcription and protein biosynthesis. This information is protected by DNA repair mechanisms and propagated through DNA replication. Many viruses have an RNA genome, such as HIV, which uses reverse transcription to create a DNA template from its viral RNA genome. RNA in ribozymes such as spliceosomes and ribosomes is similar to enzymes as it can catalyze chemical reactions. Individual nucleosides are made by attaching a nucleobase to a ribose sugar. These bases are heterocyclic rings containing nitrogen, classified as purines or pyrimidines. Nucleotides also act as coenzymes in metabolic-group-transfer reactions.

Coenzymes

Metabolism involves a vast array of chemical reactions, but most fall under a few basic types of reactions that involve the transfer of functional groups of atoms and their bonds within molecules. This common chemistry allows cells to use a small set of metabolic intermediates to carry chemical groups between different reactions. These group-transfer intermediates are called coenzymes. Each class of group-transfer reactions is carried out by a particular coenzyme, which is the substrate for a set of enzymes that produce it, and a set of enzymes that consume it. These coenzymes are therefore continuously made, consumed and then recycled.

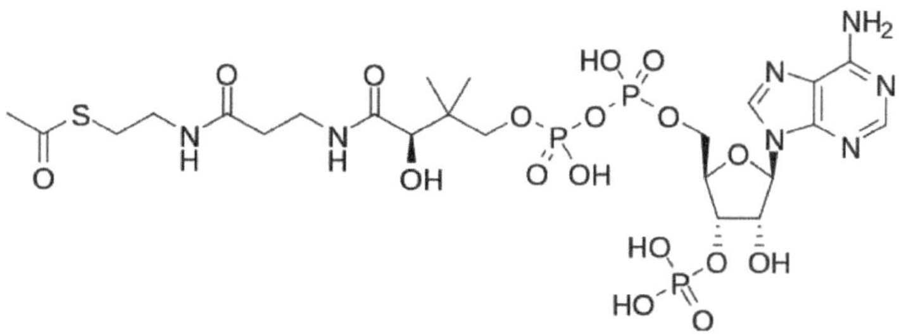

Structure of the coenzyme acetyl-CoA.The transferable acetyl group is bonded to the sulfur atom at the extreme left.

One central coenzyme is adenosine triphosphate (ATP), the universal energy currency of cells. This nucleotide is used to transfer chemical energy between different chemical reactions. There is only a small amount of ATP in cells, but as it is continuously regenerated, the human body can use about its own weight in ATP per day. ATP acts as a bridge between catabolism and anabolism. Catabolism breaks down molecules, and anabolism puts them together. Catabolic reactions generate ATP, and anabolic reactions consume it. It also serves as a carrier of phosphate groups in phosphorylation reactions.

A vitamin is an organic compound needed in small quantities that cannot be made in cells. In human nutrition, most vitamins function as coenzymes after modification; for example, all water-soluble vitamins are phosphorylated or are coupled to nucleotides when they are used in cells. Nicotinamide adenine dinucleotide (NAD^+), a derivative of vitamin B_3 (niacin), is an important coenzyme that acts as a hydrogen acceptor. Hundreds of separate types of dehydrogenases remove electrons from their substrates and reduce NAD^+ into NADH. This reduced form of the coenzyme is then a substrate for any of the reductases in the cell that need to reduce their substrates. Nicotinamide adenine dinucleotide exists in two related forms in the cell, NADH and NADPH. The NAD^+/NADH form is more important in catabolic reactions, while $NADP^+$/NADPH is used in anabolic reactions.

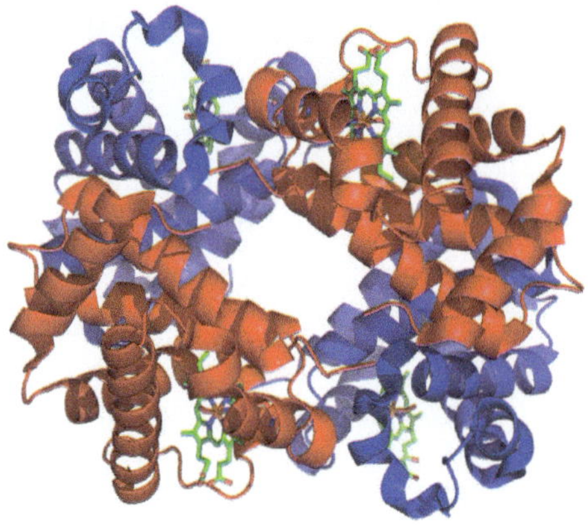

Structure of hemoglobin. The protein subunits are in red and blue, and the iron-containing heme groups in green. From PDB: 1GZX.

Minerals and Cofactors

Inorganic elements play critical roles in metabolism; some are abundant (e.g. sodium and potassium) while others function at minute concentrations. About 99% of a mammal's mass is made up of the elements carbon, nitrogen, calcium, sodium, chlorine, potassium, hydrogen, phosphorus, oxygen and sulfur. Organic compounds (proteins, lipids and carbohydrates) contain the majority of the carbon and nitrogen; most of the oxygen and hydrogen is present as water.

The abundant inorganic elements act as ionic electrolytes. The most important ions are sodium, potassium, calcium, magnesium, chloride, phosphate and the organic ion bicarbonate. The maintenance of precise ion gradients across cell membranes maintains osmotic pressure and pH. Ions are also critical for nerve and muscle function, as action potentials in these tissues are produced by the exchange of electrolytes between the extracellular fluid and the cell's fluid, the cytosol. Electrolytes enter and leave cells through proteins in the cell membrane called ion channels. For example, muscle contraction depends upon the movement of calcium, sodium and potassium through ion channels in the cell membrane and T-tubules.

Transition metals are usually present as trace elements in organisms, with zinc and iron being most abundant of those. These metals are used in some proteins as cofactors and are essential for the activity of enzymes such as catalase and oxygen-carrier proteins such as hemoglobin. Metal cofactors are bound tightly to specific sites in proteins; although enzyme cofactors can be modified during catalysis, they always return to their original state by the end of the reaction catalyzed. Metal micronutrients are taken up into organisms by specific transporters and bind to storage proteins such as ferritin or metallothionein when not in use.

Catabolism

Catabolism is the set of metabolic processes that break down large molecules. These include breaking down and oxidizing food molecules. The purpose of the catabolic reactions is to provide the energy and components needed by anabolic reactions. The exact nature of these catabolic reactions differ from organism to organism and organisms can be classified based on their sources of energy and carbon (their primary nutritional groups), as shown in the table below. Organic molecules are used as a source of energy by organotrophs, while lithotrophs use inorganic substrates and phototrophs capture sunlight as chemical energy. However, all these different forms of metabolism depend on redox reactions that involve the transfer of electrons from reduced donor molecules such as organic molecules, water, ammonia, hydrogen sulfide or ferrous ions to acceptor molecules such as oxygen, nitrate or sulfate. In animals these reactions involve complex organic molecules that are broken down to simpler molecules, such as carbon dioxide and water. In photosynthetic organisms such as plants and cyanobacteria, these electron-transfer reactions do not release energy, but are used as a way of storing energy absorbed from sunlight.

Classification of organisms based on their metabolism					
Energy source	sunlight	photo-			-troph
	Preformed molecules	chemo-			
Electron donor	organic compound		organo-		
	inorganic compound		litho-		
Carbon source	organic compound			hetero-	
	inorganic compound	auto-			

The most common set of catabolic reactions in animals can be separated into three main stages. In the first, large organic molecules such as proteins, polysaccharides or lipids are digested into their smaller components outside cells. Next, these smaller molecules are taken up by cells and converted to yet smaller molecules, usually acetyl coenzyme A (acetyl-CoA), which releases some energy. Finally, the acetyl group on the CoA is oxidised to water and carbon dioxide in the citric acid cycle and electron transport chain, releasing the energy that is stored by reducing the coenzyme nicotinamide adenine dinucleotide (NAD^+) into NADH.

Digestion

Macromolecules such as starch, cellulose or proteins cannot be rapidly taken up by cells and must be broken into their smaller units before they can be used in cell metabolism. Several common classes of enzymes digest these polymers. These digestive enzymes include proteases that digest proteins into amino acids, as well as glycoside hydrolases that digest polysaccharides into simple sugars known as monosaccharides.

Microbes simply secrete digestive enzymes into their surroundings, while animals only secrete these enzymes from specialized cells in their guts. The amino acids or sugars released by these extracellular enzymes are then pumped into cells by active transport proteins.

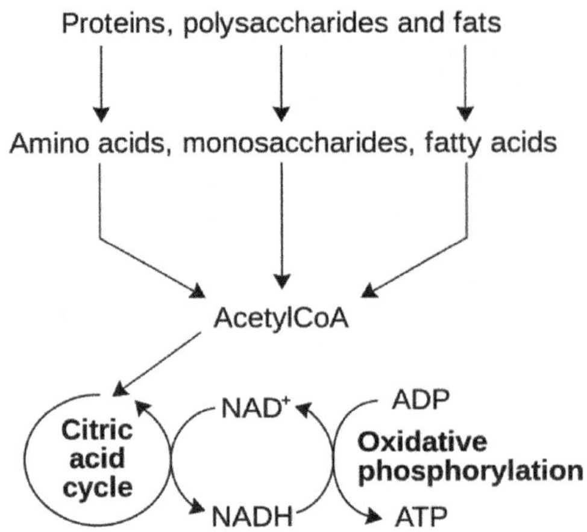

A simplified outline of the catabolism of proteins, carbohydrates and fats

Energy from Organic Compounds

Carbohydrate catabolism is the breakdown of carbohydrates into smaller units. Carbohydrates are usually taken into cells once they have been digested into monosaccharides. Once inside, the major route of breakdown is glycolysis, where sugars such as glucose and fructose are converted into pyruvate and some ATP is generated. Pyruvate is an intermediate in several metabolic pathways, but the majority is converted to acetyl-CoA and fed into the citric acid cycle. Although some more ATP is generated in the citric acid cycle, the most important product is NADH, which is made from NAD^+ as the acetyl-CoA is oxidized. This oxidation releases carbon dioxide as a waste product. In anaerobic conditions, glycolysis produces lactate, through the enzyme lactate dehydrogenase re-oxidizing NADH to NAD+ for re-use in glycolysis. An alternative route for glucose breakdown is the pentose phosphate pathway, which reduces the coenzyme NADPH and produces pentose sugars such as ribose, the sugar component of nucleic acids.

Fats are catabolised by hydrolysis to free fatty acids and glycerol. The glycerol enters glycolysis and the fatty acids are broken down by beta oxidation to release acetyl-CoA, which then is fed into the citric acid cycle. Fatty acids release more energy upon oxidation than carbohydrates because carbohydrates contain more oxygen in their structures. Steroids are also broken down by some bacteria in a process similar to beta oxidation, and this breakdown process involves the release of significant amounts of acetyl-CoA, propionyl-CoA, and pyruvate, which can all be used by the cell for energy. *M. tuberculosis* can also grow on the lipid cholesterol as a sole source of carbon, and genes involved in the cholesterol use pathway(s) have been validated as important during various stages of the infection lifecycle of *M. tuberculosis*.

Amino acids are either used to synthesize proteins and other biomolecules, or oxidized to urea and carbon dioxide as a source of energy. The oxidation pathway starts with the removal of the amino group by a transaminase. The amino group is fed into the urea cycle, leaving a deaminated carbon skeleton in the form of a keto acid. Several of these keto acids are intermediates in the citric acid cycle, for example the deamination of glutamate forms α-ketoglutarate. The glucogenic amino acids can also be converted into glucose, through gluconeogenesis.

Energy Transformations

Oxidative Phosphorylation

In oxidative phosphorylation, the electrons removed from organic molecules in areas such as the protagon acid cycle are transferred to oxygen and the energy released is used to make ATP. This is done in eukaryotes by a series of proteins in the membranes of mitochondria called the electron transport chain. In prokaryotes, these proteins are found in the cell's inner membrane. These proteins use the energy released from passing electrons from reduced molecules like NADH onto oxygen to pump protons across a membrane.

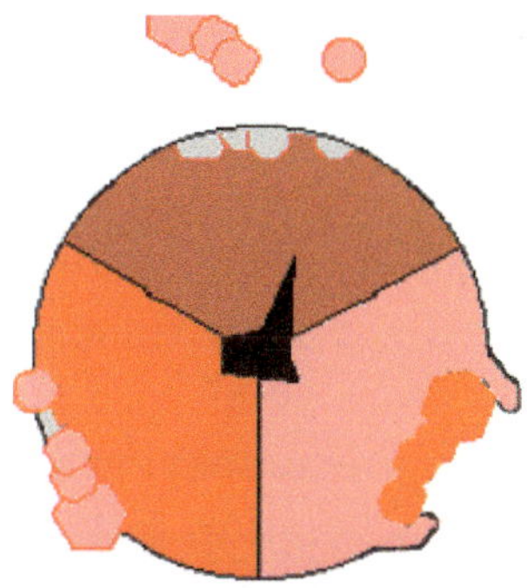

Mechanism of ATP synthase. ATP is shown in red, ADP and phosphate in pink and the rotating stalk subunit in black.

Pumping protons out of the mitochondria creates a proton concentration difference across the membrane and generates an electrochemical gradient. This force drives protons back into the mitochondrion through the base of an enzyme called ATP synthase. The flow of protons makes the stalk subunit rotate, causing the active site of the synthase domain to change shape and phosphorylate adenosine diphosphate – turning it into ATP.

Energy from Inorganic Compounds

Chemolithotrophy is a type of metabolism found in prokaryotes where energy is obtained from the oxidation of inorganic compounds. These organisms can use hydrogen, reduced sulfur compounds (such as sulfide, hydrogen sulfide and thiosulfate), ferrous iron (FeII) or ammonia as sources of reducing power and they gain energy from the oxidation of these compounds with electron acceptors such as oxygen or nitrite. These microbial processes are important in global biogeochemical cycles such as acetogenesis, nitrification and denitrification and are critical for soil fertility.

Energy from Light

The energy in sunlight is captured by plants, cyanobacteria, purple bacteria, green sulfur bacteria and some protists. This process is often coupled to the conversion of carbon dioxide into organic compounds, as part of photosynthesis, which is discussed below. The energy capture and carbon fixation systems can however operate separately in prokaryotes, as purple bacteria and green sulfur bacteria can use sunlight as a source of energy, while switching between carbon fixation and the fermentation of organic compounds.

In many organisms the capture of solar energy is similar in principle to oxidative phosphorylation, as it involves the storage of energy as a proton concentration gradient. This proton motive force then drives ATP synthesis. The electrons needed to drive this electron transport chain come from light-gathering proteins called photosynthetic reaction centres or rhodopsins. Reaction centers are classed into two types depending on the type of photosynthetic pigment present, with most photosynthetic bacteria only having one type, while plants and cyanobacteria have two.

In plants, algae, and cyanobacteria, photosystem II uses light energy to remove electrons from water, releasing oxygen as a waste product. The electrons then flow to the cytochrome b6f complex, which uses their energy to pump protons across the thylakoid membrane in the chloroplast. These protons move back through the membrane as they drive the ATP synthase, as before. The electrons then flow through photosystem I and can then either be used to reduce the coenzyme $NADP^+$, for use in the Calvin cycle, which is discussed below, or recycled for further ATP generation.

Anabolism

Anabolism is the set of constructive metabolic processes where the energy released by catabolism is used to synthesize complex molecules. In general, the complex molecules that make up cellular structures are constructed step-by-step from small and simple precursors. Anabolism involves three basic stages. First, the production of precursors such as amino acids, monosaccharides, isoprenoids and nucleotides, secondly, their activation into reactive forms using energy from ATP, and thirdly, the assembly of these precursors into complex molecules such as proteins, polysaccharides, lipids and nucleic acids.

Organisms differ in how many of the molecules in their cells they can construct for themselves. Autotrophs such as plants can construct the complex organic molecules in cells such as polysaccharides and proteins from simple molecules like carbon dioxide and water. Heterotrophs, on the other hand, require a source of more complex substances, such as monosaccharides and amino acids, to produce these complex molecules. Organisms can be further classified by ultimate source of their energy: photoautotrophs and photoheterotrophs obtain energy from light, whereas chemoautotrophs and chemoheterotrophs obtain energy from inorganic oxidation reactions.

Carbon Fixation

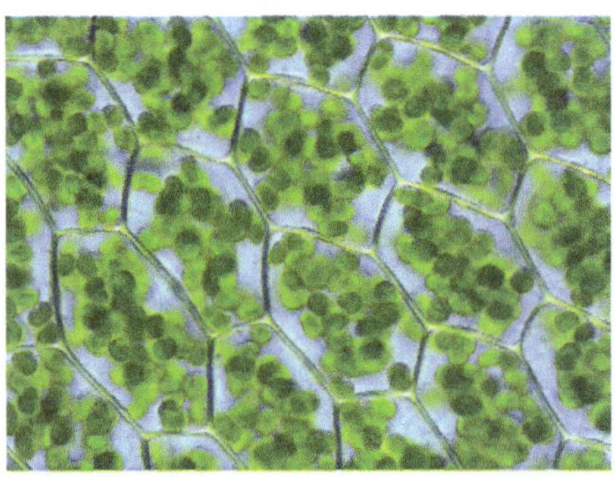

Plant cells (bounded by purple walls) filled with chloroplasts (green), which are the site of photosynthesis

Photosynthesis is the synthesis of carbohydrates from sunlight and carbon dioxide (CO_2). In plants, cyanobacteria and algae, oxygenic photosynthesis splits water, with oxygen produced as a waste product. This process uses the ATP and NADPH produced by the photosynthetic reaction centres, as described above, to convert CO_2 into glycerate 3-phosphate, which can then be converted into glucose. This carbon-fixation reaction is carried out by the enzyme RuBisCO as part of the Calvin – Benson cycle. Three types of photosynthesis occur in plants, C3 carbon fixation, C4 carbon fixation and CAM photosynthesis. These differ by the route that carbon dioxide takes to the Calvin cycle, with C3 plants fixing CO_2 directly, while C4 and CAM photosynthesis incorporate the CO_2 into other compounds first, as adaptations to deal with intense sunlight and dry conditions.

In photosynthetic prokaryotes the mechanisms of carbon fixation are more diverse. Here, carbon dioxide can be fixed by the Calvin – Benson cycle, a reversed citric acid cycle, or the carboxylation of acetyl-CoA. Prokaryotic chemoautotrophs also fix CO_2 through the Calvin – Benson cycle, but use energy from inorganic compounds to drive the reaction.

Carbohydrates and Glycans

In carbohydrate anabolism, simple organic acids can be converted into monosaccharides such as glucose and then used to assemble polysaccharides such as starch. The generation of glucose from compounds like pyruvate, lactate, glycerol, glycerate 3-phosphate and amino acids is called gluconeogenesis. Gluconeogenesis converts pyruvate to glucose-6-phosphate through a series of intermediates, many of which are shared with glycolysis. However, this pathway is not simply glycolysis run in reverse, as several steps are catalyzed by non-glycolytic enzymes. This is important as it allows the formation and breakdown of glucose to be regulated separately, and prevents both pathways from running simultaneously in a futile cycle.

Although fat is a common way of storing energy, in vertebrates such as humans the fatty acids in these stores cannot be converted to glucose through gluconeogenesis as these organisms cannot convert acetyl-CoA into pyruvate; plants do, but animals do not, have the necessary enzymatic machinery. As a result, after long-term starvation, vertebrates need to produce ketone bodies from fatty acids to replace glucose in tissues such as the brain that cannot metabolize fatty acids. In other organisms such as plants and bacteria, this metabolic problem is solved using the glyoxylate cycle, which bypasses the decarboxylation step in the citric acid cycle and allows the transformation of acetyl-CoA to oxaloacetate, where it can be used for the production of glucose.

Polysaccharides and glycans are made by the sequential addition of monosaccharides by glycosyltransferase from a reactive sugar-phosphate donor such as uridine diphosphate glucose (UDP-glucose) to an acceptor hydroxyl group on the growing polysaccharide. As any of the hydroxyl groups on the ring of the substrate can be acceptors, the polysaccharides produced can have straight or branched structures. The polysaccharides produced can have structural or metabolic functions themselves, or be transferred to lipids and proteins by enzymes called oligosaccharyltransferases.

Fatty Acids, Isoprenoids and Steroids

Fatty acids are made by fatty acid synthases that polymerize and then reduce acetyl-CoA units. The acyl chains in the fatty acids are extended by a cycle of reactions that add the acyl group, reduce it to an alcohol, dehydrate it to an alkene group and then reduce it again to an alkane group. The enzymes of fatty acid biosynthesis are divided into two groups: in animals and fungi, all these fatty acid synthase reactions are carried out by a single multifunctional type I protein, while in plant plastids and bacteria separate type II enzymes perform each step in the pathway.

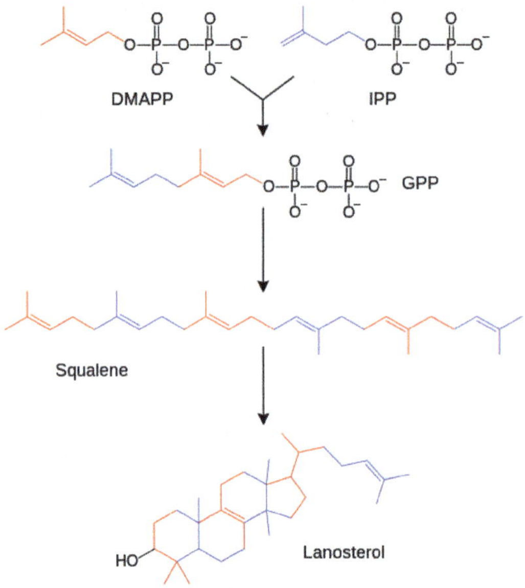

Simplified version of the steroid synthesis pathway with the intermediates isopentenyl pyrophosphate (IPP), dimethylallyl pyrophosphate (DMAPP), geranyl pyrophosphate (GPP) and squalene shown. Some intermediates are omitted for clarity.

Terpenes and isoprenoids are a large class of lipids that include the carotenoids and form the largest class of plant natural products. These compounds are made by the assembly and modification of isoprene units donated from the reactive precursors isopentenyl pyrophosphate and dimethylallyl pyrophosphate. These precursors can be made in different ways. In animals and archaea, the mevalonate pathway produces these compounds from acetyl-CoA, while in plants and bacteria the non-mevalonate pathway uses pyruvate and glyceraldehyde 3-phosphate as substrates. One important reaction that uses these activated isoprene donors is steroid biosynthesis. Here, the isoprene units are joined together to make squalene and then folded up and formed into a set of rings to make lanosterol. Lanosterol can then be converted into other steroids such as cholesterol and ergosterol.

Proteins

Organisms vary in their ability to synthesize the 20 common amino acids. Most bacteria and plants can synthesize all twenty, but mammals can only synthesize eleven nonessential amino acids, so nine essential amino acids must be obtained from food. Some simple parasites, such as the bacteria *Mycoplasma pneumoniae*, lack all amino acid synthesis and take their amino acids directly from their hosts. All amino acids are synthesized from intermediates in glycolysis, the citric acid cycle, or the pentose phosphate pathway. Nitrogen is provided by glutamate and glutamine. Amino acid synthesis depends on the formation of the appropriate alpha-keto acid, which is then transaminated to form an amino acid.

Amino acids are made into proteins by being joined together in a chain of peptide bonds. Each different protein has a unique sequence of amino acid residues: this is its primary structure. Just as the letters of the alphabet can be combined to form an almost endless variety of words, amino acids can be linked in varying sequences to form a huge variety of proteins. Proteins are made from amino acids that have been activated by attachment to a transfer RNA molecule through an ester bond. This aminoacyl-tRNA precursor is produced in an ATP-dependent reaction carried out by an aminoacyl tRNA synthetase. This aminoacyl-tRNA is then a substrate for the ribosome, which joins the amino acid onto the elongating protein chain, using the sequence information in a messenger RNA.

Nucleotide Synthesis and Salvage

Nucleotides are made from amino acids, carbon dioxide and formic acid in pathways that require large amounts of metabolic energy. Consequently, most organisms have efficient systems to salvage preformed nucleotides. Purines are synthesized as nucleosides (bases attached to ribose). Both adenine and guanine are made from the precursor nucleoside inosine monophosphate, which is synthesized using atoms from the amino acids glycine, glutamine, and aspartic acid, as well as formate transferred from the coenzyme tetrahydrofolate. Pyrimidines, on the other hand, are synthesized from the base orotate, which is formed from glutamine and aspartate.

Xenobiotics and Redox Metabolism

All organisms are constantly exposed to compounds that they cannot use as foods and would be harmful if they accumulated in cells, as they have no metabolic function. These potentially damaging compounds are called xenobiotics. Xenobiotics such as synthetic drugs, natural poisons and antibiotics are detoxified by a set of xenobiotic-metabolizing enzymes. In humans, these include cytochrome P450 oxidases, UDP-glucuronosyltransferases, and glutathione *S*-transferases. This system of enzymes acts in three stages to firstly oxidize the xenobiotic (phase I) and then conjugate water-soluble groups onto the molecule (phase II). The modified water-soluble xenobiotic can then be pumped out of cells and in multicellular organisms may be further metabolized before being excreted (phase III). In ecology, these reactions are particularly important in microbial biodegradation of pollutants and the bioremediation of contaminated land and oil spills. Many of these microbial reactions are shared with multicellular organisms, but due to the incredible diversity of types of microbes these organisms are able to deal with a far wider range of xenobiotics than multicellular organisms, and can degrade even persistent organic pollutants such as organochloride compounds.

A related problem for aerobic organisms is oxidative stress. Here, processes including oxidative phosphorylation and the formation of disulfide bonds during protein folding produce reactive oxygen species such as hydrogen peroxide. These damaging oxidants are removed by antioxidant metabolites such as glutathione and enzymes such as catalases and peroxidases.

Thermodynamics of Living Organisms

Living organisms must obey the laws of thermodynamics, which describe the transfer of heat and work. The second law of thermodynamics states that in any closed system, the amount of entropy (disorder) cannot decrease. Although living organisms' amazing complexity appears to contradict this law, life is possible as all organisms are open systems that exchange matter and energy with their surroundings. Thus living systems are not in equilibrium, but instead are dissipative systems that maintain their state of high complexity by causing a larger increase in the entropy of their environments. The metabolism of a cell achieves this by coupling the spontaneous processes of catabolism to the non-spontaneous processes of anabolism. In thermodynamic terms, metabolism maintains order by creating disorder.

Regulation and Control

As the environments of most organisms are constantly changing, the reactions of metabolism must be finely regulated to maintain a constant set of conditions within cells, a condition called homeostasis. Metabolic regulation also allows organisms to respond to signals and interact actively with their environments. Two closely linked concepts are important for understanding how metabolic pathways are controlled. Firstly, the *regulation* of an enzyme in a pathway is how its activity is increased and decreased in response to signals. Secondly, the *control* exerted by this enzyme is the effect that these changes in its activity have on the overall rate of the pathway (the flux through the pathway). For example, an enzyme may show large changes in activity (*i.e.* it is highly regulated) but if these changes have little effect on the flux of a metabolic pathway, then this enzyme is not involved in the control of the pathway.

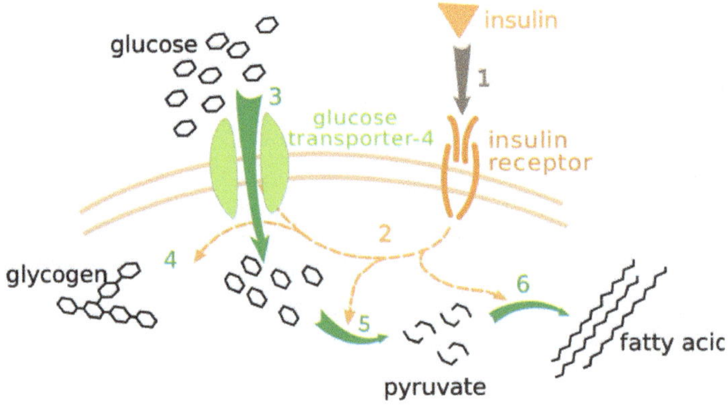

Effect of insulin on glucose uptake and metabolism. Insulin binds to its receptor (1), which in turn starts many protein activation cascades (2). These include: translocation of Glut-4 transporter to the plasma membrane and influx of glucose (3), glycogen synthesis (4), glycolysis (5) and fatty acid synthesis (6).

There are multiple levels of metabolic regulation. In intrinsic regulation, the metabolic pathway self-regulates to respond to changes in the levels of substrates or products; for example, a decrease in the amount of product can increase the flux through the pathway to compensate. This type of regulation often involves allosteric regulation of the activities of multiple enzymes in the pathway. Extrinsic control involves a cell in a multicellular organism changing its metabolism in response to signals from other cells. These signals are usually in the form of soluble messengers such as hormones and growth factors and are detected by specific receptors on the cell surface. These signals are then transmitted inside the cell by second messenger systems that often involved the phosphorylation of proteins.

A very well understood example of extrinsic control is the regulation of glucose metabolism by the hormone insulin. Insulin is produced in response to rises in blood glucose levels. Binding of the hormone to insulin receptors on cells then activates a cascade of protein kinases that cause the cells to take up glucose and convert it into storage molecules such as fatty acids and glycogen. The metabolism of glycogen is controlled by activity of phosphorylase, the enzyme that breaks down glycogen, and glycogen synthase, the enzyme that makes it. These enzymes are regulated in a reciprocal fashion, with phosphorylation inhibiting glycogen synthase, but activating phosphorylase. Insulin causes glycogen synthesis by activating protein phosphatases and producing a decrease in the phosphorylation of these enzymes.

Evolution

The central pathways of metabolism described above, such as glycolysis and the citric acid cycle, are present in all three domains of living things and were present in the last universal ancestor. This universal ancestral cell was prokaryotic and probably a methanogen that had extensive amino acid, nucleotide, carbohydrate and lipid metabolism. The retention of these ancient pathways during later evolution may be the result of these reactions having been an optimal solution to their particular metabolic problems, with pathways such as glycolysis and the citric acid cycle producing their end products highly efficiently and in a minimal number of steps. The first pathways of enzyme-based metabolism may have been parts of purine nucleotide metabolism, while previous metabolic pathways were a part of the ancient RNA world.

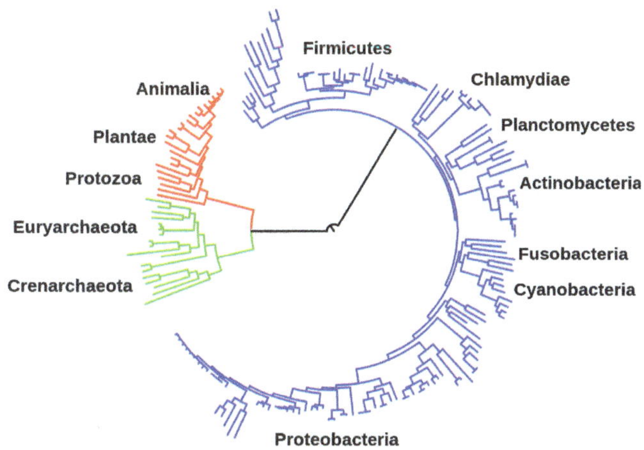

Evolutionary tree showing the common ancestry of organisms from all three domains of life. Bacteria are colored blue, eukaryotes red, and archaea green. Relative positions of some of the phyla included are shown around the tree.

Many models have been proposed to describe the mechanisms by which novel metabolic pathways evolve. These include the sequential addition of novel enzymes to a short ancestral pathway, the duplication and then divergence of entire pathways as well as the recruitment of pre-existing enzymes and their assembly into a novel reaction pathway. The relative importance of these mechanisms is unclear, but genomic studies have shown that enzymes in a pathway are likely to have a shared ancestry, suggesting that many pathways have evolved in a step-by-step fashion with novel functions created from pre-existing steps in the pathway. An alternative model comes from studies that trace the evolution of proteins' structures in metabolic networks, this has suggested that enzymes are pervasively recruited, borrowing enzymes to perform similar functions in different metabolic pathways (evident in the MANET database) These recruitment processes result in an evolutionary enzymatic mosaic. A third possibility is that some parts of metabolism might exist as "modules" that can be reused in different pathways and perform similar functions on different molecules.

As well as the evolution of new metabolic pathways, evolution can also cause the loss of metabolic functions. For example, in some parasites metabolic processes that are not essential for survival are lost and preformed amino acids, nucleotides and carbohydrates may instead be scavenged from the host. Similar reduced metabolic capabilities are seen in endosymbiotic organisms.

Investigation and Manipulation

Classically, metabolism is studied by a reductionist approach that focuses on a single metabolic pathway. Particularly valuable is the use of radioactive tracers at the whole-organism, tissue and cellular levels, which define the paths from precursors to final products by identifying radioactively labelled intermediates and products. The enzymes that catalyze these chemical reactions can then be purified and their kinetics and responses to inhibitors investigated. A parallel approach is to identify the small molecules in a cell or tissue; the complete set of these molecules is called the metabolome. Overall, these studies give a good view of the structure and function of simple metabolic pathways, but are inadequate when applied to more complex systems such as the metabolism of a complete cell.

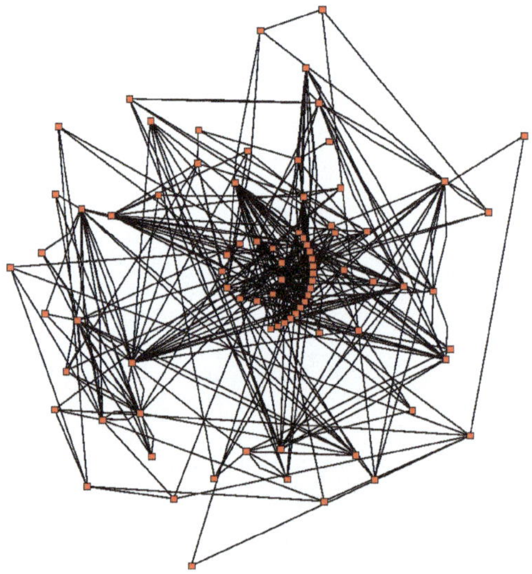

Metabolic network of the *Arabidopsis thaliana* citric acid cycle. Enzymes and metabolites are shown as red squares and the interactions between them as black lines.

An idea of the complexity of the metabolic networks in cells that contain thousands of different enzymes is given by the figure showing the interactions between just 43 proteins and 40 metabolites to the right: the sequences of genomes provide lists containing anything up to 45,000 genes. However, it is now possible to use this genomic data to reconstruct complete networks of biochemical reactions and produce more holistic mathematical models that may explain and predict their behavior. These models are especially powerful when used to integrate the pathway and metabolite data obtained through classical methods with data on gene expression from proteomic and DNA microarray studies. Using these techniques, a model of human metabolism has now been produced, which will guide future drug discovery and biochemical research. These models are now used in network analysis, to classify human diseases into groups that share common proteins or metabolites.

Bacterial metabolic networks are a striking example of bow-tie organization, an architecture able to input a wide range of nutrients and produce a large variety of products and complex macromolecules using a relatively few intermediate common currencies.

A major technological application of this information is metabolic engineering. Here, organisms such as yeast, plants or bacteria are genetically modified to make them more useful in biotechnology and aid the production of drugs such as antibiotics or industrial chemicals such as 1,3-propanediol and shikimic acid. These genetic modifications usually aim to reduce the amount of energy used to produce the product, increase yields and reduce the production of wastes.

History

The first documented references of metabolism were made by Ibn al-Nafis in his 1260 AD work titled Al-Risalah al-Kamiliyyah fil Siera al-Nabawiyyah (The Treatise of Ka-mil on the Prophet's Biography) which included the following phrase "Both the body and its parts are in a continuous state of dissolution and nourishment, so they are inevitably under-going permanent change." The history of the scientific study of metabolism spans several centuries and has moved from examining whole animals in early studies, to examining individual metabolic reactions in modern biochemistry. The first controlled experiments in human metabolism were published by Santorio Santorio in 1614 in his book *Ars de statica medicina*. He described how he weighed himself before and after eating, sleep, working, sex, fasting, drinking, and excreting. He found that most of the food he took in was lost through what he called "insensible perspiration".

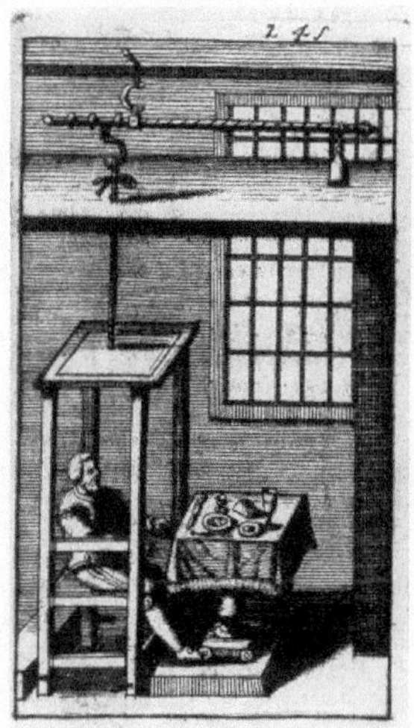

Santorio Santorio in his steelyard balance, from *Ars de statica medicina*, first published 1614

In these early studies, the mechanisms of these metabolic processes had not been identified and a vital force was thought to animate living tissue. In the 19th century, when studying the fermentation of sugar to alcohol by yeast, Louis Pasteur concluded that fermentation was catalyzed by substances within the yeast cells he called "ferments". He wrote that "alcoholic fermentation is an act correlated with the life and organization of the yeast cells, not with the death or putrefaction of the cells." This discovery, along with the publication by Friedrich Wöhler in 1828 of a paper on the chemical synthesis of urea, and is notable for being the first organic compound prepared from wholly inorganic precursors. This proved that the organic compounds and chemical reactions found in cells were no different in principle than any other part of chemistry.

It was the discovery of enzymes at the beginning of the 20th century by Eduard Buchner that separated the study of the chemical reactions of metabolism from the biological study of cells, and marked the beginnings of biochemistry. The mass of biochemical knowledge grew rapidly throughout the early 20th century. One of the most prolific of these modern biochemists was Hans Krebs who made huge contributions to the study of metabolism. He discovered the urea cycle and later, working with Hans Kornberg, the citric acid cycle and the glyoxylate cycle. Modern biochemical research has been greatly aided by the development of new techniques such as chromatography, X-ray diffraction, NMR spectroscopy, radioisotopic labelling, electron microscopy and molecular dynamics simulations. These techniques have allowed the discovery and detailed analysis of the many molecules and metabolic pathways in cells.

Metabolic Equivalent

The Metabolic Equivalent of Task (MET), or simply metabolic equivalent, is a physiological measure expressing the energy cost of physical activities and is defined as the ratio of metabolic rate (and therefore the rate of energy consumption) during a specific physical activity to a reference metabolic rate, set by convention to 3.5 ml $O_2 \cdot kg^{-1} \cdot min$ equivalently:

$$1\ \mathrm{MET} = 1\frac{\mathrm{kcal}}{\mathrm{kg} * h} = 4.184\frac{\mathrm{kJ}}{\mathrm{kg} * h} = 1.162\frac{\mathrm{W}}{\mathrm{kg}}$$

1 MET is also defined as 58.2 W/m^2 (18.4 Btu/h·ft^2), which is equal to the rate of energy produced per unit surface area of an average person seated at rest. The surface area of an average person is 1.8 m^2 (19 ft^2). Metabolic rate is usually expressed in terms of unit area of the total body surface (ANSI/ASHRAE Standard 55).

Originally, 1 MET was considered as the Resting Metabolic Rate (RMR) obtained during quiet sitting. MET values of activities range from 0.9 (sleeping) to 23 (running at 22.5 km/h or a 4:17 mile pace).

Although the RMR of any person may deviate from the reference value, MET can be thought of as an index of the intensity of activities: for example, an activity with a MET value of 2, such as walking at a slow pace (e.g., 3 km/h) would require twice the energy that an average person consumes at rest (e.g., sitting quietly).

MET is used as a means of expressing the intensity and energy expenditure of activities in a way comparable among persons of different weight. Actual energy expenditure (e.g., in calories or joules) during an activity depends on the person's body mass; therefore, the energy cost of the same activity will be different for persons of different weight. However, since the RMR is also dependent on body mass in a similar way, it is assumed that the ratio of this energy cost to the RMR of each person will remain more or less stable for the specific activity and thus independent of each person's weight.

The 1 MET reference value of 1 kcal·kg^{-1}·h^{-1}, is used by convention and refers to a typical metabolism at rest of an "average" individual. It must not be confused or misused as an approximation of Basal Metabolic Rate (BMR), which is the minimum metabolic rate obtained under specified conditions. This is illustrated by the fact that sleeping has a MET of 0.9, while an individual's normal sleeping metabolism may be greater than the BMR.

Compendium of Physical Activities

The *Compendium of Physical Activities* was developed for use in epidemiologic studies to standardize the assignment of MET intensities in physical activity questionnaires. Dr. Bill Haskell from Stanford University conceptualized the compendium and developed a prototype for the document. The compendium was used first in the *Survey of Activity, Fitness, and Exercise* (SAFE study - 1987 to 1989) to code and score physical activity records. Since then, the compendium has been used in studies worldwide to assign intensity units to physical activity questionnaires and to develop innovative ways to assess energy expenditure in physical activity studies. The compendium was published in 1993 and updated in 2000 and 2011.

Scope of Usage of The MET Concept

Epidemiology and Public Health

MET (Metabolic Equivalent): The ratio of the work metabolic rate to the resting metabolic rate. One MET is defined as 1 kcal/kg/hour and is roughly equivalent to the energy cost of sitting quietly. A MET also is defined as oxygen uptake in ml/kg/min with one MET equal to the oxygen cost of sitting quietly, equivalent to 3.5 ml/kg/min.

The MET concept was primarily designed to be used in epidemiological surveys, where survey respondents answer the amount of time they spend for specific physical activities.

Moreover, MET is used to provide general medical thresholds and guidelines to a population. A MET is the ratio of the rate of energy expended during an activity to the rate of energy expended at rest. For example, 1 MET is the rate of energy expenditure while at rest. A 4 MET activity expends 4 times the energy used by the body at rest. If a person does a 4 MET activity for 30 minutes, he or she has done 4 x 30 = 120 MET-minutes (or 2.0 MET-hours) of physical activity. A person could also achieve 120 MET-minutes by doing an 8 MET activity for 15 minutes.

Physical activity	MET
Light intensity activities	< 3
sleeping	0.9
watching television	1.0
writing, desk work, typing	1.5
walking, 1.7 mph (2.7 km/h), level ground, strolling, very slow	2.3
walking, 2.5 mph (4 km/h)	2.9
Moderate intensity activities	3 to 6
bicycling, stationary, 50 watts, very light effort	3.0
walking 3.0 mph (4.8 km/h)	3.3
calisthenics, home exercise, light or moderate effort, general	3.5
walking 3.4 mph (5.5 km/h)	3.6
bicycling, <10 mph (16 km/h), leisure, to work or for pleasure	4.0

bicycling, stationary, 100 watts, light effort	5.5
sexual activity	5.8
Vigorous intensity activities	> 6
jogging, general	7.0
calisthenics (e.g. pushups, situps, pullups, jumping jacks), heavy, vigorous effort	8.0
running jogging, in place	8.0
rope jumping	10.0

Limitations in The Usage of Met to Calculate Actual Energy Expenditure

Published MET values (or exercise calorie calculators on web sites, which are based on such values) for specific activities are experimentally and statistically derived from a sample of persons and are indicative averages. The level of intensity at which a specific person performs a specific physical activity (e.g., the pace of walking, the speed of running, etc.) will deviate from the representative experimental conditions used for the calculation of the standard MET values. Moreover, as is explained in the following, the actual energy expenditure and the RMR will differ according to the person's overall fitness level and other factors.

The same holds for MET (or kcal) values indicated in modern fitness exercise equipment, which are based on statistical models and are of indicative value only. In this case, even if the MET value indicated is a better statistical prediction than published tables, there is no way to account for the person's actual RMR and thus energy expenditure (e.g., Kcal). In short, a person can use the MET concept to plan or monitor physical activity levels or get an indication of the aerobic intensity and order of magnitude of energy expenditure for a specific activity, but not use the MET concept to calculate actual energy expenditure or a daily energy input-output balance.

More specifically, from a strictly scientific point of view, statistically estimated predictions, such as MET or BMI, are inaccurate when used for specific persons, and MET values must be treated as indicative only, taking into account that both RMR and actual energy consumption are highly dependent on physical and environmental factors such as adiposity, physical fitness level, cardiovascular health, or even ambient temperature.

Moreover, even the definition of MET is problematic when used for specific persons. By convention, 1 MET is considered equivalent to the consumption of 3.5 ml $O_2 \cdot kg^{-1} \cdot min^{-1}$ (or 3.5 ml of oxygen per kilogram of body mass per minute) and is roughly equivalent to the expenditure of 1 kcal per kilogram of body weight per hour. This value was first experimentally derived from the resting oxygen consumption of a particular subject (a healthy 40-year-old, 70 kg man) and must therefore be treated as a convention. Since the RMR of a person depends mainly on lean body mass (and not total weight) and other physiological factors such as health status, age, etc., actual RMR (and thus 1-MET energy equivalents) may vary significantly from the kcal/(kg·h) rule of thumb. RMR measurements by calorimetry in medical surveys have shown that the conventional 1-MET value overestimates the actual resting O_2 consumption and energy expenditures by about 20% to 30% on the average, whereas body composition (ratio of body fat to lean body mass) accounted for most of the variance.

Basal Metabolic Rate

Basal metabolic rate (BMR) is the minimal rate of energy expenditure per unit time by endothermic animals at rest. It is reported in energy units per unit time ranging from watt (Joule/second) to ml O_2/min or Joule per hour per kg body mass J/(h.kg)). Proper measurement requires a strict set of criteria be met. These criteria include being in a physically and psychologically undisturbed state, in a thermally neutral environment, while in the post-absorptive state (i.e., not actively digesting food). In bradymetabolic animals, such as fish and reptiles, the equivalent term standard metabolic rate (SMR) is used. It follows the same criteria as BMR, but requires the documentation of the temperature at which the metabolic rate was measured. This makes BMR a variant of standard metabolic rate measurement that excludes the temperature data, a practice that has led to problems in defining "standard" rates of metabolism for many mammals.

Metabolism refers to the processes that the body needs to function. Basal Metabolic Rate is the amount of energy expressed in calories that a person needs to keep the body functioning at rest. Some of those processes are breathing, blood circulation, controlling body temperature, cell growth, brain and nerve function, and contraction of muscles. Basal metabolic rate (BMR) affects the rate that a person burns calories and ultimately whether that individual maintains, gains, or loses weight. The basal metabolic rate accounts for about 60 to 75% of the daily calorie expenditure by individuals. It is influenced by several factors. BMR typically declines by 1-2% per decade after age 20, mostly due to loss of fat-free mass, although the variability between individuals is high.

Description

The body's generation of heat is known as thermogenesis and it can be measured to determine the amount of energy expended. BMR generally decreases with age and with the decrease in lean body mass (as may happen with aging). Increasing muscle mass has the effect of increasing BMR. Aerobic (resistance) fitness level, a product of cardiovascular exercise, while previously thought to have effect on BMR, has been shown in the 1990s not to correlate with BMR when adjusted for fat-free body mass. But anaerobic exercise does increase resting energy consumption. Illness, previously consumed food and beverages, environmental temperature, and stress levels can affect one's overall energy expenditure as well as one's BMR.

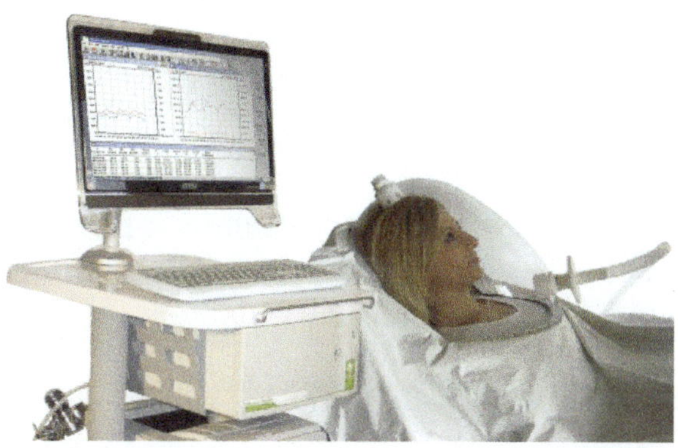

Indirect calorimetry laboratory with canopy hood (dilution technique)

BMR is measured under very restrictive circumstances when a person is awake. An accurate BMR measurement requires that the person's sympathetic nervous system not be stimulated, a condition which requires complete rest. A more common measurement, which uses less strict criteria, is resting metabolic rate (RMR).

BMR may be measured by gas analysis through either direct or Indirect Calorimetry, though a rough estimation can be acquired through an equation using age, sex, height, and weight. Studies of energy metabolism using both methods provide convincing evidence for the validity of the respiratory quotient (R.Q.), which measures the inherent composition and utilization of carbohydrates, fats and proteins as they are converted to energy substrate units that can be used by the body as energy.

Nutrition and Dietary Considerations

Basal metabolism is usually by far the largest component of total caloric expenditure. However, the Harris–Benedict equations are only approximate and variation in BMR (reflecting varying body composition), in physical activity levels, and in energy expended in thermogenesis make it difficult to estimate the dietary consumption any particular individual needs in order to maintain body weight.

Physiology

The early work of the scientists J. Arthur Harris and Francis G. Benedict showed that approximate values for BMR could be derived using body surface area (computed from height and weight), age, and sex, along with the oxygen and carbon dioxide measures taken from calorimetry. Studies also showed that by eliminating the sex differences that occur with the accumulation of adipose tissue by expressing metabolic rate per unit of "fat-free" or lean body mass, the values between sexes for basal metabolism are essentially the same. Exercise physiology textbooks have tables to show the conversion of height and body surface area as they relate to weight and basal metabolic values.

The primary organ responsible for regulating metabolism is the hypothalamus. The hypothalamus is located on the diencephalon and forms the floor and part of the lateral walls of the third ventricle of the cerebrum. The chief functions of the hypothalamus are:

1. control and integration of activities of the autonomic nervous system (ANS)
    - The ANS regulates contraction of smooth muscle and cardiac muscle, along with secretions of many endocrine organs such as the thyroid gland (associated with many metabolic disorders).
    - Through the ANS, the hypothalamus is the main regulator of visceral activities, such as heart rate, movement of food through the gastrointestinal tract, and contraction of the urinary bladder.
2. production and regulation of feelings of rage and aggression
3. regulation of body temperature
4. regulation of food intake, through two centers:

- The feeding center or hunger center is responsible for the sensations that cause us to seek food. When sufficient food or substrates have been received and leptin is high, then the satiety center is stimulated and sends impulses that inhibit the feeding center. When insufficient food is present in the stomach and ghrelin levels are high, receptors in the hypothalamus initiate the sense of hunger.

- The thirst center operates similarly when certain cells in the hypothalamus are stimulated by the rising osmotic pressure of the extracellular fluid. If thirst is satisfied, osmotic pressure decreases.

All of these functions taken together form a survival mechanism that causes us to sustain the body processes that BMR measures.

BMR Estimation Formulas

Several prediction equations exist. Historically, the most notable one was the Harris-Benedict equation, which was created in 1919.

In each of the formulas:

- P is total heat production at complete rest,
- m is mass (kg),
- h is height (cm), and
- a is age (years),

The Original Harris-Benedict Equation:

- $$P = \left(\frac{13.7516m}{1\,\text{kg}} + \frac{5.0033h}{1\,\text{cm}} - \frac{6.7550a}{1\,\text{year}} + 66.4730 \right) \frac{\text{kcal}}{\text{day}}$$

- $$P = \left(\frac{9.5634m}{1\,\text{kg}} + \frac{1.8496h}{1\,\text{cm}} - \frac{4.6756a}{1\,\text{year}} + 655.0955 \right) \frac{\text{kcal}}{\text{day}}$$ [6

The difference in BMR for men and women is mainly due to differences in body weight. For example, a 55-year-old woman weighing 130 lb (59 kg) and 5 feet 6 inches (168 cm) tall would have a BMR of 1272 kcal per day or 53 kcal/h (61.3 watts).and with the difference in BMR for men and women being mainly due to differences in body weight.

In 1984, the original Harris-Benedict equations were revised using new data. In comparisons with actual expenditure, the revised equations were found to be more accurate.

The Revised Harris-Benedict Equation:

- $$P = \left(\frac{13.397m}{1\text{kg}} + \frac{4.799h}{1\text{cm}} - \frac{5.677a}{1\text{year}} + 88.362 \right) \frac{\text{kcal}}{\text{day}}$$
- $$P = \left(\frac{9.247m}{1\text{kg}} + \frac{3.098h}{1\text{cm}} - \frac{4.330a}{1\text{year}} + 447.593 \right) \frac{\text{kcal}}{\text{day}}$$

It was the best prediction equation until 1990, when Mifflin *et al.* introduced the equation:

The Mifflin St Jeor Equation:

- P = (10.0 m 1 kg + 6.25 h 1 cm − 5.0 a 1 year + s) kcal day

  $$P = \left(\frac{10.0m}{1\text{kg}} + \frac{6.25h}{1\text{cm}} - \frac{5.0a}{1\text{year}} + s \right) \frac{\text{kcal}}{\text{day}}$$, where s is +5 for males and −161 for fe males.

According to this formula, the woman in the example above has a BMR of 1204 kcal per day. During the last 100 years, lifestyles have changed and Frankenfield *et al.* showed it to be about 5% more accurate.

These formulas are based on body weight, which does not take into account the difference in metabolic activity between lean body mass and body fat. Other formulas exist which take into account lean body mass, two of which are the Katch-McArdle formula, and Cunningham formula. The Katch-McArdle formula is used to predict Resting Daily Energy Expenditure (RDEE). The Cunningham formula is commonly attributed as being used to predict RMR instead of BMR, however the formulas provided by Katch-McArdle and Cunningham are the same.

The Katch-McArdle Formula (Resting Daily Energy Expenditure):

- P = 370 + (21.6 . L B M) $P = 370 + (21.6 \cdot LBM)$, where LBM is the lean body mass in kg.

According to this formula, if the woman in the example has a body fat percentage of 30%, her RDEE (the authors use the term of basal and resting metabolism interchangeably) would be 1263 kcal per day.

Causes of Individual Differences in BMR

The basal metabolic rate varies between individuals. One study of 150 adults representative of the population in Scotland reported basal metabolic rates from as low as 1027 kcal per day (4301 kJ/day) to as high as 2499 kcal/day (10455 kJ/day); with a mean BMR of 1500 kcal/day (6279 kJ/day). Statistically, the researchers calculated that 62.3% of this variation was explained by differences in fat free mass. Other factors explaining the variation included fat mass (6.7%), age (1.7%), and experimental error including within-subject difference (2%). The rest of the variation (26.7%) was unexplained. This remaining difference was not explained by sex nor by differing tissue size of highly energetic organs such as the brain.

Differences in BMR have been observed when comparing subjects with *the same* lean body mass. In one study, when comparing individuals with the same lean body mass, the top 5% of BMRs are 28-32% higher than the lowest 5% BMR. Additionally, this study reports a case where two individuals with the same lean body mass of 43 kg had BMRs of 1075 kcal/day (4.5 MJ/day) and 1790 kcal/day (7.5 MJ/day). This difference of 715 kcal/day (67%) is equivalent to one of the individuals completing a 10 kilometer run every day. However, this study did not account for the sex, height, fasting-state, or body fat percentage of the subjects.

Biochemistry

About 70% of a human's total energy expenditure is due to the basal life processes within the organs of the body (see table). About 20% of one's energy expenditure comes from physical activity and another 10% from thermogenesis, or digestion of food (*postprandial thermogenesis*). All of these processes require an intake of oxygen along with coenzymes to provide energy for survival (usually from macronutrients like carbohydrates, fats, and proteins) and expel carbon dioxide, due to processing by the Krebs cycle.

Energy expenditure breakdown	
Liver	27%
Brain	19%
Skeletal Muscle	18%
Kidneys	10%
Heart	7%
Other organs	19%

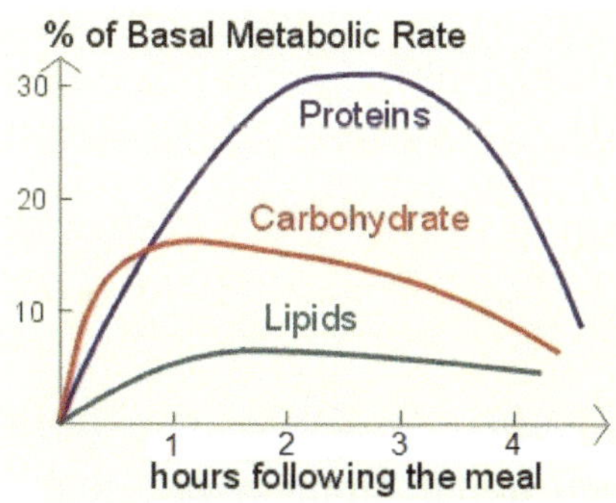

Postprandial thermogenesis increases in basal metabolic rate occur at different degrees depending on consumed food composition.

For the BMR, most of the energy is consumed in maintaining fluid levels in tissues through osmoregulation, and only about one-tenth is consumed for mechanical work, such as digestion, heartbeat, and breathing.

What enables the Krebs cycle to perform metabolic changes to fats, carbohydrates, and proteins is energy, which can be defined as the ability or capacity to do work. The breakdown of large molecules into smaller molecules—associated with release of energy—is catabolism. The building up process is termed anabolism. The breakdown of proteins into amino acids is an example of catabolism, while the formation of proteins from amino acids is an anabolic process.

Exergonic reactions are energy-releasing reactions and are generally catabolic. Endergonic reactions require energy and include anabolic reactions and the contraction of muscle. Metabolism is the total of all catabolic, exergonic, anabolic, endergonic reactions.

Adenosine Triphosphate (ATP) is the intermediate molecule that drives the exergonic transfer of energy to switch to endergonic anabolic reactions used in muscle contraction. This is what causes muscles to work which can require a breakdown, and also to build in the rest period, which occurs during the strengthening phase associated with muscular contraction. ATP is composed of adenine, a nitrogen containing base, ribose, a five carbon sugar (collectively called adenosine), and three phosphate groups. ATP is a high energy molecule because it stores large amounts of energy in the chemical bonds of the two terminal phosphate groups. The breaking of these chemical bonds in the Krebs Cycle provides the energy needed for muscular contraction.

Glucose

Because the ratio of hydrogen to oxygen atoms in all carbohydrates is always the same as that in water—that is, 2 to 1—all of the oxygen consumed by the cells is used to oxidize the carbon in the carbohydrate molecule to form carbon dioxide. Consequently, during the complete oxidation of a glucose molecule, six molecules of carbon dioxide and six molecules of water are produced and six molecules of oxygen are consumed.

The overall equation for this reaction is:

$$C_6H_{12}O_6 + 6\ O_2 \rightarrow 6\ CO_2 + 6\ H_2O$$

(38 ATP molecules)

Because the gas exchange in this reaction is equal, the respiratory quotient (R.Q.) for carbohydrate is unity or 1.0:

$$R.Q. = 6\ CO_2 / 6\ O_2 = 1.0$$

Fats

The chemical composition for fats differs from that of carbohydrates in that fats contain considerably fewer oxygen atoms in proportion to atoms of carbon and hydrogen. When listed on nutritional information tables, fats are generally divided into six categories: total fats, saturated fatty acid, polyunsaturated fatty acid, monounsaturated fatty acid, dietary cholesterol, and trans fatty acid. From a basal metabolic or resting metabolic perspective, more energy is needed to burn a saturated fatty acid than an unsaturated fatty acid. The fatty acid molecule is broken down and categorized based on the number of carbon atoms in its molecular structure. The chemical equation for metabolism of the twelve to sixteen carbon atoms in a saturated fatty acid molecule shows the difference between metabolism of carbohydrates and fatty acids. Palmitic acid is a commonly studied example of the saturated fatty acid molecule.

The overall equation for the substrate utilization of palmitic acid is:

$$C_{16}H_{32}O_2 + 23\ O_2 \rightarrow 16\ CO_2 + 16\ H_2O$$

Thus the R.Q. for palmitic acid is 0.696:

$$R.Q. = 16\ CO_2\ /\ 23\ O_2 = 0.696$$

Proteins

Proteins are composed of carbon, hydrogen, oxygen, and nitrogen arranged in a variety of ways to form a large combination of amino acids. Unlike fat the body has no storage deposits of protein. All of it is contained in the body as important parts of tissues, blood hormones, and enzymes. The structural components of the body that contain these amino acids are continually undergoing a process of breakdown and replacement. The respiratory quotient for protein metabolism can be demonstrated by the chemical equation for oxidation of albumin:

$$C_{72}H_{112}N_{18}O_{22}S + 77\ O_2 \rightarrow 63\ CO_2 + 38\ H_2O + SO_3 + 9\ CO(NH_2)_2$$

The R.Q. for albumin is $63\ CO_2 / 77\ O_2 = 0.818$

The reason this is important in the process of understanding protein metabolism is that the body can blend the three macronutrients and based on the mitochondrial density, a preferred ratio can be established which determines how much fuel is utilized in which packets for work accomplished by the muscles. Protein catabolism (breakdown) has been estimated to supply 10% to 15% of the total energy requirement during a two-hour aerobic training session. This process could severely degrade the protein structures needed to maintain survival such as contractile properties of proteins in the heart, cellular mitochondria, myoglobin storage, and metabolic enzymes within muscles.

The oxidative system (aerobic) is the primary source of ATP supplied to the body at rest and during low intensity activities and uses primarily carbohydrates and fats as substrates. Protein is not normally metabolized significantly, except during long term starvation and long bouts of exercise (greater than 90 minutes.) At rest approximately 70% of the ATP produced is derived from fats and 30% from carbohydrates. Following the onset of activity, as the intensity of the exercise increases, there is a shift in substrate preference from fats to carbohydrates. During high intensity aerobic exercise, almost 100% of the energy is derived from carbohydrates, if an adequate supply is available.

Aerobic Vs. Anaerobic Exercise

Studies published in 1992 and 1997 indicate that the level of aerobic fitness of an individual does not have any correlation with the level of resting metabolism. Both studies find that aerobic fitness levels do not improve the predictive power of fat free mass for resting metabolic rate.

Anaerobic exercise, such as weight lifting, builds additional muscle mass. Muscle contributes to the fat-free mass of an individual and therefore effective results from anaerobic exercise will increase BMR. However, the actual effect on BMR is controversial and difficult to enumerate. Various studies suggest that the resting metabolic rate of trained muscle is around 55kJ per kilogram, per day. Even a substantial increase in muscle mass, say 5 kg, would make only a minor impact on BMR.

Longevity

In 1926, Raymond Pearl proposed that longevity varies inversely with basal metabolic rate (the "rate of living hypothesis"). Support for this hypothesis comes from the fact that mammals with larger body size have longer maximum life spans (large animals do have higher total metabolic rates, but the metabolic rate at the cellular level is much lower, and the breathing rate and heartbeat are slower in larger animals) and the fact that the longevity of fruit flies varies inversely with ambient temperature. Additionally, the life span of houseflies can be extended by preventing physical activity. This theory has been bolstered by several new studies linking lower basal metabolic rate to increased life expectancy, across the animal kingdom—including humans. Calorie restriction and reduced thyroid hormone levels, both of which decrease the metabolic rate, have been associated with higher longevity in animals.

However, the ratio of total daily energy expenditure to resting metabolic rate can vary between 1.6 and 8.0 between species of mammals. Animals also vary in the degree of coupling between oxidative phosphorylation and ATP production, the amount of saturated fat in mitochondrial membranes, the amount of DNA repair, and many other factors that affect maximum life span.

Organism Longevity and Basal Metabolic Rate

In allometric scaling, maximum potential life span (MPLS) is directly related to metabolic rate (MR), where MR is the recharge rate of a biomass made up of covalent bonds. That biomass (W) is subjected to deterioration over time from thermodynamic, entropic pressure. Metabolism is essentially understood as redox coupling, and has nothing to do with thermogenesis. Metabolic efficiency (ME) is then expressed as the efficiency of this coupling, a ratio of amperes captured and used by biomass, to the amperes available for that purpose. MR is measured in watts, W is measured in grams. These factors are combined in a power law, an elaboration on Kleiber's law relating MR to W and MPLS, that appears as $MR = W(4ME-1)/4ME$. When ME is 100%, $MR = W^{3/4}$; this is popularly known as quarter power scaling, a version of allometric scaling that is premised upon unrealistic estimates of biological efficiency.

The equation reveals that as ME drops below 20%, for $W <$ one gram, MR/MPLS increases so dramatically as to endow W with virtual immortality by 16%. The smaller W is to begin with, the more dramatic is the increase in MR as ME diminishes. All of the cells of an organism fit into this range, i.e., less than one gram, and so this MR will be referred to as BMR.

But the equation reveals that as ME increases over 25%, BMR approaches zero. The equation also shows that for all $W >$ one gram, where W is the organization of all of the BMRs of the organism's structure, but also includes the activity of the structure, as ME increases over 25%, MR/MPLS increases rather than decreases, as it does for BMR. An MR made up of an organization of BMRs will be referred to as an FMR. As ME decreases below 25%, FMR diminishes rather than increases as it does for BMR.

The antagonism between FMR and BMR is what marks the process of aging of biomass W in energetic terms. The ME for the organism is the same as that for the cells, such that the success of the organism's ability to find food (and lower its ME), is key to maintaining the BMR of the cells driven, otherwise, by starvation, to approaching zero; while at the same time a lower ME diminishes the FMR/MPLS of the organism.

Medical Considerations

A person's metabolism varies with their physical condition and activity. Weight training can have a longer impact on metabolism than aerobic training, but there are no known mathematical formulas that can exactly predict the length and duration of a raised metabolism from trophic changes with anabolic neuromuscular training.

A decrease in food intake will typically lower the metabolic rate as the body tries to conserve energy. Researcher Gary Foster, Ph.D., estimates that a very low calorie diet of fewer than 800 calories a day would reduce the metabolic rate by more than 10 percent.

The metabolic rate can be affected by some drugs, such as antithyroid agents, drugs used to treat hyperthyroidism, such as propylthiouracil and methimazole, bring the metabolic rate down to normal and restore euthyroidism. Some research has focused on developing anti-obesity drugs to raise the metabolic rate, such as drugs to stimulate thermogenesis in skeletal muscle.

The metabolic rate may be elevated in stress, illness, and diabetes. Menopause may also affect metabolism.

Cardiovascular Implications

Heart rate is determined by the medulla oblongata and part of the pons, two organs located inferior to the hypothalamus on the brain stem. Heart rate is important for basal metabolic rate and resting metabolic rate because it drives the blood supply, stimulating the Krebs cycle. During exercise that achieves the anaerobic threshold, it is possible to deliver substrates that are desired for optimal energy utilization. The anaerobic threshold is defined as the energy utilization level of heart rate exertion that occurs without oxygen during a standardized test with a specific protocol for accuracy of measurement, such as the Bruce Treadmill protocol. With four to six weeks of targeted training the body systems can adapt to a higher perfusion of mitochondrial density for increased oxygen availability for the Krebs cycle, or tricarboxylic cycle, or the glycolitic cycle. This in turn leads to a lower resting heart rate, lower blood pressure, and increased resting or basal metabolic rate.

By measuring heart rate we can then derive estimations of what level of substrate utilization is actually causing biochemical metabolism in our bodies at rest or in activity. This in turn can help a person to maintain an appropriate level of consumption and utilization by studying a graphical representation of the anaerobic threshold. This can be confirmed by blood tests and gas analysis using either direct or indirect calorimetry to show the effect of substrate utilization. The measures of basal metabolic rate and resting metabolic rate are becoming essential tools for maintaining a healthy body weight.

Metabolic Age

Metabolic Age refers to a number calculated by comparing your Basal Metabolic Rate to the Basal Metabolic Rate average of your chronological age group.

This measurement is one among many which can be used to assess health, and people should avoid putting too much weight on it as it is a purely theoretical construct with no clinical studies; a more complete assessment of physical health can be obtained from a doctor, who may also have suggestions to improve health.

The hypothesis is that if someone's metabolic age is lower than his or her actual age, it suggests that the body is in good health, while a metabolic age higher than the actual age indicates that someone may be experiencing health problems.

Chronological age is your age in calendar years. Basal metabolic rate is the amount of energy consumed per unit of time when all environmental factors are considered neutral, the digestive system is in a post-absorptive state (meaning that the digestive system is inactive, which requires about twelve hours of fasting in humans), and the energy expenditure is only sufficient to support normal functioning of the vital organs, the heart, lungs, nervous system, kidneys, liver, intestine, sex organs, muscles, and skin. Formulas for estimating basal metabolic rate take into account age, weight, height, activity level, body fat mass, and lean body mass.

All the components in the body require various levels of energy to be maintained. Body fat requires much less energy than lean muscle, as lean muscle is much more metabolically active and therefore requires more energy expenditure to remain in homeostasis. If comparing two individuals, with all variables being equal, the person with more lean muscle mass will have a higher basal metabolic rate, and therefore, a lower metabolic age in comparison to those with the identical chronological age.

An individual's metabolic age will vary depending how his or her calculated basal metabolic rate compares to others of the same chronological age. Metabolic age is a new term used in the health and fitness industry to describe overall fitness and metabolic activity. Examining metabolic age will give insights to the overall level of health and wellness in comparison to those of the same age. Improving personal fitness is a main concern of most health-conscious individuals.:

VO_2 max

VO_2 max (also maximal oxygen consumption, maximal oxygen uptake, peak oxygen uptake or maximal aerobic capacity) is the maximum rate of oxygen consumption as measured during incremental exercise, most typically on a motorized treadmill. Maximal oxygen consumption reflects the aerobic physical fitness of the individual, and is an important determinant of their endurance capacity during prolonged, sub-maximal exercise. The name is derived from V - volume, O_2 - oxygen, max - maximum.

VO_2 max is expressed either as an absolute rate in (for example) litres of oxygen per minute (L/min) or as a relative rate in (for example) millilitres of oxygen per kilogram of body mass per minute (e.g., mL/(kg·min)). The latter expression is often used to compare the performance of endurance sports athletes. However, VO_2 max generally does not vary linearly with body mass, either among individuals within a species or among species, so comparisons of the performance capacities of individuals or species that differ in body size must be done with appropriate statistical procedures, such as analysis of covariance.

Measuring VO_2 Max

Accurately measuring VO_2 max involves a physical effort sufficient in duration and intensity to fully tax the aerobic energy system. In general clinical and athletic testing, this usually involves a graded exercise test (either on a treadmill or on a cycle ergometer) in which exercise intensity is progressively increased while measuring:

- ventilation and
- oxygen and carbon dioxide concentration of the inhaled and exhaled air.

VO_2 max is reached when oxygen consumption remains at a steady state despite an increase in workload.

Fick Equation

VO_2 max is properly defined by the Fick equation:

$VO_2 \text{ max} = Q \times (C_aO_2 - C_vO_2)$, when these values are obtained during an exertion at a maximal effort.

where Q is the cardiac output of the heart, C_aO_2 is the arterial oxygen content, and C_vO_2 is the venous oxygen content.

$(C_aO_2 - C_vO_2)$ is also known as the arteriovenous oxygen difference.

Estimation of Vo_2 Max

Tests measuring VO_2 max can be dangerous in individuals who are not considered normal healthy subjects, as any problems with the respiratory and cardiovascular systems will be greatly exacerbated in clinically ill patients. Thus, many protocols for estimating VO_2 max have been developed for those for whom a traditional VO_2 max test would be too risky. These generally are similar to a VO_2 max test, but do not reach the maximum of the respiratory and cardiovascular systems and are called sub-maximal tests.

Uth–Sørensen–Overgaard–Pedersen Estimation

Another estimate of VO_2 max for humans, based on maximum and resting heart rates, was created by a group of researchers from Denmark. It is given by:

VO_2 max ≈ 15.3 × HR max HR min $$VO_2 \text{ max} \approx 15.3 \times \frac{HR_{max}}{HR_{min}}$$

This equation uses the ratio of maximum heart rate (HR_{max}) to resting heart rate (HR_{rest}) to predict VO_2 max, and is measured in units of mL/kg/minute.

Cooper Test

Kenneth H. Cooper conducted a study for the United States Air Force in the late 1960s. One of the results of this was the Cooper test in which the distance covered running in 12 minutes is measured. Based on the measured distance, an estimate of VO_2 max [in mL/(kg·min)] is:

V O 2 m a x ≈ d 12 − 504.9 44.73 $$VO_2 \text{ max} \approx \frac{d_{12} - 504.9}{44.73}$$

where d_{12} is distance (in metres) covered in 12 minutes

An alternative equation is:

V O 2 m a x ≈ (35.97 * d m i l e s 12) − 11.29 $$VO_2 \text{ max} \approx (35.97 * dmiles_{12}) - 11.29$$

where d_{12} is distance (in miles) covered in 12 minutes,

Multi-stage Fitness Test

There are several other reliable tests and VO_2 max calculators to estimate VO_2 max, most notably the multi-stage fitness test (or *beep* test), based on the research paper by Leger and Lambert, "A Maximal Multi-Stage 20-m Shuttle Run Test to predict VO2 Max".

Rockport Fitness Walking Test

Estimation of VO_2 max from a timed one-mile track walk with duration t, incorporating gender, age, body weight in pounds (BW), and heart rate (HR) at the end of the mile. The factor x is 6.3150 for males, 0 for females. BW is in lbs, time is in minutes.

$$VO_2 \text{ max} \approx 132.853 - 0.0769BW - 0.3877\text{age} - 3.2649t - 0.1565HR + x$$

VO_2 Max Levels

"Maximal oxygen uptake (VO_2 max) is widely accepted as the single best measure of cardiovascular fitness and maximal aerobic power. Absolute values of VO_2 max are typically 40-60% higher in men than in women."

The average untrained healthy male will have a VO_2 max of approximately 35–40 mL/(kg·min). The average untrained healthy female will score a VO_2 max of approximately 27–31 mL/(kg·min).

These scores can improve with training and decrease with age, though the degree of trainability also varies very widely: conditioning may double VO_2 max in some individuals, and will never improve it in others. In one study, 10% of participants showed no benefit after completing a 20-week conditioning program, although the other 90% of the test subjects all showed substantial improvements in fitness to varying degree.

In sports where endurance is an important component in performance, such as cycling, rowing, cross-country skiing, swimming and running, world-class athletes typically have high VO_2 maxima. Elite male runners can consume up to 85 mL/(kg·min), and female elite runners can consume about 77 mL/(kg·min). Five time Tour de France winner Miguel Indurain is reported to have had a VO_2 max of 88.0 at his peak, while cross-country skier Bjørn Dæhlie measured at 96 mL/(kg·min). Dæhlie›s result was achieved out of season, and physiologist Erlend Hem who was responsible for the testing stated that he would not discount the possibility of the skier passing 100 mL/(kg·min) at his absolute peak. Norwegian cyclist Oskar Svendsen is thought to have recorded the highest VO_2 max of 97.5 mL/(kg·min), a "sensational" value in itself, made more remarkable by his young age (18 years old at the time). To put this into perspective, thoroughbred horses have a VO_2 max of around 180 mL/(kg·min). Siberian dogs running in the Iditarod Trail Sled Dog Race have VO_2 max values as high as 240 mL/(kg·min).

The highest values in absolute terms for humans are often found in rowers, as their much greater bulk makes up for a slightly lower VO_2 max per kg. Elite oarsmen measured in 1984 had VO_2 max values of 6.1±0.6 L/min and oarswomen 4.1±0.4 L/min. Rowers are interested in both absolute values of VO_2 max and in lung capacity, and the fact that they are measured in similar units means that the two are often confused. British rower Sir Matthew Pinsent is variously reported to have had a VO_2 of 7.5 L/min or 8.5 L/min, although the latter may represent confusion with his lung capacity of 8.5 litres. New Zealand sculler Rob Waddell has one of the highest absolute VO2 max levels ever tested.

Factors Affecting VO_2 Max

The factors affecting VO_2 are often divided into supply and demand. Supply is the transport of oxygen from the lungs to the mitochondria (including lung diffusion, stroke volume, blood volume, and capillary density of the skeletal muscle) while demand is the rate at which the mitochondria can reduce oxygen in the process of oxidative phosphorylation. Of these, the supply factor is often considered to be the limiting one. However, it has also been argued that while trained subjects probably are supply limited, untrained subjects can indeed have a demand limitation.

Tim Noakes, a professor of exercise and sports science at the University of Cape Town, describes a number of factors that may affect VO_2 max: age, sex, fitness and training, changes in altitude, and action of the ventilatory muscles. Noakes also asserts that VO_2 max is a relatively poor predictor of performance in runners due to variations in running economy and fatigue resistance during prolonged exercise.

Cardiac output, pulmonary diffusion capacity, oxygen carrying capacity, and other peripheral limitations like muscle diffusion capacity, mitochondrial enzymes, and capillary density are all examples of VO_2 max determinants. The body works as a system. If one of these factor is sub-par, then the whole system loses its normal capacity to function properly.

The drug erythropoietin (EPO) can boost VO_2 max by a significant amount in both humans and other mammals. This makes EPO attractive to athletes in endurance sports, such as professional cycling. By 1998 it had become widespread in cycling and led to the Festina affair as well as being mentioned ubiquitously in the USADA 2012 report on the US Postal team. Greg LeMond has suggested establishing a baseline for riders' VO_2 max (and other attributes) to detect abnormal performance increases.

References

- Friedrich C (1998). "Physiology and genetics of sulfur-oxidizing bacteria". Adv Microb Physiol. Advances in Microbial Physiology. 39: 235–89. doi:10.1016/S0065-2911(08)60018-1. ISBN 978-0-12-027739-1.
- Nelson, David L.; Michael M. Cox (2005). Lehninger Principles of Biochemistry. New York: W. H. Freeman and company. p. 841. ISBN 0-7167-4339-6.
- Guyton, Arthur C.; John E. Hall (2006). Textbook of Medical Physiology. Philadelphia: Elsevier. pp. 855–6. ISBN 0-7216-0240-1.
- Koch A (1998). "How did bacteria come to be?". Adv Microb Physiol. Advances in Microbial Physiology. 40: 353–99. doi:10.1016/S0065-2911(08)60135-6. ISBN 978-0-12-027740-7.
- McArdle, W (2006). Essentials of Exercise Physiology. Lippincott Williams & Wilkins. p. 266. ISBN 9780495014836.
- Lisa Gordon-Davis (2004). Hospitality Industry Handbook on Nutrition and Menu Planning. Juta and Company Ltd. p. 112. ISBN 978-0-7021-5578-9.
- "Arteriovenous oxygen difference". Sports Medicine, Sports Science and Kinesiology. Net Industries and its Licensors. 2011. Retrieved 30 April 2011.

7

Aspects Related to Exercise Physiology

Exercise intensity is the amount of energy spent while exercising, and every individual has a different exercise intensity. A typical measure of exercise intensity is the heart rate. Muscle contraction determines the flow of blood inside the body. All the aspects of exercise physiology have been carefully analyzed in this chapter.

Exercise Trends

Worldwide there has been a large shift towards less physically demanding work. This has been accompanied by increasing use of mechanized transportation, a greater prevalence of labor saving technology in the home, and less active recreational pursuits. At least 31% of the world's population does not get sufficient physical exercise. This is true in almost all developed and developing countries, and among children. Some experts refer to sitting as "the new smoking" because of its negative effects on overall health.

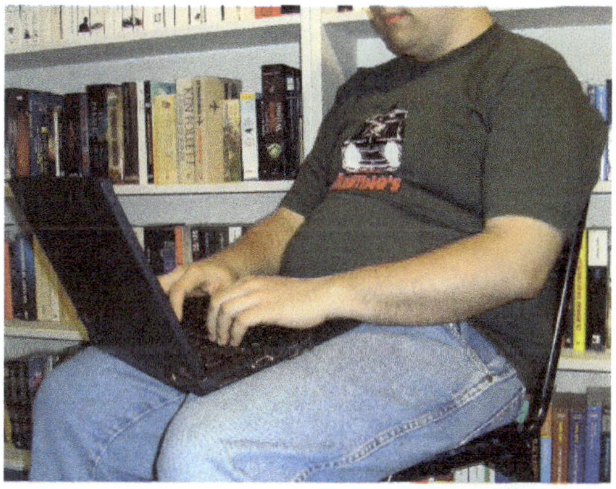

Increases in sedentary behaviors such as overuse of electronics may lead to a decrease of physical activity

These exercise trends are contributing to the rising rates of chronic diseases including: obesity, heart disease, stroke and high cholesterol. Active transport (walking, bicycling, etc.) has been found to be inversely related to obesity in Europe, North America, and Australia. Thus exercise has been associated with a decrease in mortality.

Causes of Lack of Exercise

One of the causes most prevalent in the developing world is urbanization. As more of the population moves to cities, population over-crowding, increased poverty, increased levels of crime, high-density traffic, low air quality and lack of parks, sidewalks and recreational sports facilities leads to a less active lifestyle.

Physical inactivity is increasing or high among many groups in the population including: young people, women, and the elderly.

A 2005 population study in south Brazil showed physical inactivity during leisure time to be more prevalent among females and those living with a partner; with a positive correlation associated with age and number of cigarettes smoked, and a negative correlation (decreased levels of physical inactivity) associated with years of formal education, body mass index, and increasing socioeconomic status.

Studies in children and adults have found an association between the number of hours of television watched and the prevalence of obesity. A 2008 meta analysis found that 63 of 73 studies (86%) showed an increased rate of childhood obesity with increased media exposure, and rates increasing proportionally to time spent watching television.

Another cause in the case of children is that physical activity in activities from self-propelled transport, to school physical education, and organized sports is declining in many countries.

Symptoms

Noncommunicable diseases, partly due to a lack of exercise, are currently the greatest public health problem in most countries around the world. Each year at least 1.9 million people die as a result of physical inactivity, which makes inactivity one of the leading preventable causes of death worldwide.

Countries

Australia

Australian children between 1961 and 2002 have had a marked decline in their aerobic fitness.

Canada

Obese people are less active than their normal weight counterparts. In Canada, 27.0% of sedentary men are obese as opposed to 19.6% of active men. Lean people are more fidgety than their obese counterparts; this relationship is maintained even if normal weight people eat more or the obese person loses weight.

National data indicates that only 10% of Canadian youth are meeting the guideline for screen time of less than 2 hours per day. As well, although 2/3 of families live close enough for their children to bike or walk to school, only 1/3 report actually walking to school and 80% report never having cycled to school.

Asia and China

A study from China found urbanization reduces daily energy expenditure by about 300–400 kcal and going to work by car or bus reduced it by a further 200 kcal.

A rapid decline in physical activity has occurred between the 1980s and the 2000s. The decline in physical activity is attributed to increasing technology in the workplace and changing leisure activities. In 1989 65% of Chinese had jobs that required heavy labor. This decreased to 51% in the year 2000.

Among Asian children between 1917 and 2003 little change has been seen in power and speed however endurance has decreased substantially in the last 10–15 years.

Finland

In Finland leisure-time physical activity has increased, while occupational and commuting physical activity has decreased from 1972 to 2002. Leisure-time physical activity increased from 66% (1972) to 77% (2002) in men and from 49% (1972)to 76% (2002) in women. Physically demanding work decreased from 60% (1972) to 38% (2002) in men and from 47% (1972) to 25% (2002) in women. Daily commuting activity decreased from 30% (1972) to 10% (2002) in men and from 34% (1972) to 22% (2002) in women.

Netherlands

As of 2007 walking and cycling as a means of transport In the Netherlands has been stable since 1994. The average Dutch citizen in the year 2007 walked 240 km (150 mi) and cycled 908 km (564 mi) per year.

South America

Over 60% of the population of Brazil, Chile, and Peru do not meet the recommended levels of physical activity needed to maintain health. A study of a southern Brazilian population found that >80% of the population was physically inactive.

Sweden

A study of Swedish males found a significant decrease in total physical exercise even though recreational exercise has increased. This was due to a decrease in work place exercise and physical exercise in transportation.

United States

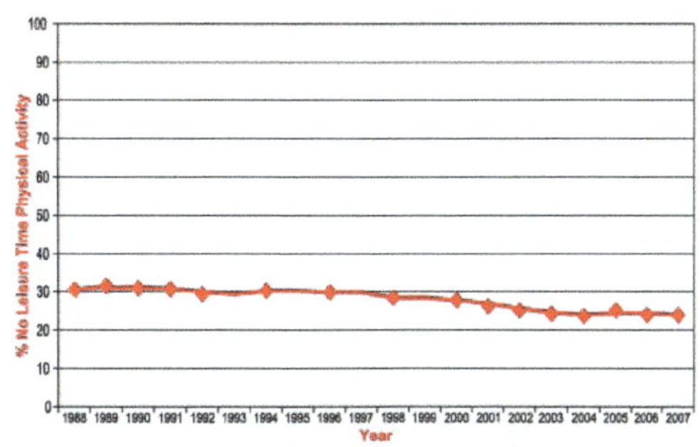

Graph showing the trend in the proportion of the U.S. population which reported no leisure-time physical activity, 1988 - 2007.

Americans have become less physically active overall between 1955 and 2005. While the rate of leisure-time physical activity has not changed significantly there has been a decrease in work-related activity, human powered transportation, activity in the home, and increasing sedentary activity. During 2000 and 2005 the number of adults who were never physically active increased from 9.4% to 10.3%

while the number who were engaged in the highest level of physical activity decreased from 18.7% to 16.7%. Pertaining to leisure-time physical activity, people involved in no activity increased from 38.5% to 40.0% while those who spent most of their day sitting increased from 36.8% to 39.9%.

In 2000 the CDC estimated that more than 40% of the US population was sedentary, another 30% was active but not sufficiently and less than 30% had an adequate level of physical activity. There has been a trend toward decreased physical activity in part due to increasingly mechanized forms of work, changing modes of transportation, and increasing urbanization. Obesity rates have increased in relation to expanding suburbs. This has been attributed to increased time spent commuting, leading to less exercise and less meal preparation at home. In the time between 1983 and 1990 the number of trips taken by foot decreased from 9% down to 7%. Driving one's children to school has become increasingly popular. In the USA the proportion of children who walk or bike to school declined between 1969 (42%) and 2001 (16%) resulting in less exercise.

UK

In England both walking and cycling have declined since 1975 being replaced by motorized transport. The average British citizen in the year 2005 walked 317 km (197 mi) per year, a fall of 106 km (66 mi) since 1975.

Solutions to Address The Lack of Exercise

Many measures have been attempted to address low levels of physical activity. Some of these include: Walking bus, Riding school bus, Mall walking, and Girls on the Run.

Exercise Intensity

Exercise intensity refers to how much energy is expended when exercising. Perceived intensity varies with each person. It has been found that intensity has an effect on what fuel the body uses and what kind of adaptations the body makes after exercise. Intensity is the amount of physical power (expressed as a percentage of the maximal oxygen consumption) that the body uses when performing an activity. For example, exercise intensity defines how hard the body has to work to walk a mile in 20 minutes.

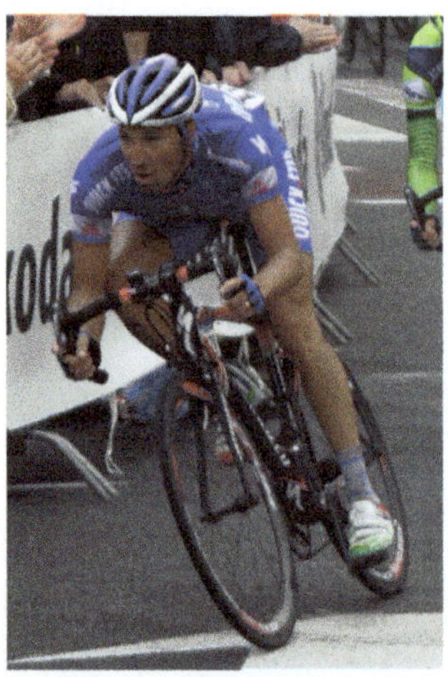

Measures of Intensity

Heart Rate is typically used as a measure of exercise intensity. Heart rate can be an indicator of the challenge to the cardiovascular system that the exercise represents.

The most precise measure of intensity is oxygen consumption (VO_2). VO_2 represents the overall metabolic challenge that an exercise imposes. There is a direct linear relationship between intensity of aerobic exercise and VO_2. Our maximum intensity is a reflection of our maximal oxygen consumption (VO_2 max). Such a measurement represents a cardiovascular fitness level.

VO_2 is measured in METs (mL/kg/min). One MET, which is equal to 3.5 ml/kg per minute, is considered to be the average resting energy expenditure of a typical human being. Intensity of exercise can be expressed as multiples of resting energy expenditure. An intensity of exercise equivalent to 6 METs means that the energy expenditure of the exercise is six times the resting energy expenditure.

Intensity of exercise can be expressed in absolute or relative terms. For example, two individuals with different measures of VO_2 max, running at 7 mph are running at the same absolute intensity (miles/hour) but a different relative intensity (% of VO_2 max expended). The individual with the higher VO_2 max is running at a lower intensity at this pace than the individual with the lower VO_2 max is.

Some studies measure exercise intensity by having subjects perform exercise trials to determine peak power output, which may be measured in watts, heart rate, or (on a cycle) average cadence (cycling). This approach attempts to gauge overall workload.

Intensity Levels

Exercise is categorized into three different intensity levels. These levels include low, moderate, and vigorous and are measured by the metabolic equivalent of task (aka metabolic equivalent or METs). The effects of exercise are different at each intensity level (i.e. training effect). Recommendations to lead a healthy lifestyle vary for individuals based on age, weight, and existing activity levels. "Published guidelines for healthy adults state that 20-60 minutes of medium intensity continuous or intermittent aerobic activity 3-5 times per week is needed for developing and maintaining cardiorespiratory fitness, body composition, and muscular strength."

Physical Activity	MET
Light Intensity Activities	< 3
sleeping	0.9
watching television	1.0
writing, desk work, typing	1.8
walking, 1.7 mph (2.7 km/h), level ground, strolling, very slow	2.3
walking, 2.5 mph (4 km/h)	2.9
Moderate Intensity Activities	3 to 6
bicycling, stationary, 50 watts, very light effort	3.0
walking 3.0 mph (4.8 km/h)	3.3
calisthenics, home exercise, light or moderate effort, general	3.5

walking 3.4 mph (5.5 km/h)	3.6
bicycling, <10 mph (16 km/h), leisure, to work or for pleasure	4.0
bicycling, stationary, 100 watts, light effort	5.5
Vigorous Intensity Activities	> 6
jogging, general	7.0
calisthenics (e.g. pushups, situps, pullups, jumping jacks), heavy, vigorous effort	8.0
running jogging, in place	8.0
rope jumping	10.0

Fuel Used

The body uses different amounts of energy substrates (carbohydrates or fats) depending on the intensity of the exercise and the heart rate of the exerciser. Protein is a third energy substrate, but it contributes minimally and is therefore discounted in the percent contribution graphs reflecting different intensities of exercise. The fuel provided by the body dictates an individual's capacity to increase the intensity level of a given activity. In other words, the intensity level of an activity determines the order of fuel recruitment. Specifically, exercise physiology dictates that low intensity, long duration exercise provides a larger percentage of fat contribution in the calories burned because the body does not need to quickly and efficiently produce energy (i.e., adenosine triphosphate) to maintain the activity. On the other hand, high intensity activity utilizes a larger percentage of carbohydrates in the calories expended because its quick production of energy makes it the preferred energy substrate for high intensity exercise. High intensity activity also yields a higher total caloric expenditure.

This table outlines the estimated distribution of energy consumption at different intensity levels for a healthy 20-year-old with a Max Heart Rate (MHR) of 200.

Intensity (%MHR)	**Heart Rate (bpm)**	% Carbohydrate	% Fat
65-70	130-140	15	85
70-75	140-150	35	65
75-80	150-160	65	35
80-85	160-170	80	20
85-90	170-180	90	10
90-95	180-190	95	5
100	190-200	100	-

These estimates are valid only when glycogen reserves are able to cover the energy needs. If a person depletes glycogen reserves after a long workout (a phenomenon known as "hitting the wall") or during a low carbohydrate diet, the body will shift into ketosis and use mostly fat and muscle for energy. Intermittent fasting can be used to train the body to shift easily into ketosis.

Heart Rate

Heart rate is the speed of the heartbeat measured by the number of contractions of the heart per minute (bpm). The heart rate can vary according to the body's physical needs, including the need to absorb oxygen and excrete carbon dioxide. It is usually equal or close to the pulse measured at any peripheral point. Activities that can provoke change include physical exercise, sleep, anxiety, stress, illness, and ingestion of drugs.

The normal resting adult human heart rate ranges from 60–100 bpm. Tachycardia is a fast heart rate, defined as above 100 bpm at rest. Bradycardia is a slow heart rate, defined as below 60 bpm at rest. During sleep a slow heartbeat with rates around 40–50 bpm is common and is considered normal. When the heart is not beating in a regular pattern, this is referred to as an arrhythmia. Abnormalities of heart rate sometimes indicate disease.

Physiology

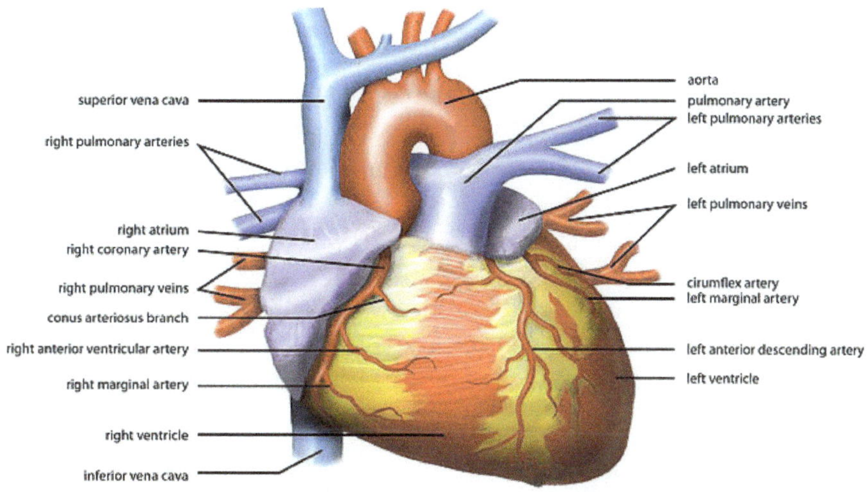

The Human Heart

While heart rhythm is regulated entirely by the sinoatrial node under normal conditions, heart rate is regulated by sympathetic and parasympathetic input to the sinoatrial node. The accelerans nerve provides sympathetic input to the heart by releasing norepinephrine onto the cells of the sinoatrial node (SA node), and the vagus nerve provides parasympathetic input to the heart by releasing acetylcholine onto sinoatrial node cells. Therefore, stimulation of the accelerans nerve increases heart rate, while stimulation of the vagus nerve decreases it.

Due to individuals having a constant blood volume, one of the physiological ways to deliver more oxygen to an organ is to increase heart rate to permit blood to pass by the organ more often. Normal resting heart rates range from 60–100 bpm. Bradycardia is defined as a resting heart rate below 60 bpm. However, heart rates from 50 to 60 bpm are common among healthy people and do not necessarily require special attention. Tachycardia is defined as a resting heart rate above 100 bpm, though persistent rest rates between 80–100 bpm, mainly if they are present during sleep, may be signs of hyperthyroidism or anemia.

- Central nervous system stimulants such as substituted amphetamines increase heart rate.
- Central nervous system depressants or sedatives decrease the heart rate (apart from some particularly strange ones with equally strange effects, such as ketamine which can cause - amongst many other things - stimulant-like effects such as tachycardia).

There are many ways in which the heart rate speeds up or slows down. Most involve stimulant-like endorphins and hormones being released in the brain, many of which are those that are 'forced'/'enticed' out by the ingestion and processing of drugs.

Influences from The Central Nervous System

Cardiovascular Centres

The heart rate is rhythmically generated by the sinoatrial node. It is also influenced by central factors through sympathetic and parasympathetic nerves. Nervous influence over the heartrate is centralized within the two paired cardiovascular centres of the medulla oblongata. The cardioaccelerator regions stimulate activity via sympathetic stimulation of the cardioaccelerator nerves, and the cardioinhibitory centers decrease heart activity via parasympathetic stimulation as one component of the vagus nerve. During rest, both centers provide slight stimulation to the heart, contributing to autonomic tone. This is a similar concept to tone in skeletal muscles. Normally, vagal stimulation predominates as, left unregulated, the SA node would initiate a sinus rhythm of approximately 100 bpm.

Both sympathetic and parasympathetic stimuli flow through the paired cardiac plexus near the base of the heart. The cardioaccelerator center also sends additional fibers, forming the cardiac nerves via sympathetic ganglia (the cervical ganglia plus superior thoracic ganglia T1–T4) to both the SA and AV nodes, plus additional fibers to the atria and ventricles. The ventricles are more richly innervated by sympathetic fibers than parasympathetic fibers. Sympathetic stimulation causes the release of the neurotransmitter norepinephrine (also known as noradrenaline) at the neuromuscular junction of the cardiac nerves. This shortens the repolarization period, thus speeding the rate of depolarization and contraction, which results in an increased heartrate. It opens chemical or ligand-gated sodium and calcium ion channels, allowing an influx of positively charged ions.

Norepinephrine binds to the beta–1 receptor. High blood pressure medications are used to block these receptors and so reduce the heart rate.

Parasympathetic stimulation originates from the cardioinhibitory region with impulses traveling via the vagus nerve (cranial nerve X). The vagus nerve sends branches to both the SA and AV nodes, and to portions of both the atria and ventricles. Parasympathetic stimulation releases the neurotransmitter acetylcholine (ACh) at the neuromuscular junction. ACh slows HR by opening chemical- or ligand-gated potassium ion channels to slow the rate of spontaneous depolarization, which extends repolarization and increases the time before the next spontaneous depolarization occurs. Without any nervous stimulation, the SA node would establish a sinus rhythm of approximately 100 bpm. Since resting rates are considerably less than this, it becomes evident that parasympathetic stimulation normally slows HR. This is similar to an individual driving a car with one foot on the brake pedal. To speed up, one need merely remove one's foot from the brake and let the engine increase speed. In the case of the heart, decreasing parasympathetic stimulation decreases the release of ACh, which allows HR to increase up to approximately 100 bpm. Any increases beyond this rate would require sympathetic stimulation.

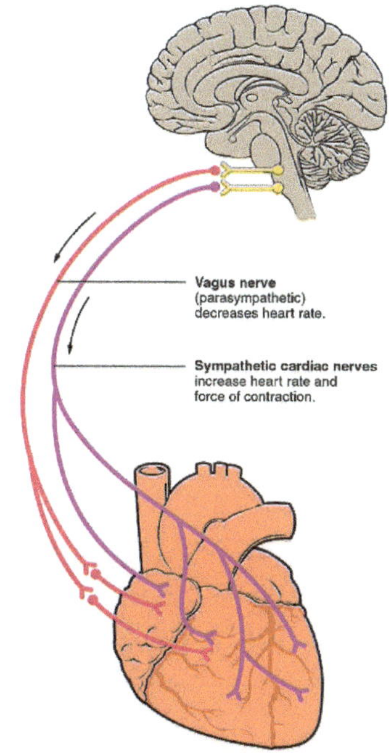

Autonomic Innervation of the Heart - Cardioaccelerator and cardioinhibitory areas are components of the paired cardiac centers located in the medulla oblongata of the brain. They innervate the heart via sympathetic cardiac nerves that increase cardiac activity and vagus (parasympathetic) nerves that slow cardiac activity.

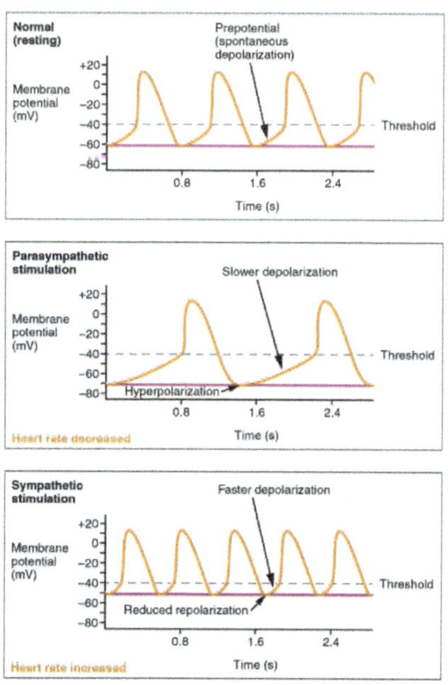

Effects of Parasympathetic and Sympathetic Stimulation on Normal Sinus Rhythm - The wave of depolarization in a normal sinus rhythm shows a stable resting HR. Following parasympathetic stimulation, HR slows. Following sympathetic stimulation, HR increases.

Input to The Cardiovascular Centres

The cardiovascular centres receive input from a series of visceral receptors with impulses traveling through visceral sensory fibers within the vagus and sympathetic nerves via the cardiac plexus. Among these receptors are various proprioreceptors, baroreceptors, and chemoreceptors, plus stimuli from the limbic system which normally enable the precise regulation of heart function, via cardiac reflexes. Increased physical activity results in increased rates of firing by various proprioreceptors located in muscles, joint capsules, and tendons. The cardiovascular centres monitor these increased rates of firing, suppressing parasympathetic stimulation or increasing sympathetic stimulation as needed in order to increase blood flow.

Similarly, baroreceptors are stretch receptors located in the aortic sinus, carotid bodies, the venae cavae, and other locations, including pulmonary vessels and the right side of the heart itself. Rates of firing from the baroreceptors represent blood pressure, level of physical activity, and the relative distribution of blood. The cardiac centers monitor baroreceptor firing to maintain cardiac homeostasis, a mechanism called the baroreceptor reflex. With increased pressure and stretch, the rate of baroreceptor firing increases, and the cardiac centers decrease sympathetic stimulation and increase parasympathetic stimulation. As pressure and stretch decrease, the rate of baroreceptor firing decreases, and the cardiac centers increase sympathetic stimulation and decrease parasympathetic stimulation.

There is a similar reflex, called the atrial reflex or Bainbridge reflex, associated with varying rates of blood flow to the atria. Increased venous return stretches the walls of the atria where specialized baroreceptors are located. However, as the atrial baroreceptors increase their rate of firing and as they stretch due to the increased blood pressure, the cardiac center responds by increasing sympathetic stimulation and inhibiting parasympathetic stimulation to increase HR. The opposite is also true.

Increased metabolic byproducts associated with increased activity, such as carbon dioxide, hydrogen ions, and lactic acid, plus falling oxygen levels, are detected by a suite of chemoreceptors innervated by the glossopharyngeal and vagus nerves. These chemoreceptors provide feedback to the cardiovascular centers about the need for increased or decreased blood flow, based on the relative levels of these substances.

The limbic system can also significantly impact HR related to emotional state. During periods of stress, it is not unusual to identify higher than normal HRs, often accompanied by a surge in the stress hormone cortisol. Individuals experiencing extreme anxiety may manifest panic attacks with symptoms that resemble those of heart attacks. These events are typically transient and treatable. Meditation techniques have been developed to ease anxiety and have been shown to lower HR effectively. Doing simple deep and slow breathing exercises with one's eyes closed can also significantly reduce this anxiety and HR.

Factors Influencing Heart Rate

Using a combination of autorhythmicity and innervation, the cardiovascular center is able to provide relatively precise control over the heart rate, but other factors can impact on this. These include hormones, notably epinephrine, norepinephrine, and thyroid hormones; levels of various ions including calcium, potassium, and sodium; body temperature; hypoxia; and pH balance.

Table 1: Major factors increasing heart rate and force of contraction

Factor	Effect
Cardioaccelerator nerves	Release of norepinephrine
Proprioreceptors	Increased rates of firing during exercise
Chemoreceptors	Decreased levels of O_2; increased levels of H^+, CO_2, and lactic acid
Baroreceptors	Decreased rates of firing, indicating falling blood volume/ pressure
Limbic system	Anticipation of physical exercise or strong emotions
Catecholamines	Increased epinephrine and norepinephrine
Thyroid hormones	Increased T3 and T4
Calcium	Increased Ca^{2+}
Potassium	Decreased K^+
Sodium	Decreased Na^+
Body temperature	Increased body temperature
Nicotine and caffeine	Stimulants, increasing heart rate

Table 2: Factors decreasing heart rate and force of contraction

Factor	Effect
Cardioinhibitor nerves (vagus)	Release of acetylcholine
Proprioreceptors	Decreased rates of firing following exercise
Chemoreceptors	Increased levels of O_2; decreased levels of H^+ and CO_2
Baroreceptors	Increased rates of firing, indicating higher blood volume/ pressure
Limbic system	Anticipation of relaxation
Catecholamines	Decreased epinephrine and norepinephrine
Thyroid hormones	Decreased T3 and T4
Calcium	Decreased Ca^{2+}
Potassium	Increased K^+
Sodium	Decreased Na^+
Body temperature	Decrease in body temperature

Epinephrine and Norepinephrine

The catecholamines, epinephrine and norepinephrine, secreted by the adrenal medulla form one component of the extended fight-or-flight mechanism. The other component is sympathetic stimulation. Epinephrine and norepinephrine have similar effects: binding to the beta-1 adrenergic receptors, and opening sodium and calcium ion chemical- or ligand-gated channels. The rate of depolarization is increased by this additional influx of positively charged ions, so the threshold is reached more quickly and the period of repolarization is shortened. However, massive releases of these hormones coupled with sympathetic stimulation may actually lead to arrhythmias. There is no parasympathetic stimulation to the adrenal medulla.

Thyroid Hormones

In general, increased levels of the thyroid hormones (thyroxine(T4) and triiodothyronine (T3)), increase the heart rate; excessive levels can trigger tachycardia. The impact of thyroid hormones is typically of a much longer duration than that of the catecholamines. The physiologically active form of triiodothyronine, has been shown to directly enter cardiomyocytes and alter activity at the level of the genome. It also impacts the beta adrenergic response similar to epinephrine and norepinephrine.

Calcium

Calcium ion levels greatly impact on heartrate and contractility; increased levels cause an increase in both. High levels of calcium ions result in (hypercalcemia) and excessive levels can induce cardiac arrest. Drugs known as calcium channel blockers slow HR by binding to these channels and blocking or slowing the inward movement of calcium ions.

Caffeine and Nicotine

Caffeine and nicotine are both stimulants of the nervous system and of the cardiac centres causing an increased heart rate. Caffeine works by increasing the rates of depolarization at the SA node, whereas nicotine stimulates the activity of the sympathetic neurons that deliver impulses to the heart. Both stimulants are legal and unregulated, and are known to be very addictive.

Factors Decreasing Heart Rate

The heart rate can be slowed by altered sodium and potassium levels, hypoxia, acidosis, alkalosis, and hypothermia. The relationship between electrolytes and HR is complex, but maintaining electrolyte balance is critical to the normal wave of depolarization. Of the two ions, potassium has the greater clinical significance. Initially, both hyponatremia (low sodium levels) and hypernatremia (high sodium levels) may lead to tachycardia. Severely high hypernatremia may lead to fibrillation, which may cause CO to cease. Severe hyponatremia leads to both bradycardia and other arrhythmias. Hypokalemia (low potassium levels) also leads to arrhythmias, whereas hyperkalemia (high potassium levels) causes the heart to become weak and flaccid, and ultimately to fail.

Heart muscle relies exclusively on aerobic metabolism for energy. Hypoxia (an insufficient supply of oxygen) leads to decreasing HRs, since metabolic reactions fueling heart contraction are restricted.

Acidosis is a condition in which excess hydrogen ions are present, and the patient's blood expresses a low pH value. Alkalosis is a condition in which there are too few hydrogen ions, and the patient's blood has an elevated pH. Normal blood pH falls in the range of 7.35–7.45, so a number lower than this range represents acidosis and a higher number represents alkalosis. Enzymes, being the regulators or catalysts of virtually all biochemical reactions - are sensitive to pH and will change shape slightly with values outside their normal range. These variations in pH and accompanying slight physical changes to the active site on the enzyme decrease the rate of formation of the enzyme-substrate complex, subsequently decreasing the rate of many enzymatic reactions, which can have complex effects on HR. Severe changes in pH will lead to denaturation of the enzyme.

The last variable is body temperature. Elevated body temperature is called hyperthermia, and suppressed body temperature is called hypothermia. Slight hyperthermia results in increasing HR and strength of contraction. Hypothermia slows the rate and strength of heart contractions. This distinct slowing of the heart is one component of the larger diving reflex that diverts blood to essential organs while submerged. If sufficiently chilled, the heart will stop beating, a technique that may be employed during open heart surgery. In this case, the patient's blood is normally diverted to an artificial heart-lung machine to maintain the body's blood supply and gas exchange until the surgery is complete, and sinus rhythm can be restored. Excessive hyperthermia and hypothermia will both result in death, as enzymes drive the body systems to cease normal function, beginning with the central nervous system.

Heart Rates in Different Circumstances

Heart rate is not a stable value and it increases or decreases in response to the body's need in a way to maintain an equilibrium (basal metabolic rate) between requirement and delivery of oxygen and nutrients. The normal SA node firing rate is affected by autonomic nervous system activity: sympathetic stimulation increases and parasympathetic stimulation decreases the firing rate. A number of different metrics are used to describe heart rate.

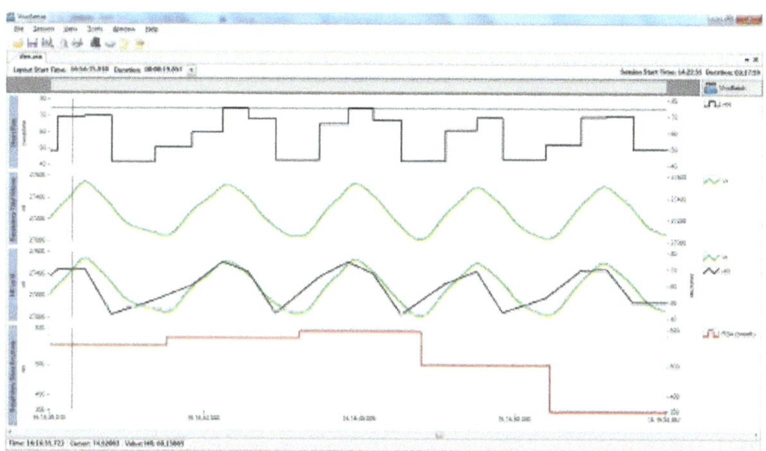

Heart rate (HR) (top trace) and tidal volume (Vt) (lung volume, second trace) plotted on the same chart, showing how heart rate increases with inspiration and decreases with expiration.

Resting Heart Rate

The basal or resting heart rate (HR_{rest}) is defined as the heart rate when a person is awake, in a neutrally temperate environment, and has not been subject to any recent exertion or stimulation, such as stress or surprise. The typical resting heart rate in adults is 60–100 beats per minute (bpm). This is the firing rate of the heart's sinoatrial node, where the faster pacemaker cells driving the self-generated rhythmic firing and responsible for the heart's autorhythmicity are located. For endurance athletes at the elite level, it is not unusual to have a resting heart rate between 33 and 50 bpm.

Target Heart Rate

For healthy people, the *Target Heart Rate* or *Training Heart Rate* (THR) is a desired range of heart rate reached during aerobic exercise which enables one's heart and lungs to receive the most benefit from a workout. This theoretical range varies based mostly on age; however, a person's physical condition, sex, and previous training also are used in the calculation. Below are two ways to calculate one's THR. In each of these methods, there is an element called "intensity" which is expressed as a percentage. The THR can be calculated as a range of 65–85% intensity. However, it is crucial to derive an accurate HR_{max} to ensure these calculations are meaningful.

Example for someone with a HR_{max} of 180 (age 40, estimating HR_{max} As 220 – age):

$$65\%\text{ Intensity: } (220 - (\text{age} = 40)) \times 0.65 \rightarrow 117\text{ bpm}$$

$$85\%\text{ Intensity: } (220 - (\text{age} = 40)) \times 0.85 \rightarrow 153\text{ bpm}$$

Karvonen Method

The *Karvonen method* factors in resting heart rate (HR_{rest}) to calculate target heart rate (THR), using a range of 50–85% intensity:

$$THR = ((HR_{max} - HR_{rest}) \times \%\text{ intensity}) + HR_{rest}$$

Example for someone with a HR_{max} of 180 and a HR_{rest} of 70:

$$50\%\text{ Intensity: } ((180 - 70) \times 0.50) + 70 = 125\text{ bpm}$$

$$85\%\text{ Intensity: } ((180 - 70) \times 0.85) + 70 = 163\text{ bpm}$$

Zoladz Method

An alternative to the Karvonen method is the *Zoladz method,* which derives exercise zones by subtracting values from HR_{max}:

$$THR = HR_{max} - \text{Adjuster} \pm 5\text{ bpm}$$

$$\text{Zone 1 Adjuster} = 50\text{ bpm}$$

$$\text{Zone 2 Adjuster} = 40\text{ bpm}$$

$$\text{Zone 3 Adjuster} = 30\text{ bpm}$$

$$\text{Zone 4 Adjuster} = 20\text{ bpm}$$

$$\text{Zone 5 Adjuster} = 10\text{ bpm}$$

Example for someone with a HR_{max} of 180:

$$\text{Zone 1(easy exercise): } 180 - 50 \pm 5 \rightarrow 125 - 135\text{ bpm}$$

$$\text{Zone 4(tough exercise): } 180 - 20 \pm 5 \rightarrow 155 - 165\text{ bpm}$$

Maximum Heart Rate

The *maximum heart rate* (HR_{max}) is the highest heart rate an individual can achieve without severe problems through exercise stress, and generally decreases with age. Since HR_{max} varies by individual, the most accurate way of measuring any single person's HR_{max} is via a cardiac stress test. In this test, a person is subjected to controlled physiologic stress (generally by treadmill) while being monitored by an ECG. The intensity of exercise is periodically increased until certain changes in heart function are detected on the ECG monitor, at which point the subject is directed to stop. Typical duration of the test ranges ten to twenty minutes.

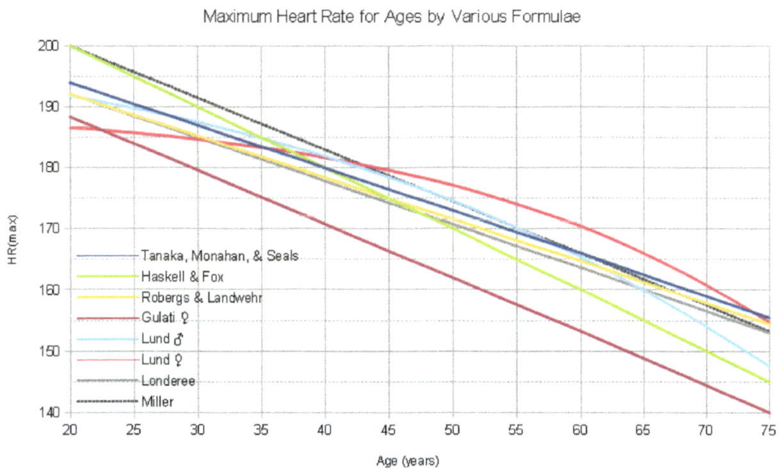

The various formulae provide slightly different numbers for the maximum heart rates by age.

Adults who are beginning a new exercise regimen are often advised to perform this test only in the presence of medical staff due to risks associated with high heart rates. For general purposes, a formula is often employed to estimate a person's maximum heart rate. However, these predic-tive formulas have been criticized as inaccurate because they generalized population-averages and usually focus on a person's age. It is well-established that there is a "poor relationship between maximal heart rate and age" and large standard deviations relative to predicted heart rates.

A number of formulas are used to estimate HR_{max}

Tanaka, Monahan, & Seals

From Tanaka, Monahan, & Seals (2001):

- $HR_{max} = 208 - (0.7 \times \text{age})$

Their meta-analysis (of 351 prior studies involving 492 groups and 18,712 subjects) and laboratory study (of 514 healthy subjects) concluded that, using this equation, HRmax was very strongly correlated to age (r = −0.90). The regression equation that was obtained in the laboratory-based study (209 – 0.7 x age), was virtually identical to that of the meta-study. The results showed HRmax to be independent of gender and independent of wide variations in habitual physical activity levels. This study found a standard deviation of ~10 beats per minute for individuals of any age, meaning the HRmax formula given has an accuracy of ±20 beats per minute.

In 2007, researchers at the Oakland University analyzed maximum heart rates of 132 individuals recorded yearly over 25 years, and produced a linear equation very similar to the Tanaka formula, $HR_{max} = 206.9 - (0.67 \times \text{age})$, and a nonlinear equation, $HR_{max} = 191.5 - (0.007 \times \text{age}^2)$. The linear equation had a confidence interval of ±5–8 bpm and the nonlinear equation had a tighter range of ±2–5 bpm. Also a third nonlinear equation was produced: $HR_{max} = 163 + (1.16 \times \text{age}) - (0.018 \times \text{age}^2)$.

Haskell and Fox

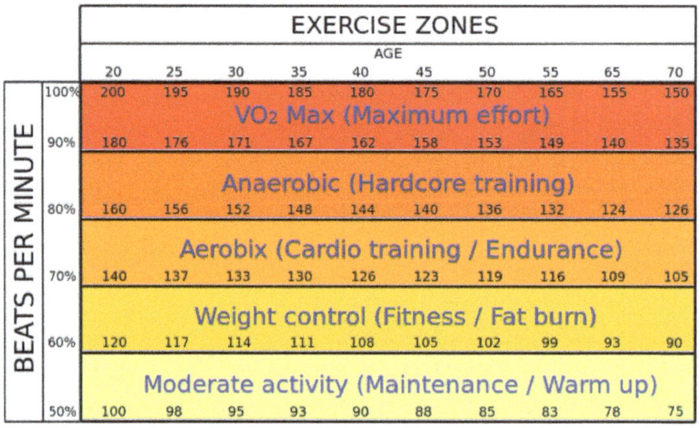

Fox and Haskell formula; widely used.

Notwithstanding the research of Tanaka, Monahan, & Seals, the most widely cited formula for HR_{max} (which contains no reference to any standard deviation) is still:

$$HR_{max} = 220 - \text{age}$$

Although attributed to various sources, it is widely thought to have been devised in 1970 by Dr. William Haskell and Dr. Samuel Fox. Inquiry into the history of this formula reveals that it was not developed from original research, but resulted from observation based on data from approximately 11 references consisting of published research or unpublished scientific compilations. It gained widespread use through being used by Polar Electro in its heart rate monitors, which Dr. Haskell has "laughed about", as the formula "was never supposed to be an absolute guide to rule people's training."

While it is the most common (and easy to remember and calculate), this particular formula is not considered by reputable health and fitness professionals to be a good predictor of HR_{max}. Despite the widespread publication of this formula, research spanning two decades reveals its large inherent error, S_{xy} = 7–11 bpm. Consequently, the estimation calculated by $HR_{max} = 220 - \text{age}$ has neither the accuracy nor the scientific merit for use in exercise physiology and related fields.

Robergs and Landwehr

A 2002 study of 43 different formulas for HR_{max} published in the Journal of Exercise Psychology concluded that:

1. no "acceptable" formula currently existed (they used the term "acceptable" to mean acceptable for both prediction of VO_2, and prescription of exercise training HR ranges)

2. the least objectionable formula was:

   $HR_{max} = 205.8 - (0.685 \times age)$

   This had a standard deviation that, although large (6.4 bpm), was considered acceptable for prescribing exercise training HR ranges.

Gulati (For Women)

Research conducted at Northwestern University by Martha Gulati, et al., in 2010 suggested a maximum heart rate formula for women:

$$HR_{max} = 206 - (0.88 \times age)$$

Gellish

A 2008 study from Lund, Sweden gives reference values (obtained during bicycle ergometry) for men:

$$HR_{max} = 203.7 / (1 + \exp(0.033 \times (age - 104.3)))$$

and for women:

$$HR_{max} = 190.2 / (1 + \exp(0.0453 \times (age - 107.5)))$$

Other Formulae

- $HR_{max} = 206.3 - (0.711 \times age)$

  (Often attributed to "Londeree and Moeschberger from the University of Missouri")

- $HR_{max} = 217 - (0.85 \times age)$

  (Often attributed to "Miller et al. from Indiana University")

Limitations

Maximum heart rates vary significantly between individuals. Even within a single elite sports team, such as Olympic rowers in their 20s, maximum heart rates have been reported as varying from 160 to 220. Such a variation would equate to a 60 or 90 year age gap in the linear equations above, and would seem to indicate the extreme variation about these average figures.

Figures are generally considered averages, and depend greatly on individual physiology and fitness. For example, an endurance runner's rates will typically be lower due to the increased size of the heart required to support the exercise, while a sprinter's rates will be higher due to the improved response time and short duration. While each may have predicted heart rates of 180 (= 220 – age), these two people could have actual HR_{max} 20 beats apart (e.g., 170-190).

Further, note that individuals of the same age, the same training, in the same sport, on the same team, can have actual HR_{max} 60 bpm apart (160–220): the range is extremely broad, and some say "The heart rate is probably the least important variable in comparing athletes."

Heart Rate Reserve

Heart rate reserve ($HR_{reserve}$) is the difference between a person's measured or predicted maximum heart rate and resting heart rate. Some methods of measurement of exercise intensity measure percentage of heart rate reserve. Additionally, as a person increases their cardiovascular fitness, their HR_{rest} will drop, that the heart rate reserve will increase. Percentage of $HR_{reserve}$ is equivalent to percentage of VO_2 reserve.

$$HR_{reserve} = HR_{max} - HR_{rest}$$

This is often used to gauge exercise intensity (first used in 1957 by Karvonen).

Karvonen's study findings have been questioned, due to the following:

- The study did not use VO_2 data to develop the equation.
- Only six subjects were used, and the correlation between the percentages of $HR_{reserve}$ and VO_2 max was not statistically significant.

Heart Rate Recovery

Heart rate recovery ($HR_{recovery}$) is the reduction in heart rate at peak exercise and the rate as measured after a cool-down period of fixed duration. A greater reduction in heart rate after exercise during the reference period is associated with a higher level of cardiac fitness.

Heart rates that do not drop by more than 12 bpm one minute after stopping exercise are associated with an increased risk of death. Investigators of the Lipid Research Clinics Prevalence Study, which included 5,000 subjects, found that patients with an abnormal $HR_{recovery}$ (defined as a decrease of 42 beats per minutes or less at two minutes post-exercise) had a mortality rate 2.5 times greater than patients with a normal recovery. Another study by Nishime et al. and featuring 9,454 patients followed for a median period of 5.2 years found a four-fold increase in mortality in subjects with an abnormal $HR_{recovery}$ (≤12 bpm reduction one minute after the cessation of exercise). Shetler et al. studied 2,193 patients for thirteen years and found that a $HR_{recovery}$ of ≤22 bpm after two minutes "best identified high-risk patients". They also found that while $HR_{recovery}$ had significant prognostic value it had no diagnostic value.

Development

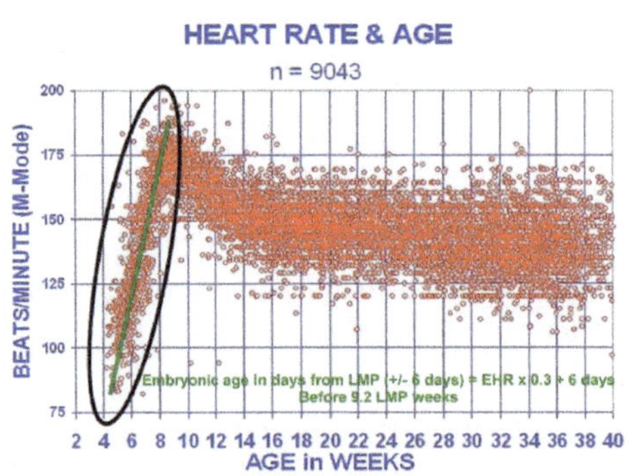

At 21 days after conception, the human heart begins beating at 70 to 80 beats per minute and accelerates linearly for the first month of beating.

The Human Heart Beats More Than 3.5 Billion Times in An Average Lifetime.

The heartbeat of a human embryo begins at approximately 21 days after conception, or five weeks after the last normal menstrual period (LMP), which is the date normally used to date pregnancy in the medical community. The electrical depolarizations that trigger cardiac myocytes to contract arise spontaneously within the myocyte itself. The heartbeat is initiated in the pacemaker regions and spreads to the rest of the heart through a conduction pathway. Pacemaker cells develop in the primitive atrium and the sinus venosus to form the sinoatrial node and the atrioventricular node respectively. Conductive cells develop the bundle of His and carry the depolarization into the lower heart.

The human heart begins beating at a rate near the mother's, about 75-80 beats per minute (BPM). The embryonic heart rate then accelerates linearly for the first month of beating, peaking at 165-185 BPM during the early 7th week, (early 9th week after the LMP). This acceleration is approximately 3.3 BPM per day, or about 10 BPM every three days, an increase of 100 BPM in the first month.

After peaking at about 9.2 weeks after the LMP, it decelerates to about 150 BPM (+/-25 BPM) during the 15th week after the LMP. After the 15th week the deceleration slows reaching an average rate of about 145 (+/-25 BPM) BPM at term. The regression formula which describes this acceleration before the embryo reaches 25 mm in crown-rump length or 9.2 LMP weeks is:

$$\text{Age in days} = \text{EHR}(0.3) + 6$$

There is No Difference in Male and Female Heart Rates before Birth.

Clinical Significance

Measurement

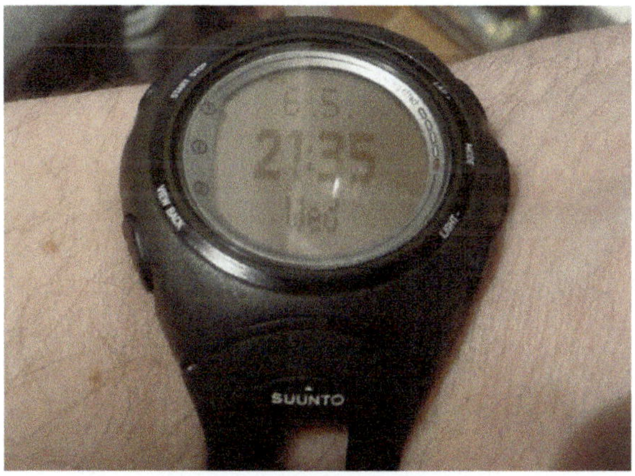

Wrist heart rate monitor

Manual Measurement

Heart rate is measured by finding the pulse of the heart. This pulse rate can be found at any point on the body where the artery's pulsation is transmitted to the surface by pressuring it with the index and middle fingers; often it is compressed against an underlying structure like bone. (A good area is on the neck, under the corner of the jaw.) The thumb should not be used for measuring another person's heart rate, as its strong pulse may interfere with the correct perception of the target pulse.

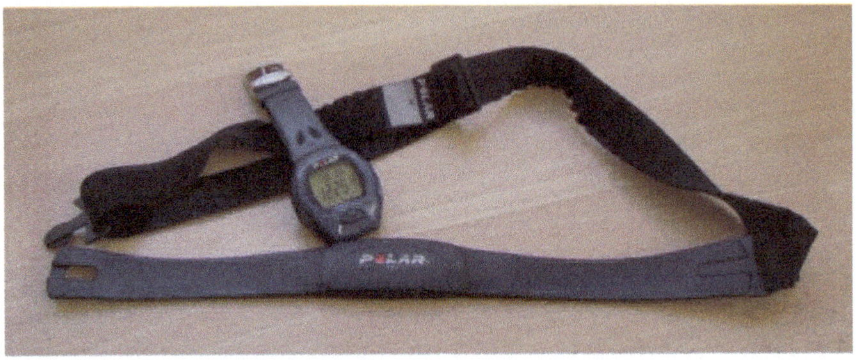

Heart rate monitor with a wrist receiver

The radial artery is the easiest to use to check the heart rate. However, in emergency situations the most reliable arteries to measure heart rate are carotid arteries. This is important mainly in patients with atrial fibrillation, in whom heart beats are irregular and stroke volume is largely different from one beat to another. In those beats following a shorter diastolic interval left ventricle doesn't fill properly, stroke volume is lower and pulse wave is not strong enough to be detected by palpation on a distal artery like the radial artery. It can be detected, however, by doppler.

Possible points for measuring the heart rate are:

1. The ventral aspect of the wrist on the side of the thumb (radial artery).
2. The ulnar artery.
3. The neck (carotid artery).
4. The inside of the elbow, or under the biceps muscle (brachial artery).
5. The groin (femoral artery).
6. Behind the medial malleolus on the feet (posterior tibial artery).
7. Middle of dorsum of the foot (dorsalis pedis).
8. Behind the knee (popliteal artery).
9. Over the abdomen (abdominal aorta).
10. The chest (apex of the heart), which can be felt with one's hand or fingers. It is also possible to auscultate the heart using a stethoscope.
11. The temple (superficial temporal artery).
12. The lateral edge of the mandible (facial artery).
13. The side of the head near the ear (posterior auricular artery).

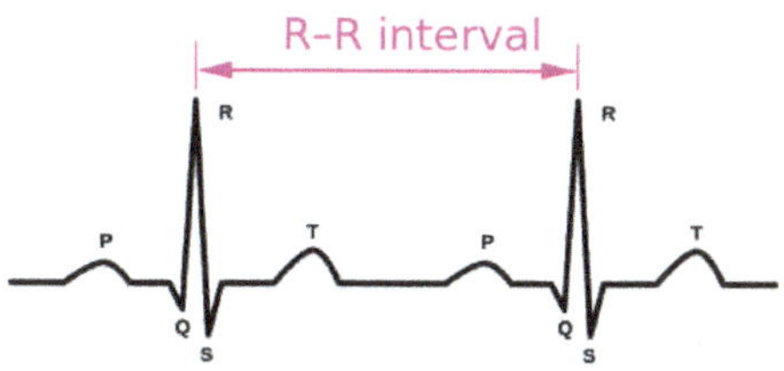

ECG-RRinterval

Electronic Measurement

A more precise method of determining heart rate involves the use of an electrocardiograph, or ECG (also abbreviated EKG). An ECG generates a pattern based on electrical activity of the heart, which closely follows heart function. Continuous ECG monitoring is routinely done in many clinical settings, especially in critical care medicine. On the ECG, instantaneous heart rate is calculated using the R wave-to-R wave (RR) interval and multiplying/dividing in order to derive heart rate in heartbeats/min. Multiple methods exist:

- HR = 1,500/(RR interval in millimeters)
- HR = 60/(RR interval in seconds)
- HR = 300/number of "large" squares between successive R waves.

Heart rate monitors allow measurements to be taken continuously and can be used during exercise when manual measurement would be difficult or impossible (such as when the hands are being used). Various commercial heart rate monitors are also available. Some monitors, used during sport, consist of a chest strap with electrodes. The signal is transmitted to a wrist receiver for display.

Alternative methods of measurement include pulse oximetry and seismocardiography.

Tachycardia

Tachycardia is a resting heart rate more than 100 beats per minute. This number can vary as smaller people and children have faster heart rates than average adults.

Physiological conditions where tachycardia occurs:

1. Exercise
2. Pregnancy
3. Emotional conditions such as anxiety or stress.

Pathological conditions where tachycardia occurs:

1. Sepsis
2. Fever

3. Anemia
4. Hypoxia
5. Hyperthyroidism
6. Hypersecretion of catecholamines
7. Cardiomyopathy
8. Valvular heart diseases
9. Acute Radiation Syndrome

Bradycardia

Bradycardia was defined as a heart rate less than 60 beats per minute when textbooks asserted that the normal range for heart rates was 60–100 BPM. The normal range has since been revised in textbooks to 50–90 BPM for a human at total rest. Setting a lower threshold for bradycardia prevents misclassification of fit individuals as having a pathologic heart rate. The normal heart rate number can vary as children and adolescents tend to have faster heart rates than average adults. Bradycardia may be associated with medical conditions such as hypothyroidism.

Trained athletes tend to have slow resting heart rates, and resting bradycardia in athletes should not be considered abnormal if the individual has no symptoms associated with it. For example, Miguel Indurain, a Spanish cyclist and five time Tour de France winner, had a resting heart rate of 28 beats per minute, one of the lowest ever recorded in a healthy human. Daniel Green achieved the world record for the slowest heartbeat in a healthy human with a heart rate of just 26 bpm in 2014.

Arrhythmia

Arrhythmias are abnormalities of the heart rate and rhythm (sometimes felt as palpitations). They can be divided into two broad categories: fast and slow heart rates. Some cause few or minimal symptoms. Others produce more serious symptoms of lightheadedness, dizziness and fainting.

Correlation With Cardiovascular Mortality Risk

A number of investigations indicate that faster resting heart rate has emerged as a new risk factor for mortality in homeothermic mammals, particularly cardiovascular mortality in human beings. Faster heart rate may accompany increased production of inflammation molecules and increased production of reactive oxygen species in cardiovascular system, in addition to increased mechanical stress to the heart. There is a correlation between increased resting rate and cardiovascular risk. This is not seen to be "using an allotment of heart beats" but rather an increased risk to the system from the increased rate.

An Australian-led international study of patients with cardiovascular disease has shown that heart beat rate is a key indicator for the risk of heart attack. The study, published in *The Lancet* (September 2008) studied 11,000 people, across 33 countries, who were being treated for heart problems. Those patients whose heart rate was above 70 beats per minute had significantly higher incidence of heart attacks, hospital admissions and the need for surgery. Higher heart rate is thought to be correlated with an increase in heart attack and about a 46 percent increase in hospitalizations for non-fatal or fatal heart attack."

Standard textbooks of physiology and medicine mention that heart rate (HR) is readily calculated from the ECG as follows:

> HR = 1,500/RR interval in millimeters, HR = 60/RR interval in seconds, or HR = 300/number of large squares between successive R waves. In each case, the authors are actually referring to instantaneous HR, which is the number of times the heart would beat if successive RR intervals were constant. However, because the above formula is almost always mentioned, students determine HR this way without looking at the ECG any further.

A very slow heart rate (bradycardia) may be associated with heart block. It may also arise from autonomous nervous system impairment.

Muscle Contraction

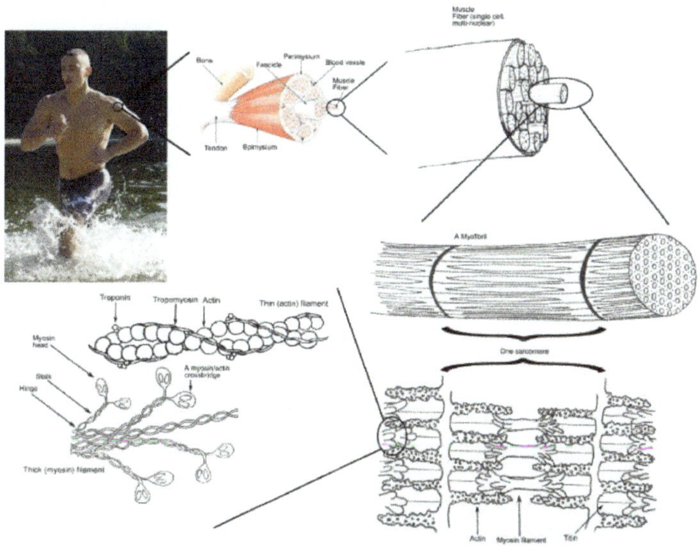

Hierarchical organization of skeletal muscle

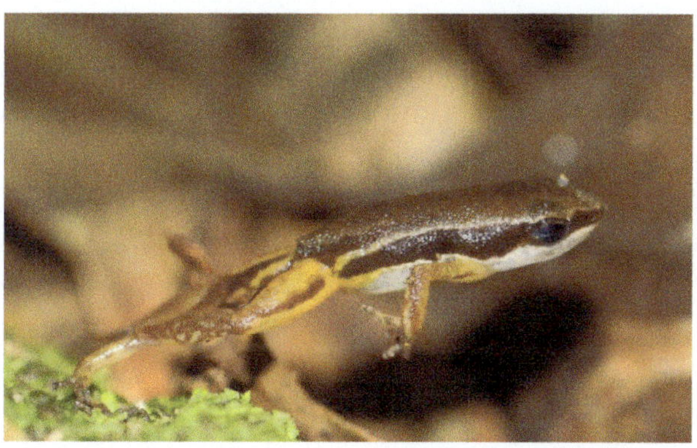
Contractions of skeletal muscles allow vertebrate animals such as frogs to move

Muscle Contractions Underlie Movement

Muscle contraction is the activation of tension-generating sites within muscle fibers. In physiology, muscle contraction does not mean muscle shortening because muscle tension can be produced without changes in muscle length such as holding a heavy book or a dumbbell at the same position. The termination of muscle contraction is followed by muscle relaxation, which is a return of the muscle fibers to their low tension-generating state.

Muscle contractions can be described based on two variables: length and tension. A muscle contraction is described as isometric if the muscle tension changes but the muscle length remains the same. In contrast, a muscle contraction is isotonic if muscle length changes but the muscle tension remains the same. If the muscle length shortens, the contraction is concentric; if the muscle length lengthens, the contraction is eccentric. In natural movements that underlie locomotor activity, muscle contractions are multifaceted as they are able to produce changes in length and tension in a time-varying manner. Therefore, neither length nor tension is likely to remain the same in muscles that contract during locomotor activity.

In vertebrates, skeletal muscle contractions are neurogenic as they require synaptic input from motor neurons to produce muscle contractions. A single motor neuron is able to innervate multiple muscle fibers, thereby causing the fibers to contract at the same time. Once innervated, the protein filaments within each skeletal muscle fiber slide past each other to produce a contraction, which is explained by the sliding filament theory. The contraction produced can be described as a twitch, summation, or tetanus, depending on the frequency of action potentials. In skeletal muscles, muscle tension is at its greatest when the muscle is stretched to an intermediate length as described by the length-tension relationship.

Smooth and cardiac muscle contractions are myogenic and can be modulated by the autonomic nervous system. The mechanisms of contraction in these muscle tissues are similar to those in skeletal muscle tissues.

Types

Muscle contractions can be described based on two variables: force and length. Force itself can be differentiated as either tension or load. Muscle tension is the force exerted by the muscle on an object whereas a load is the force exerted by an object on the muscle. When muscle tension changes without any corresponding changes in muscle length, the muscle contraction is described as isometric. If the muscle length changes while muscle tension remains the same, then the muscle contraction is isotonic. In an isotonic contraction, the muscle length can either shorten to produce a concentric contraction or lengthen to produce an eccentric contraction. Furthermore, if the muscle length shortens, the contraction is concentric. But if the muscle length lengthens, then the contraction is eccentric. In natural movements that underlie locomotor activity, muscle contractions are multifaceted as they are able to produce changes in length and tension in a time-varying manner. Therefore, neither length nor tension is likely to remain constant when the muscle is active during locomotor activity.

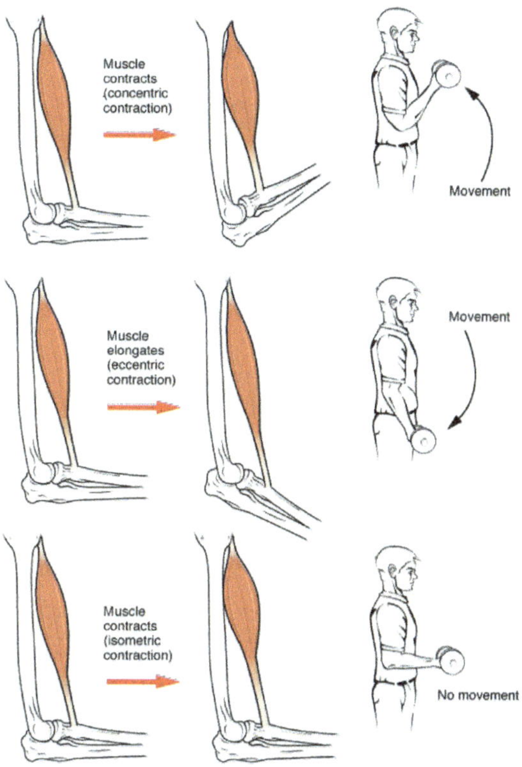

Types of muscle contractions

Isometric Contraction

An isometric contraction of a muscle generates tension without changing length. An example can be found when the muscles of the hand and forearm grip an object; the joints of the hand do not move, but muscles generate sufficient force to prevent the object from being dropped.

Isotonic Contraction

In isotonic contraction, the tension in the muscle remains constant despite a change in muscle length. This occurs when a muscle's force of contraction matches the total load on the muscle.

Concentric Contraction

In concentric contraction, muscle tension is sufficient to overcome the load, and the muscle shortens as it contracts. This occurs when the force generated by the muscle exceeds the load opposing its contraction.

During a concentric contraction, a muscle is stimulated to contract according to the sliding filament theory. This occurs throughout the length of the muscle, generating a force at the origin and insertion, causing the muscle to shorten and changing the angle of the joint. In relation to the elbow, a concentric contraction of the biceps would cause the arm to bend at the elbow as the hand moved from the leg to the shoulder (a biceps curl). A concentric contraction of the triceps would change the angle of the joint in the opposite direction, straightening the arm and moving the hand towards the leg.

Eccentric Contraction

In *eccentric contraction*, the tension generated is insufficient to overcome the external load on the muscle and the muscle fibers lengthen as they contract. Rather than working to pull a joint in the direction of the muscle contraction, the muscle acts to decelerate the joint at the end of a movement or otherwise control the repositioning of a load. This can occur involuntarily (e.g., when attempting to move a weight too heavy for the muscle to lift) or voluntarily (e.g., when the muscle is 'smoothing out' a movement). Over the short-term, strength training involving both eccentric and concentric contractions appear to increase muscular strength more than training with concentric contractions alone. However, exercise-induced muscle damage is also greater during lengthening contractions.

During an eccentric contraction of the biceps muscle, the elbow starts the movement while bent and then straightens as the hand moves away from the shoulder. During an eccentric contraction of the triceps muscle, the elbow starts the movement straight and then bends as the hand moves towards the shoulder. Desmin, titin, and other z-line proteins are involved in eccentric contractions, but their mechanism is poorly understood in comparison to crossbridge cycling in concentric contractions.

Though the muscle is doing a negative amount of mechanical work, (work is being done *on* the muscle), chemical energy (in fat, glucose or ATP) is nevertheless consumed, although less than would be consumed during a concentric contraction of the same force. For example, one expends more energy going up a flight of stairs than going down the same flight.

Muscles undergoing heavy eccentric loading suffer greater damage when overloaded (such as during muscle building or strength training exercise) as compared to concentric loading. When eccentric contractions are used in weight training, they are normally called *negatives*. During a concentric contraction, muscle fibers slide across each other, pulling the Z-lines together. During an eccentric contraction, the filaments slide past each other the opposite way, though the actual movement of the myosin heads during an eccentric contraction is not known. Exercise featuring a heavy eccentric load can actually support a greater weight (muscles are approximately 40% stronger during eccentric contractions than during concentric contractions) and also results in greater muscular damage and delayed onset muscle soreness one to two days after training. Exercise that incorporates both eccentric and concentric muscular contractions (i.e., involving a strong contraction and a controlled lowering of the weight) can produce greater gains in strength than concentric contractions alone. While unaccustomed heavy eccentric contractions can easily lead to overtraining, moderate training may confer protection against injury.

Eccentric Contractions in Movement

Eccentric contractions normally occur as a braking force in opposition to a concentric contraction to protect joints from damage. During virtually any routine movement, eccentric contractions assist in keeping motions smooth, but can also slow rapid movements such as a punch or throw. Part of training for rapid movements such as pitching during baseball involves reducing eccentric braking allowing a greater power to be developed throughout the movement.

Eccentric contractions are being researched for their ability to speed rehabilitation of weak or injured tendons. Achilles tendinitis and patellar tendonitis (also known as jumper's knee or patellar tendonosis) have been shown to benefit from high-load eccentric contractions.

Vertebrate Animals

In vertebrate animals, there are three types of muscle tissues: skeletal, smooth, and cardiac. Skeletal muscle constitutes the majority of muscle mass in the body and is responsible for locomotor activity. Smooth muscle forms blood vessels, gastrointestinal tract, and other areas in the body that produce sustained contractions. Cardiac muscle make up the heart, which pumps blood. Skeletal and cardiac muscles are called striated muscle because of their striped appearance under a microscope, which is due to the highly organized alternating pattern of A bands and I bands.

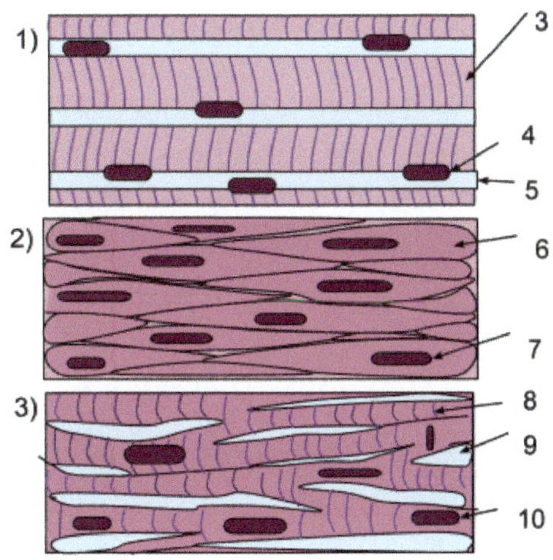

In vertebrate animals, there are three types of muscle tissues: 1) skeletal, 2) smooth, and 3) cardiac

Skeletal Muscle

Excluding reflexes, all skeletal muscles contractions occur as a result of conscious effort originating in the brain. The brain sends electrochemical signals through the nervous system to the motor neuron that innervates several muscle fibers. In the case of some reflexes, the signal to contract can originate in the spinal cord through a feedback loop with the grey matter. Other actions such as locomotion, breathing, and chewing have a reflex aspect to them: the contractions can be initiated both consciously or unconsciously.

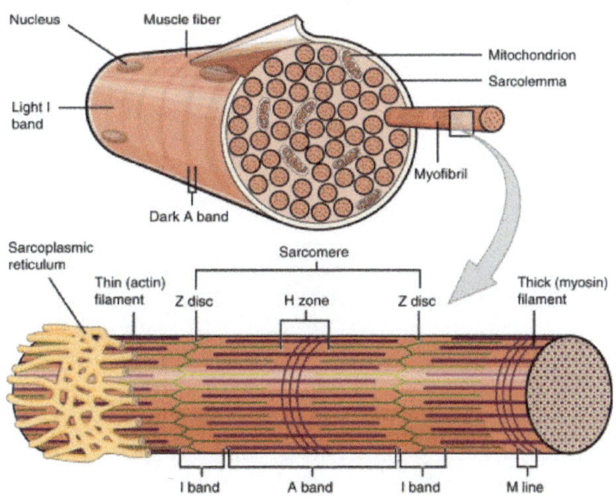

Organization of skeletal muscle

Neuromuscular Junction

A neuromuscular junction is a chemical synapse formed by the contact between a motor neuron and a muscle fiber. It is the site in which a motor neuron transmits a signal to a muscle fiber to initiate muscle contraction. The sequence of events that results in the depolarization of the muscle fiber at the neuromuscular junction begins when an action potential is initiated in the cell body of a motor neuron, which is then propagated by saltatory conduction along its axon toward the neuromuscular junction. Once it reaches the terminal bouton, the action potential causes a Ca2+ ion influx into the terminal by way of the voltage-gated calcium channels. The Ca2+ influx causes synaptic vesicles containing the neurotransmitter acetylcholine to fuse with the plasma membrane, releasing acetylcholine into the synaptic cleft between the motor neuron terminal and the neuromuscular junction of the skeletal muscle fiber. Acetylcholine diffuses across the synapse and binds to and activates nicotinic acetylcholine receptors on the neuromuscular junction. Activation of the nicotinic receptor opens its intrinsic sodium/potassium channel, causing sodium to rush in and potassium to trickle out. As a result, the sarcolemma reverses polarity and its voltage quickly jumps from the resting membrane potential of -90mV to as high as +75mV as sodium enters. The membrane potential then becomes hyperpolarized when potassium exits and is then adjusted back to the resting membrane potential. This rapid fluctuation is called the end-plate potential The voltage-gated ion channels of the sarcolemma next to the end plate open in response to the end plate potential. These voltage-gated channels are sodium and potassium specific and only allow one through. This wave of ion movements creates the action potential that spreads from the motor end plate in all directions. If action potentials stop arriving, then acetylcholine ceases to be released from the terminal bouton. The remaining acetylcholine in the synaptic cleft is either degraded by active acetylcholine esterase or reabsorbed by the synaptic knob and none is left to replace the degraded acetylcholine.

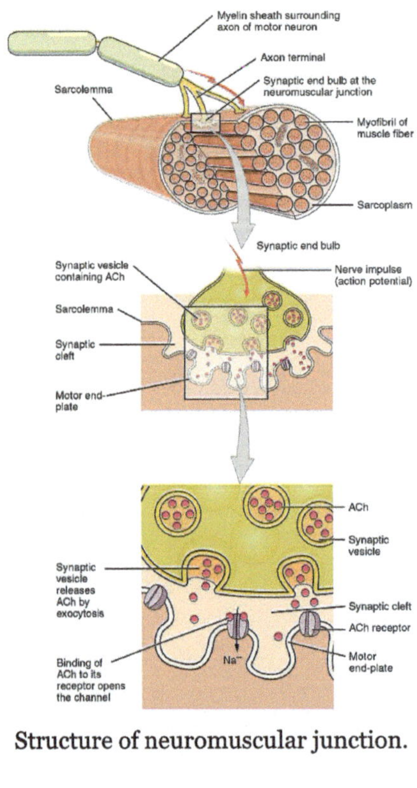

Structure of neuromuscular junction.

Excitation-contraction Coupling

Excitation–contraction coupling is the process by which a muscular action potential in the muscle fiber causes the myofibrils to contract. In skeletal muscle, excitation–contraction coupling relies on a direct coupling between key proteins, the sarcoplasmic reticulum (SR) calcium release channel (identified as the ryanodine receptor, RyR) and voltage-gated L-type calcium channels (identified as dihydropyridine receptors, DHPRs). DHPRs are located on the sarcolemma (which includes the surface sarcolemma and the transverse tubules), while the RyRs reside across the SR membrane. The close apposition of a transverse tubule and two SR regions containing RyRs is described as a triad and is predominantly where excitation–contraction coupling takes place. Excitation–contraction coupling occurs when depolarization of skeletal muscle cell results in a muscle action potential, which spreads across the cell surface and into the muscle fiber's network of T-tubules, thereby depolarizing the inner portion of the muscle fiber. Depolarization of the inner portions activates dihydropyridine receptors in the terminal cisternae, which are in close proximity to ryanodine receptors in the adjacent sarcoplasmic reticulum. The activated dihydropyridine receptors physically interact with ryanodine receptors to activate them via foot processes (involving conformational changes that allosterically activates the ryanodine receptors). As the ryanodine receptors open, Ca2+is released from the sarcoplasmic reticulum into the local junctional space, which then diffuses into the bulk cytoplasm to cause a calcium spark. Note that the sarcoplasmic reticulum has a large calcium buffering capacity partially due to a calcium-binding protein called calsequestrin. The near synchronous activation of thousands of calcium sparks by the action potential causes a cell-wide increase in calcium giving rise to the upstroke of the calcium transient. The Ca2+released into the cytosol binds to Troponin C by the actin filaments, to allow crossbridge cycling, producing force and, in some situations, motion. The sarco/endoplasmic reticulum calcium-ATPase (SERCA) actively pumps Ca2+back into the sarcoplasmic reticulum. As Ca2+declines back to resting levels, the force declines and relaxation occurs.

Sliding Filament Theory

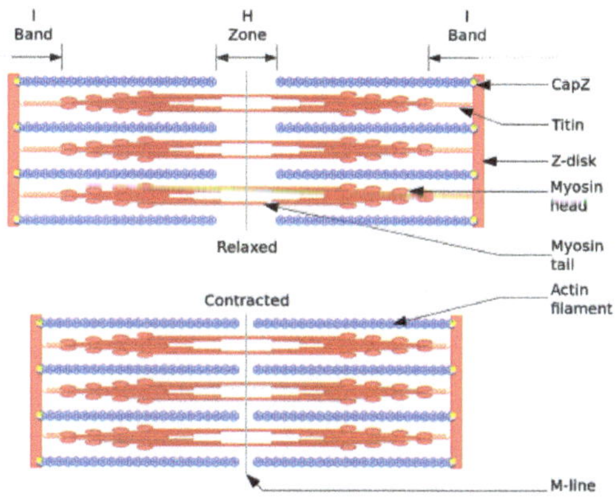

Sliding filament theory: A sarcomere in relaxed (above) and contracted (below) positions

The sliding filament theory describes a process used by muscles to contract. It is a cycle of repetitive events that cause a thin filament to slide over a thick filament and generate tension in the muscle. It was independently developed by Andrew Huxley and Rolf Niedergerke and by Hugh Huxley and Jean Hanson in 1954. Physiologically, this contraction is not uniform across the sarcomere; the central position of the thick filaments becomes unstable and can shift during contraction. However the actions of elastic proteins such as titin are hypothesised to maintain uniform tension across the sarcomere and pull the thick filament into a central position.

Crossbridge Cycling

Crossbridge cycling is a sequence of molecular events that underlies the sliding filament theory. A crossbridge is a myosin projection, consisting of two myosin heads, that extends from the thick filaments. Each myosin head has two binding sites: one for ATP and another for actin. The binding of ATP to a myosin head detaches myosin from actin, thereby allowing myosin to bind to another actin molecule. Once attached, the ATP is hydrolyzed by myosin, which uses the released energy to move into the "cocked position" whereby it binds weakly to a part of the actin binding site. The remainder of the actin binding site is blocked by tropomyosin. With the ATP hydrolyzed, the cocked myosin head now contains ADP + P_i. Two Ca2+ions binds to troponin C on the actin filaments. The troponin-Ca2+complex causes tropomyosin to slide over and unblock the remainder of the actin binding site. Unblocking the rest of the actin binding sites allows the two myosin heads to close and myosin to bind strongly to actin. The myosin head then releases the inorganic phosphate and initiates a *power stroke,* which generates a force of 2 pN. The power stroke moves the actin filament inwards, thereby shortening the sarcomere. Myosin then releases ADP but still remains tightly bounded to actin. At the end of the power stroke, ADP is released from the myosin head, leaving myosin attached to actin in a rigor state until another ATP binds to myosin. A lack of ATP would result in the rigor state characteristic of rigor mortis. Once another ATP binds to myosin, the myosin head will again detach from actin and another crossbridges cycle occurs.

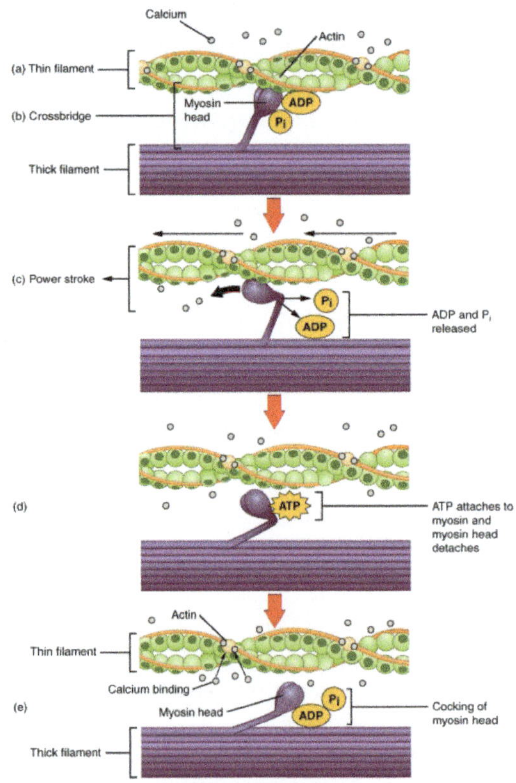

Crossbridge cycling

1in the cytoplasm. Termination of crossbridge cycling can occur when Ca2+is actively pumped back into the sarcoplasmic reticulum. When Ca2+is no longer present on the thin filament, the tropomyosin changes conformation back to its previous state so as to block the binding sites again. The myosin ceases binding to the thin filament, and the muscle relaxes. The Ca2+ions leave the troponin molecule in order to maintain the Ca2+ion concentration in the sarcoplasm. The active pumping of Ca2+ions into the sarcoplasmic reticulum creates a deficiency in the fluid around the myofibrils. This causes the removal of Ca2+ions from the troponin. Thus, the tropomyosin-troponin complex again covers the binding sites on the actin filaments and contraction ceases.

Gradation of Skeletal Muscle Contractions

Three Types of Skeletal Muscle Contractions

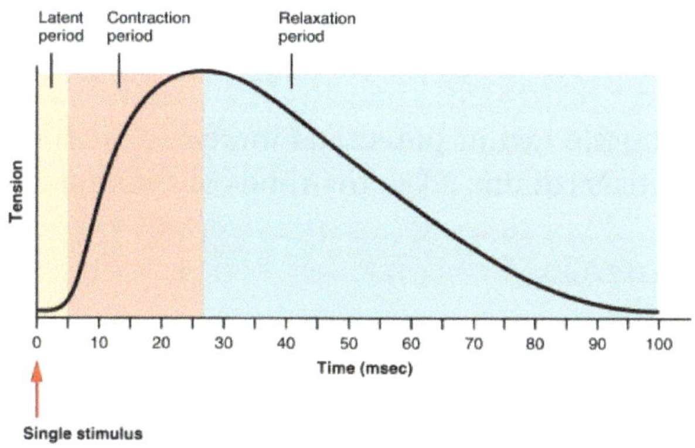

Twitch

The strength of skeletal muscle contractions can be broadly separated into twitch, summation, and tetanus. A twitch is a single contraction and relaxation cycle produced by an action potential within the muscle fiber itself. The time between a stimulus to the motor nerve and the subsequent contraction of the innervated muscle is called the latent period, which usually takes about 10 ms and is caused by the time taken for nerve action potential to propagate, the time for chemical transmission at the neuromuscular junction, then the subsequent steps in excitation-contraction coupling.

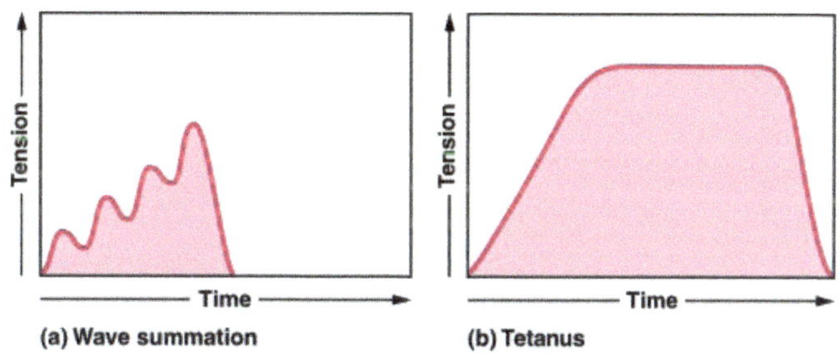

Summation and tetanus

If another muscle action potential were to be produced before the complete relaxation of a muscle twitch, then the next twitch will simply sum onto the previous twitch, thereby producing a *summation*. Summation can be achieved in two ways: *frequency summation* and *multiple fiber summation*. In frequency summation, the force exerted by the skeletal muscle is controlled by varying the frequency at which action potentials are sent to muscle fibers. Action potentials do not arrive at muscles synchronously, and, during a contraction, some fraction of the fibers in the muscle will be firing at any given time. In a typical circumstance, when a human is exerting a muscle as hard as he/she is consciously able, roughly one-third of the fibers in that muscle will be firing at once, though this ratio can be affected by various physiological and psychological factors (including Golgi tendon organs and Renshaw cells). This 'low' level of contraction is a protective mechanism to prevent avulsion of the tendon—the force generated by a 95% contraction of all fibers is sufficient to damage the body. In multiple fiber summation, if the central nervous system sends a weak signal to contract a muscle, the smaller motor units, being more excitable than the larger ones, are stimulated first. As the strength of the signal increases, more motor units are excited in addition to larger ones, with the largest motor units having as much as 50 times the contractile strength as the smaller ones. As more and larger motor units are activated, the force of muscle contraction becomes progressively stronger. A concept known as the size principle, allows for a gradation of muscle force during weak contraction to occur in small steps, which then become progressively larger when greater amounts of force are required.

Finally, if the frequency of muscle action potentials increases such that the muscle contraction reaches its peak force and plateaus at this level, then the contraction is a *tetanus*.

Length-tension Relationship

Length-tension relationship relates the strength of an isometric contraction to the length of the muscle at which the contraction occurs. Muscles operate with greatest active tension when close to an ideal length (often their resting length). When stretched or shortened beyond this (whether due to the action of the muscle itself or by an outside force), the maximum active tension generated decreases. This decrease is minimal for small deviations, but the tension drops off rapidly as the length deviates further from the ideal. Due to the presence of elastic proteins within a muscle cell (such as titin) and extracellular matrix, as the muscle is stretched beyond a given length, there is an entirely passive tension, which opposes lengthening. Combined together, there is a strong resistance to lengthening an active muscle far beyond the peak of active tension.

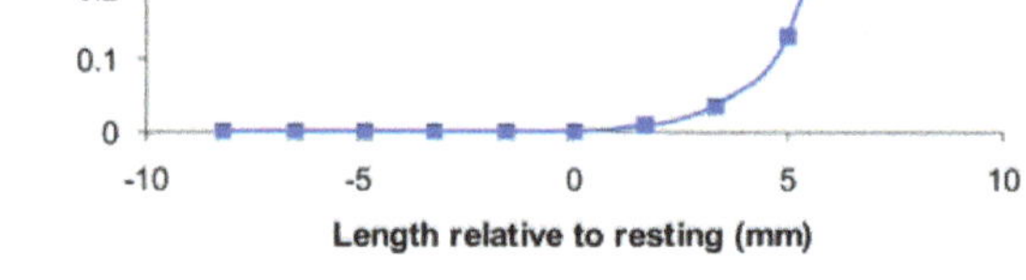

Muscle length versus isometric force

Force-velocity Relationships

Force–velocity relationship relates the speed at which a muscle changes its length (usually regulated by external forces, such as load or other muscles) to the amount of force that it generates. Force declines in a hyperbolic fashion relative to the isometric force as the shortening velocity increases, eventually reaching zero at some maximum velocity. The reverse holds true for when the muscle is stretched – force increases above isometric maximum, until finally reaching an absolute maximum. This has strong implications for the rate at which muscles can perform mechanical work (power). Since power is equal to force times velocity, the muscle generates no power at either isometric force (due to zero velocity) or maximal velocity (due to zero force). Instead, the optimal shortening velocity for power generation is approximately one-third of maximum shortening velocity.

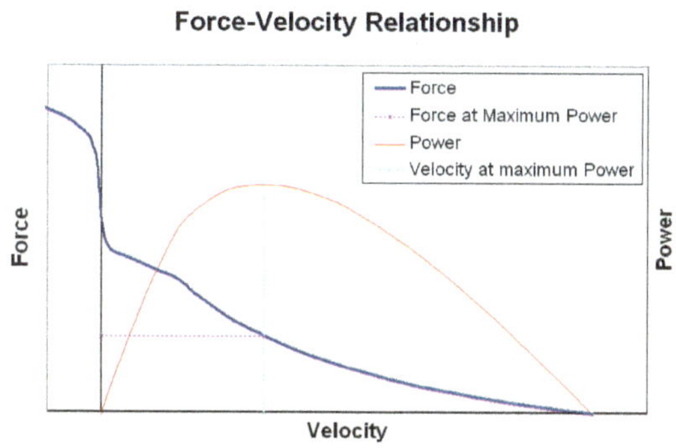

Force–velocity relationship: right of the vertical axis concentric contractions (the muscle is shortening), left of the axis eccentric contractions (the muscle is lengthened under load); power developed by the muscle in red.

These two fundamental properties of muscle have numerous biomechanical consequences, including limiting running speed, strength, and jumping distance and height.

Smooth Muscle

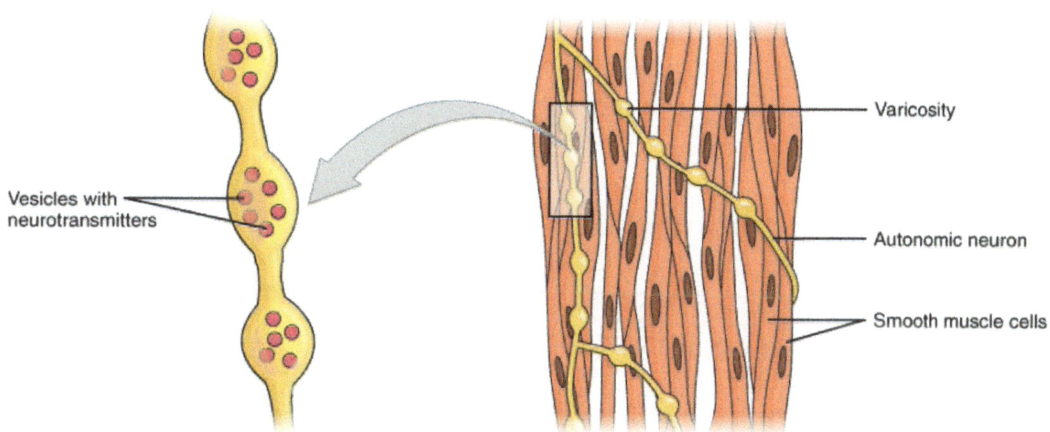

Swellings called varicosities belonging to an autonomic neuron innervate the smooth muscle cells.

Smooth muscles can be divided into two subgroups: single-unit (unitary) and multi-unit. Single-unit smooth muscle cells can be found in the gut and blood vessels. Because these cells are linked together by gap junctions, they are able to contract as a syncytium. Single-unit smooth muscle cells contract myogenically, which can be modulated by the autonomic nervous system.

Unlike single-unit smooth muscle cells, multi-unit smooth muscle cells are found in the muscle of the eye and in the base of hair follicles. Multi-unit smooth muscle cells contract by being separately stimulated by nerves of the autonomic nervous system. As such, they allow for fine control and gradual responses, much like motor unit recruitment in skeletal muscle.

Mechanisms of Smooth Muscle Contraction

The contractile activity of smooth muscle cells is influenced by multiple inputs such as spontaneous electrical activity, neural and hormonal inputs, local changes in chemical composition, and stretch. This is in contrast to the contractile activity of skeletal muscle cells, which relies on a single neural input. Some types of smooth muscle cells are able to generate their own action potentials spontaneously, which usually occur following a pacemaker potential or a slow wave potential. These action potentials are generated by the influx of extracellular Ca2+, and not Na+. Like skeletal muscles, cytosolic Ca2+ions are also required for crossbridge cycling in smooth muscle cells.

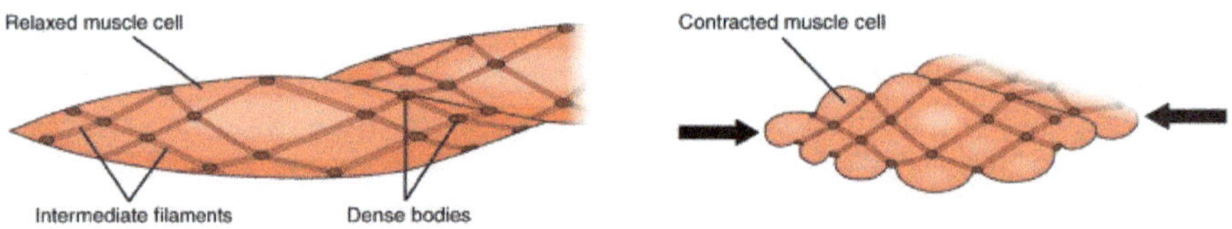

Smooth muscle contractions

The two sources for cytosolic Ca2+in smooth muscle cells are the extracellular Ca2+entering through calcium channels and the Ca2+ions that are released from the sarcoplasmic reticulum. The elevation of cytosolic Ca2+results in more Ca2+binding to calmodulin, which then binds and activates myosin light-chain kinase. The calcium-calmodulin-myosin light-chain kinase complex phosphorylates myosin on the 20 kilodalton (kDa) myosin light chains on amino acid residue-serine 19, initiating contraction and activating the myosin ATPase. Unlike skeletal muscle cells, smooth muscle cells lack troponin, even though they contain the thin filament protein tropomyosin and other notable proteins – caldesmon and calponin. Thus, smooth muscle contractions are initiated by the Ca2+-activated phosphorylation of myosin rather than Ca2+binding to the troponin complex that regulates myosin binding sites on actin like in skeletal and cardiac muscles.

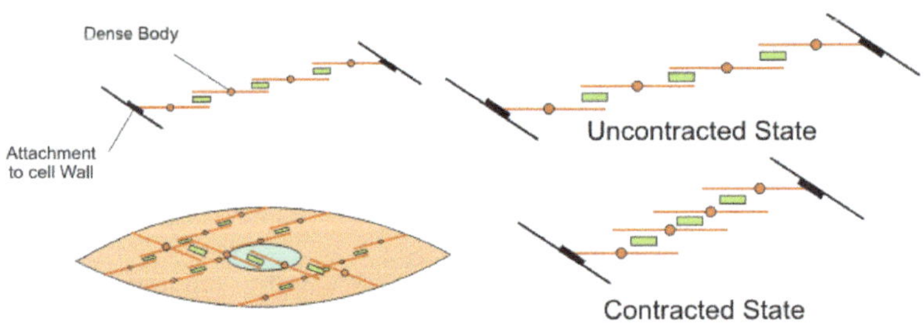

Actin-myosin filaments

Sliding filaments in contracted and uncontracted states

Termination of crossbridge cycling (and leaving the muscle in latch-state) occurs when myosin light chain phosphatase removes the phosphate groups from the myosin heads. Phosphorylation of the 20 kDa myosin light chains correlates well with the shortening velocity of smooth muscle. During this period, there is a rapid burst of energy utilization as measured by oxygen consumption. Within a few minutes of initiation, the calcium level markedly decreases, the 20 kDa myosin light chains' phosphorylation decreases, and energy utilization decreases; however, force in tonic smooth muscle is maintained. During contraction of muscle, rapidly cycling crossbridges form between activated actin and phosphorylated myosin, generating force.

It is hypothesized that the maintenance of force results from dephosphorylated "latch-bridges" that slowly cycle and maintain force. A number of kinases such as rho kinase, ZIP kinase, and protein kinase C are believed to participate in the sustained phase of contraction, and Ca2+ flux may be significant.

Neuromodulation

Although smooth muscle contractions are myogenic, the rate and strength of their contractions can be modulated by the autonomic nervous system. Postganglionic nerve fibers of parasympathetic nervous system release the neurotransmitter acetylcholine, which binds to muscarinic acetylcholine receptors (mAChRs) on smooth muscle cells. These receptors are metabotropic, or G-protein coupled receptors that initiate a second messenger cascade. Conversely, postganglionic nerve fibers of the sympathetic nervous system release the neurotransmitters epinephrine and norepinephrine, which bind to adrenergic receptors that are also metabotropic. The exact effects on the smooth muscle depend on the specific characteristics of the receptor activated—both parasympathetic input and sympathetic input can be either excitatory (contractile) or inhibitory (relaxing).

Cardiac Muscle

There are two types of cardiac muscle cells: autorhythmic and contractile. Autorhythmic muscle cells do not contract, but instead set the pace of contraction for other cardiac muscle cells, which can be modulated by the autonomic nervous system. In contrast, contractile muscle cells constitute the majority of the heart muscle and are able to contract.

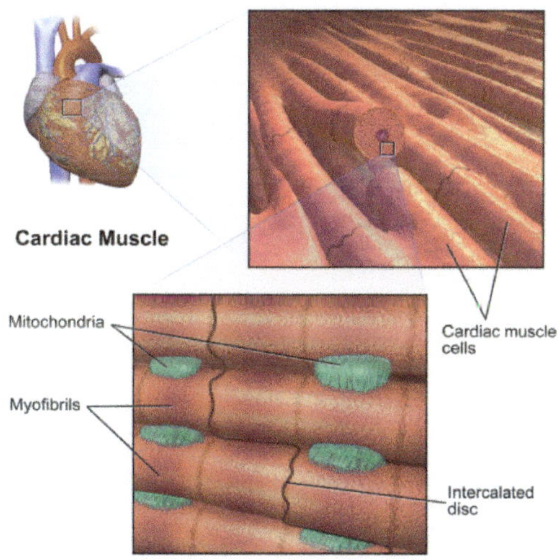

Cardiac muscle

Excitation-contraction Coupling

Unlike skeletal muscle, excitation–contraction coupling in cardiac muscle is thought to depend primarily on a mechanism called calcium-induced calcium release. Though the proteins involved are similar, the DHPR and RyR (type 2) are not physically coupled. Instead, RyRs are activated by a calcium trigger, which is brought about by the activation of DHPRs. Further, cardiac muscle tend to exhibit diad (or dyad) structures, rather than triads.

Excitation-contraction coupling in cardiac muscle cells occurs when an action potential is initiated by pacemaker cells in the Sinoatrial node or Atrioventricular node and conducted to all cells in the heart via gap junctions. The action potential travels along the surface membrane into T-tubules (the latter are not seen in all cardiac cell types) and the depolarisation causes extracellular Ca2+to enter the cell via L-type calcium channels and possibly sodium-calcium exchanger during the early part of the plateau phase. This Ca2+influx causes a small local increase in intracellular Ca2+. The increase in Ca2+is detected by ryanodine receptors in the membrane of the sarcoplasmic reticulum which releases Ca2+in a positive feedback physiological response. This positive feedback is known as calcium-induced calcium release and gives rise to calcium sparks (Ca2+sparks). The spatial and temporal summation of ~30,000 Ca2+sparks gives a cell-wide increase in cytoplasmic calcium concentration. The cytoplasmic calcium binds to Troponin C, moving the tropomyosin complex off the actin binding site allowing the myosin head to bind to the actin filament. From this point on, the contractile mechanism is essentially the same as for skeletal muscle (above). Briefly, using ATP hydrolysis, the myosin head pulls the actin filament toward the centre of the sarcomere. Intracellular calcium is taken up by the sarco/endoplasmic reticulum ATPase pump back into the sarcoplasmic reticulum ready for the next cycle to begin. Calcium is also ejected from the cell mainly by the sodium-calcium exchanger and, to a lesser extent, a plasma membrane calcium ATPase and/or taken up by the mitochondria. An enzyme, phospholamban, serves as a brake for the ATPase. At low heart rates, phospholamban is active and slows down the activity of the ATPase so that Ca2+does not have to leave the cell entirely. At high heart rates, phospholamban is phosphorylated and deactivated thus removing most Ca2+from the cell back into the sarcoplasmic reticulum. This allows the heart muscles to relax to allow for ventricular filling. Intracellular calcium concentration drops and troponin complex returns over the active site of the actin filament, ending contraction.

Invertebrate Animals

Circular and Longitudinal Muscles

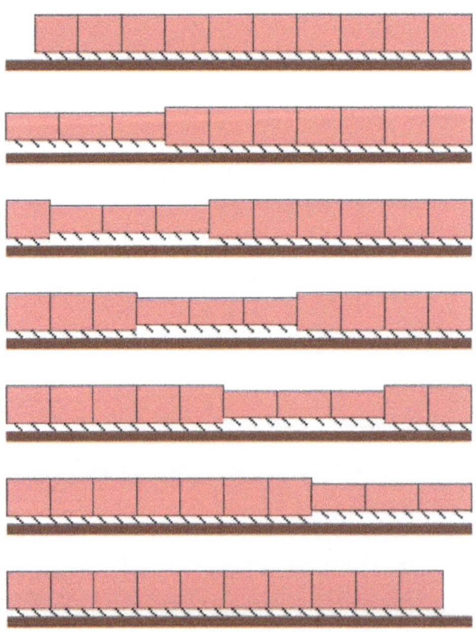

A simplified image showing earthworm movement via peristalsis

In annelids such as earthworms and leeches, circular and longitudinal muscles cells form the body wall of these animals and are responsible for their movement. In an earthworm that is moving through a soil, for example, contractions of circular and longitudinal muscles occur reciprocally while the coelomic fluid serves as a hydroskeleton by maintaining turgidity of the earthworm. When the circular muscles in the anterior segments contract, the anterior portion of animal's body begins to constrict radially, which pushes the incompressible coelomic fluid forward and increasing the length of the animal. As a result, the front end of the animal moves forward. As the front end of the earthworm becomes anchored and the circular muscles in the anterior segments become relaxed, a wave of longitudinal muscle contractions passes backwards, which pulls the rest of animal's trailing body forward. These alternating waves of circular and longitudinal contractions is called peristalsis, which underlies the creeping movement of earthworms.

Obliquely Striated Muscles

Invertebrates such as annelids, mollusks, and nematodes, possess obliquely striated muscles, which contain bands of thick and thin filaments that are arranged helically rather than transversely, like in vertebrate skeletal or cardiac muscles. In bivalves, the obliquely striated muscles can maintain tension over long periods without using too much energy. Bivalves use these muscles to keep their shells closed.

Fibrillar Muscles

Advanced insects such as wasps, flies, bees, and beetles possess fibrillar muscles that constitute the flight muscles in these animals. These flight muscles are called fibrillar muscles because they contain myofibrils that are thick and conspicuous. A remarkable feature of these muscles is that they do not require stimulation for each muscle contraction. Hence, they are sometimes called *asynchronous muscles* because the number of contractions in these muscles do not correspond (or synchronize) with the number of action potentials. For example, a wing muscle of a tethered fly may receive action potentials at a frequency of 3 Hz but it is able to beat at a frequency of 120 Hz. The high frequency beating is made possible because the muscles are connected to a resonant system, which is driven to a natural frequency of vibration.

History

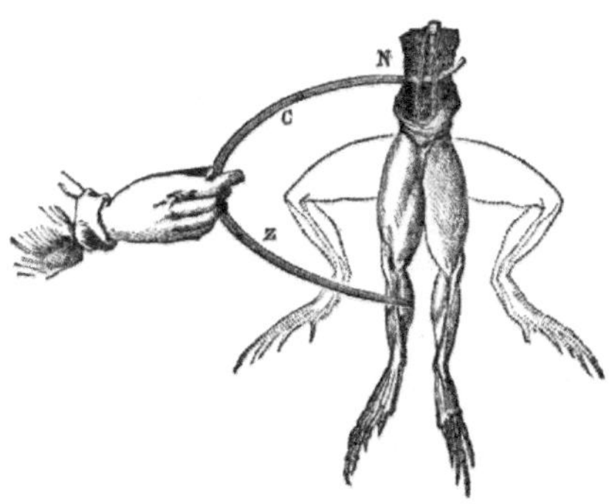

Electrodes touch a frog, and the legs twitch into the upward position

In 1780, Luigi Galvani discovered that the muscles of dead frogs' legs twitched when struck by an electrical spark. This was one of the first forays into the study of bioelectricity, a field that still studies the electrical patterns and signals in tissues such as nerves and muscles.

In 1952, the term excitation–contraction coupling was coined to describe the physiological process of converting an electrical stimulus to a mechanical response. This process is fundamental to muscle physiology, whereby the electrical stimulus is usually an action potential and the mechanical response is contraction. Excitation–contraction coupling can be dysregulated in many diseases.Though excitation–contraction coupling has been known for over half a century, it is still an active area of biomedical research. The general scheme is that an action potential arrives to depolarize the cell membrane. By mechanisms specific to the muscle type, this depolarization results in an increase in cytosolic calcium that is called a calcium transient. This increase in calcium activates calcium-sensitive contractile proteins that then use ATP to cause cell shortening.

The mechanism for muscle contraction evaded scientists for years and requires continued research and updating. The sliding filament theory was independently developed by Andrew F. Huxley and Rolf Niedergerke and by Hugh Huxley and Jean Hanson. Their findings were published as two consecutive papers published in the 22 May 1954 issue of *Nature* under the common theme "Structural Changes in Muscle During Contraction".

Myokine

A myokine is one of several hundred cytokines or other small proteins (~5–20 kDa) and proteoglycan peptides that are produced and released by muscle cells (myocytes) in response to muscular contractions. They have autocrine, paracrine and/or endocrine effects; their systemic effects occur at picomolar concentrations.

Receptors for myokines are found on muscle, fat, liver, pancreas, bone, heart, immune, and brain cells. The location of these receptors explain the fact that myokines have multiple functions. Foremost, they are involved in exercise-associated metabolic changes, as well as in the metabolic changes following training adaptation. They also participate in tissue regeneration and repair, maintenance of healthy bodily functioning, immunomodulation; and cell signaling, expression and differentiation.

History

The present definition of the term myokine is attributed to Dr. Bente Klarlund Pedersen et al., who suggested its use in 2003. In 2008, the first myokine, myostatin, was identified. The gp130 receptor cytokine IL-6 (Interleukin 6) was the first myokine found to be secreted into the blood stream in response to muscle contractions.

Repetitive Skeletal Muscle Contractions

There is an emerging understanding of skeletal muscle as a secretory organ, and of myokines as mediators of physical fitness through the practice of regular physical exercise (aerobic exercise and strength training), as well as new awareness of the anti-inflammatory and thus disease prevention aspects of exercise. Different muscle fiber types -slow twitch muscle fibers, oxidative muscle fibers, intermediate twitch muscle fibers, and fast twitch muscle fibers - release different clusters of myokines during contraction. This implies that variation of exercise types, particularly aerobic training/endurance training and muscle contraction against resistance (strength training) may offer differing myokine-induced benefits. This topic has been discussed by fitness training specialists.

"Some myokines exert their effects within the muscle itself. Thus, myostatin, LIF, IL-6 and IL-7 are involved in muscle hypertrophy and myogenesis, whereas BDNF and IL-6 are involved in AMPK-mediated fat oxidation. IL-6 also appears to have systemic effects on the liver, adipose tissue and the immune system, and mediates crosstalk between intestinal L cells and pancreatic islets. Other myokines include the osteogenic factors IGF-1 and FGF-2; FSTL-1, which improves the endothelial function of the vascular system; and the PGC-1alpha-dependent myokine irisin, which drives brown fat-like development. Studies in the past few years suggest the existence of yet unidentified factors, secreted from muscle cells, which may influence cancer cell growth and pancreas function. Many proteins produced by skeletal muscle are dependent upon contraction; therefore, physical inactivity probably leads to an altered myokine response, which could provide a potential mechanism for the association between sedentary behaviour and many chronic diseases."

"In summary, physical inactivity and muscle disuse lead to loss of muscle mass and accumulation of visceral adipose tissue and consequently to the activation of a network of inflammatory pathways, which promote development of insulin resistance, atherosclerosis, neurodegeneration and tumour growth and, thereby, promote the development of a cluster of chronic diseases. By contrast, the finding that muscles produce and release myokines provides a molecular basis for understanding how physical activity could protect against premature mortality.... Given that muscle is the largest organ in the body, the identification of the muscle secretome could set a new agenda for the scientific community. To view skeletal muscle as a secretory organ provides a conceptual basis for understanding how muscles communicate with other organs such as adipose tissue, liver, pancreas, bone and brain. Physical inactivity or muscle disuse potentially leads to an altered or impaired myokine response and/or resistance to the effects of myokines, which explains why lack of physical activity increases the risk of a whole network of diseases, including cardiovascular diseases, T2DM (Type 2 Diabetes Mellitus), cancer and osteoporosis."

Role in Regulating Heart Architecture

Heart muscle is subject to two kinds of stress: physiologic stress, i.e. exercise; and pathologic stress, i.e. disease related. Likewise, the heart has two potential responses to either stress: cardiac hypertrophy, which is a normal, physiologic, adaptive growth; or cardiac remodeling, which is an abnormal, pathologic, maladaptive growth. Upon being subjected to either stress, the heart "chooses" to turn on one of the responses and turn off the other. If it has chosen the abnormal path,i.e. remodeling, exercise can reverse this choice by turning off remodeling and turning on hypertrophy. The mechanism for reversing this choice is the microRNA miR-222 in cardiac muscle cells, which exercise up-regulates via unknown myokines. miR-222 represses genes involved in fibrosis and cell-cycle control.

Immunomodulation

Immunomodulation and immunoregulation were a particular focus of early myokine research, as, according to Dr. Bente Klarlund Pedersen and her colleagues, "the interactions between exercise and the immune system provided a unique opportunity to evaluate the role of underlying endocrine and cytokine mechanisms."

Specific Myokines

Myostatin

Both aerobic exercise and strength training (resistance exercise) attenuate myostatin expression, and myostatin inactivation potentiates the beneficial effects of endurance exercise on metabolism.

Interleukins

Aerobic exercise provokes a systemic cytokine response, including, for example, IL-6, IL-1 receptor antagonist (IL-1ra), and IL-10 (Interleukin 10). IL-6 was serendipitously discovered as a myokine because of the observation that it increased in an exponential fashion proportional to the length of exercise and the amount of muscle mass engaged in the exercise. This increase is followed by the appearance of IL-1ra and the anti-inflammatory cytokine IL-10. In general, the cytokine response to exercise and sepsis differs with regard to TNF-α. Thus, the cytokine response to exercise is not preceded by an increase in plasma-TNF-α. Following exercise, the basal plasma IL-6 concentration may increase up to 100-fold, but less dramatic increases are more frequent. The exercise-induced increase of plasma IL-6 occurs in an exponential manner and the peak IL-6 level is reached at the end of the exercise or shortly thereafter. It is the combination of mode, intensity, and duration of the exercise that determines the magnitude of the exercise-induced increase of plasma IL-6.

IL-6 had previously been classified as a proinflammatory cytokine. Therefore, it was first thought that the exercise-induced IL-6 response was related to muscle damage. However, it has become evident that eccentric exercise is not associated with a larger increase in plasma IL-6 than exercise involving concentric "nondamaging" muscle contractions. This finding clearly demonstrates that muscle damage is not required to provoke an increase in plasma IL-6 during exercise. As a matter of fact, eccentric exercise may result in a delayed peak and a much slower decrease of plasma IL-6 during recovery.

IL-6, among an increasing number of other recently identified myokines, thus remains an important topic of myokine research. It appears in muscle tissue and in the circulation during exercise at levels up to one hundred times basal rates, as noted, and is seen as having a beneficial impact on health and bodily functioning in most circumstances. P. Munoz-Canoves et al. write: "It appears consistently in the literature that IL-6, produced locally by different cell types, has a positive impact on the proliferative capacity of muscle stem cells. This physiological mechanism functions to provide enough muscle progenitors in situations that require a high number of these cells, such as during the processes of muscle regeneration and hypertrophic growth after an acute stimulus. IL-6 is also the founding member of the myokine family of muscle-produced cytokines. Indeed, muscle-produced IL-6 after repeated contractions also has important autocrine and paracrine benefits, acting as a myokine, in regulating energy metabolism, controlling, for example, metabolic functions and stimulating glucose production. It is important to note that these positive effects of IL-6 and other myokines are normally associated with its transient production and short-term action."

Interleukin 15

Interleukin-15 may play a significant role in the reduction of the volume of visceral (intra-abdominal) fat. IL-15 may accumulate within the muscle as a consequence of regular training. There is a negative association between plasma IL-15 concentration and trunk fat mass, but not limb fat mass.

Brain-derived Neurotrophic Factor

Brain-derived neurotrophic factor (BDNF) is also a myokine, though BDNF produced by contracting muscle is not released into circulation. Rather, BDNF produced in skeletal muscle appears to enhance the oxidation of fat. Skeletal muscle activation through exercise also contributes to an increase in BDNF secretion in the brain. A beneficial effect of BDNF on neuronal function has been noted in multiple studies. Dr. Pedersen writes, "Neurotrophins are a family of structurally related growth factors, including brain-derived neurotrophic factor (BDNF), which exert many of their effects on neurons primarily through Trk receptor tyrosine kinases. Of these, BDNF and its receptor TrkB are most widely and abundantly expressed in the brain. However, recent studies show that BDNF is also expressed in non-neurogenic tissues, including skeletal muscle. BDNF has been shown to regulate neuronal development and to modulate synaptic plasticity. BDNF plays a key role in regulating survival, growth and maintenance of neurons, and BDNF has a bearing on learning and memory. However, BDNF has also been identified as a key component of the hypothalamic pathway that controls body mass and energy homeostasis.

"Most recently, we have shown that BDNF appears to be a major player not only in central metabolic pathways but also as a regulator of metabolism in skeletal muscle. Hippocampal samples from Alzheimer's disease donors show decreased BDNF expression and individuals with Alzheimer's disease have low plasma levels of BDNF. Also, patients with major depression have lower levels of serum BDNF than normal control subjects. Other studies suggest that plasma BDNF is a biomarker of impaired memory and general cognitive function in ageing women and a low circulating BDNF level was recently shown to be an independent and robust biomarker of mortality risk in old women. Interestingly, low levels of circulating BDNF are also found in obese individuals and those with type 2 diabetes. In addition, we have demonstrated that there is a cerebral output of BDNF and that this is inhibited during hyperglycaemic clamp conditions in humans. This last finding may explain the concomitant finding of low circulating levels of BDNF in individuals with type 2 diabetes, and the association between low plasma BDNF and the severity of insulin resistance.

"BDNF appears to play a role in both neurobiology and metabolism. Studies have demonstrated that physical exercise may increase circulating BDNF levels in humans. To identify whether the brain is a source of BDNF during exercise, eight volunteers rowed for 4 h while simultaneous blood samples were obtained from the radial artery and the internal jugular vein. To further identify the putative cerebral region(s) responsible for BDNF release, mouse brains were dissected and analysed for BDNF mRNA expression following treadmill exercise. In humans, a BDNF release from the brain was observed at rest and increased 2- to 3-fold during exercise. Both at rest and during exercise, the brain contributed 70–80% of the circulating BDNF, while this contribution decreased following 1 h of recovery. In mice, exercise induced a 3- to 5-fold increase in BDNF mRNA expression in the hippocampus and cortex, peaking 2 h after the termination of exercise. These results suggest that the brain is a major but not the sole contributor to circulating BDNF. Moreover, the importance of the cortex and hippocampus as sources of plasma BDNF becomes even more prominent in the response to exercise."

With respect to studies of exercise and brain function, a 2010 report is of particular interest. Erickson et al. have shown that the volume of the anterior hippocampus increased by 2% in response to aerobic training in a randomized controlled trial with 120 older adults. The authors also summarize several previously-established research findings relating to exercise and brain function: (1) Aerobic exercise training increases grey and white matter volume in the prefrontal cortex of older adults and increases the functioning of key nodes in the executive control network. (2) Greater amounts of physical activity have been associated with sparing of prefrontal and temporal brain regions over a 9-y period, which reduces the risk for cognitive impairment. (3) Hippocampal and medial temporal lobe volumes are larger in higher-fit older adults (larger hippocampal volumes have been demonstrated to mediate improvements in spatial memory). (4) Exercise training increases cerebral blood volume and perfusion of the hippocampus.

Regarding the 2010 study, the authors conclude: "We also demonstrate that increased hippocampal volume is associated with greater serum levels of BDNF, a mediator of neurogenesis in the dentate gyrus. Hippocampal volume declined in the control group, but higher preintervention fitness partially attenuated the decline, suggesting that fitness protects against volume loss. Caudate nucleus and thalamus volumes were unaffected by the intervention. These theoretically important findings indicate that aerobic exercise training is effective at reversing hippocampal volume loss in late adulthood, which is accompanied by improved memory function."

Myonectin (CTRP15)

Seldin, Peterson, Byerly, Wei and Wong clarify that most myokines are also secreted by non-muscle cells. In 2012, they reported: "The expression of all myokines described to date is not restricted to skeletal muscle; they are generally expressed by a variety of cell types, and most are, in fact, expressed at much higher levels by nonmuscle tissues. Prior to (our) study, no myokine has been discovered to be preferentially expressed by skeletal muscle. While characterizing the metabolic function of the C1q/TNF-related protein (CTRP) family of proteins we recently uncovered, we identified myonectin (CTRP15) as a novel member of the family on the basis of sequence homology in the shared C1q domain, the signature that defines this protein family.... (Myonectin) is a novel nutrient-responsive myokine secreted by skeletal muscle to regulate whole-body fatty acid metabolism.... Circulating levels of myonectin were tightly regulated by the metabolic state; fasting suppressed, but refeeding dramatically increased, its mRNA and serum levels. Although mRNA and circulating levels of myonectin were reduced in a diet-induced obese state, voluntary exercise increased its expression and circulating levels. Accordingly, myonectin transcript was up-regulated by compounds (forskolin, epinephrine, ionomycin) that raise cellular cAMP or calcium levels.... In vitro results of myonectin expression in myotubes suggest that exercise-induced rises in intracellular calcium levels may also up-regulate myonectin expression in intact skeletal muscle.... Consistent with enhanced mRNA expression in skeletal muscle of mice subjected to voluntary exercise, circulating levels of myonectin also increased, suggesting a potential role of myonectin in exercise-induced physiology.

"Given that exercise induces myonectin expression in skeletal muscle, we next addressed whether short- and long-term changes in nutritional/metabolic state also regulate myonectin expression and circulating levels. Surprisingly, an overnight fast greatly suppressed myonectin expression, but a 2-h refeeding period (following an overnight fast) dramatically up-regulated its mRNA expression in skeletal muscle. Intriguingly, refeeding induced myonectin mRNA expression to a much greater extent in soleus than in plantaris muscle fiber of both male and female mice (data not shown), suggesting that myonectin expression may be regulated differentially depending on muscle fiber type. Consistent with the mRNA data, fasting reduced, but refeeding substantially increased, circulating levels of myonectin.... As compared with mice fed an isocaloric matched low-fat diet, mice fed a high-fat diet had lower myonectin mRNA and serum levels, suggesting that obesity-induced alteration in energy balance may be linked to dysregulation of myonectin-mediated processes in the obese state.... A relatively modest rise in serum myonectin levels was sufficient to lower (by >30%) nonesterified free fatty acid (NEFA) levels over time relative to vehicle-injected controls. However, no significant difference was observed in serum triacylglycerol levels between the two groups of mice. These data suggest a potential role of myonectin in regulating systemic fatty acid metabolism.... Treatment of adipocytes with recombinant myonectin (5 micrograms/ml) also enhanced fatty acid uptake to the same extent as insulin.... To determine whether myonectin-mediated enhancement of lipid uptake is specific to adipocytes, we also tested the effect of myonectin on lipid uptake in rat H4IIE hepatocytes. We observed a modest (>25%) but consistent increase in fatty acid uptake into hepatocytes stimulated with myonectin (5 micrograms/ml), an effect similar to cells treated with a saturating dose of insulin (50 nM).... Together, these results indicate that myonectin promotes lipid uptake into adipocytes and hepatocytes via transcriptional up-regulation of genes involved in fatty acid uptake....

"We provide the first characterization of myonectin, with in vitro and in vivo evidence that it is a novel myokine with important metabolic function. Unlike the other CTRPs characterized to date, myonectin (CTRP15) is expressed and secreted predominantly by skeletal muscle.... (Our) results suggest that myonectin is a nutrient-responsive metabolic regulator secreted by skeletal muscle in response to changes in cellular energy state resulting from glucose or fatty acid fluxes. Many metabolically relevant secreted proteins (e.g. adiponectin, leptin, resistin, and RBP) and the signaling pathways they regulate in tissues are known to be dysregulated in the condition of obesity. The reduction in expression and circulating levels of myonectin in the obese state may represent yet another component of the complex metabolic circuitry dysregulated by excess caloric intake. Although exercise has long been known to have profound positive impacts on systemic insulin sensitivity and energy balance, the underlying mechanisms remain incompletely understood. That voluntary exercise dramatically increases the expression and circulating levels of myonectin to promote fatty acid uptake into cells may underlie one of the beneficial effects of physical exercise.... A modest rise in the circulating levels of myonectin resulting from recombinant protein administration is sufficient to lower serum NEFA without altering serum triglyceride levels. Unlike CTRP1, CTRP3 and CTRP12, injection of recombinant myonectin into mice appears to have no glucose-lowering effect. Reduction in circulating NEFA is not due to suppression of adipose tissue lipolysis; rather, it results from increased fatty acid uptake by adipocytes and hepatocytes. Although the myonectin-mediated enhancement of lipid uptake in vitro appears modest (25–50%), in fact, the magnitude of this effect is comparable with cells stimulated with 50 nM insulin, a saturating dose that leads to maximum increase in fatty acid uptake.... In accordance with myonectin mediating its metabolic effect through a transcriptional mechanism, a reduction in circulating NEFA in mice occurred only 2 h after recombinant protein injection, a lag period presumably required for mRNA and protein synthesis."

Decorin

Decorin is an example of a proteoglycan which functions as a myokine. Kanzleiter et al have established that this myokine is secreted during muscular contraction against resistance, and plays a role in muscle growth. They reported on July 1, 2014: "The small leucine-rich proteoglycan decorin has been described as a myokine for some time. However, its regulation and impact on skeletal muscle (had) not been investigated in detail. In (our recent) study, we report decorin to be differentially expressed and released in response to muscle contraction using different approaches. Decorin is released from contracting human myotubes, and circulating decorin levels are increased in response to acute resistance exercise in humans. Moreover, decorin expression in skeletal muscle is increased in humans and mice after chronic training. Because decorin directly binds myostatin, a potent inhibitor of muscle growth, we investigated a potential function of decorin in the regulation of skeletal muscle growth. In vivo overexpression of decorin in murine skeletal muscle promoted expression of the pro-myogenic factor Mighty, which is negatively regulated by myostatin. We also found Myod1 and follistatin to be increased in response to decorin overexpression. Moreover, muscle-specific ubiquitin ligases atrogin1 and MuRF1, which are involved in atrophic pathways, were reduced by decorin overexpression. In summary, our findings suggest that decorin secreted from myotubes in response to exercise is involved in the regulation of muscle hypertrophy and hence could play a role in exercise-related restructuring processes of skeletal muscle."

Irisin

Irisin is a cleaved version of FNDC5. Boström and coworkers named the cleaved product irisin, after the Greek messenger goddess Iris. FNDC5 was initially discovered in 2002 by two independent groups of researchers.

Function of Irisin

Rana et al. reported in January 2014 that irisin (fibronectin type III domain-containing protein 5 or FNDC5), a recently described myokine hormone produced and secreted by acutely exercising skeletal muscles, is thought to bind white adipose tissue cells via undetermined receptors. Irisin has been reported to promote a brown adipose tissue-like phenotype upon white adipose tissue by increasing cellular mitochondrial density and expression of uncoupling protein-1, thereby increasing adipose tissue energy expenditure via thermogenesis. This is considered important, because excess visceral adipose tissue in particular distorts the whole body energy homeostasis, increases the risk of cardiovascular disease and raises exposure to a milieu of adipose tissue-secreted hormones (adipokines) that promote inflammation and cellular aging. The authors enquired whether the favorable impact of irisin on white adipose tissue might be associated with maintenance of telomere length, a well-established genetic marker in the aging process. They conclude that these data support the view that irisin may have a role in the modulation not only of energy balance but also the aging process.

However, exogenous irisin may aid in heightening energy expenditure, and thus in reducing obesity. Boström et al. reported on December 14, 2012: "Since the conservation of calories would likely provide an overall survival advantage for mammals, it appears paradoxical that exercise would stimulate the secretion of a polypeptide hormone that increases thermogenesis and energy expenditure. One explanation for the increased irisin expression with exercise in mouse and man may have evolved as a consequence of muscle contraction during shivering. Muscle secretion of a hormone that activates adipose thermogenesis during this process might provide a broader, more robust defense against hypothermia. The therapeutic potential of irisin is obvious. Exogenously administered irisin induces the browning of subcutaneous fat and thermogenesis, and it presumably could be prepared and delivered as an injectable polypeptide. Increased formation of brown or beige/brite fat has been shown to have anti-obesity, anti-diabetic effects in multiple murine models, and adult humans have significant deposits of UCP1-positive brown fat. (Our data show) that even relatively short treatments of obese mice with irisin improves glucose homeostasis and causes a small weight loss. Whether longer treatments with irisin and/or higher doses would cause more weight loss remains to be determined. The worldwide, explosive increase in obesity and diabetes strongly suggests exploring the clinical utility of irisin in these and related disorders. Another potentially important aspect of this work relates to other beneficial effects of exercise, especially in some diseases for which no effective treatments exist. The clinical data linking exercise with health benefits in many other diseases suggests that irisin could also have significant effects in these disorders."

While the murine findings reported by Boström et al. appear encouraging, other researchers have questioned whether irisin operates in a similar manner in humans. For example, Timmons et al. noted that over 1,000 genes are upregulated by exercise and examined how expression of FNDC5 was affected by exercise in ~200 humans. They found that it was upregulated only in highly active elderly humans, casting doubt on the conclusions of Boström et al.

Osteonectin or Secreted Protein Acidic and Rich in Cysteine (Sparc)

A novel myokine Osteonectin, or SPARC, plays a vital role in bone mineralization, cell-matrix interactions, and collagen binding. Osteonectin inhibits tumorigenesis in mice. Osteonectin can be classed as a myokine, as it was found that even a single bout of exercise increased its expression and secretion in skeletal muscle in both mice and humans.

References

- Schmidt-Nielsen, Knut (1997). Animal physiology: adaptation and environment (5th ed.). Cambridge: Cambridge Univ. Press. p. 104. ISBN 978-0-521-57098-5.
- Hall, Arthur C. Guyton, John E. (2005). Textbook of medical physiology (11th ed.). Philadelphia: W.B. Saunders. pp. 116–122. ISBN 978-0-7216-0240-0.
- Froelicher, Victor; Myers, Jonathan (2006). Exercise and the Heart (fifth ed.). Philadelphia: Elsevier. pp. ix, 108–12. ISBN 1-4160-0311-8.
- Widmaier, Eric P.; Raff, Hersel; Strang, Kevin T. (2010). "Muscle". Vander's Human Physiology: The Mechanisms of Body Function (12th ed.). New York, NY: McGraw-Hill. pp. 250–291. ISBN 0-321-98122-7.
- Silverthorn, Dee Unglaub (2016). "Muscles". Human Physiology: An Integrated Approach (7th ed.). San Francisco, CA: Pearson. pp. 377–416. ISBN 0-321-98122-7.
- Aidley, David J. (1998). "Mechanics and energetics of muscular contraction". The Physiology of Excitable Cells (4th ed.). New York, NY: Cambridge University Press. pp. 323–335. ISBN 0-521-57421-8.
- Sircar, Sabyasachi (2008). "Muscle elasticity". Principles of Medical Physiology (1st ed.). New York, NY: Thieme. p. 113. ISBN 1-588-90572-1.
- Kumar, Shrawan (2008). "Introduction and terminology". In Shrawan Kumar. Muscle strength (1st ed.). Boca

Raton, FL: CRC Press. p. 113. ISBN 0-415-36953-3.

- Biewener, Andrew A. (2003). "Muscles and skeletons: The building blocks of animal movement". Animal Locomotion. Oxford Animal Biology Series. New York, NY: Oxford University Press. pp. 15–45. ISBN 0-198-50022-X.
- Tassinary; Cacioppo (2000). "The Skeletomotor system: surface electromyography". In Cacioppo, John T.; Tassinary, Luois G.; Berntson, Gary G. Handbook of Psychophysiology (Second ed.). Cambridge: Cambridge University Press. ISBN 0-521-62634-X.
- Levitan, Irwin; Kaczmarek, Leonard (August 19, 2015). "Intercellular communication". The Neuron: Cell and Molecular Biology (4th ed.). New York, NY: Oxford Univerty Press. pp. 153–328. ISBN 0199773890.
- Hillis, David M.; Sadava, David E.; Price, Mary V. (2014). "Muscle and movement". Principles of Life (2nd ed.). Sunderland, MA: Sinauer Associates. pp. 681–698. ISBN 1-464-10947-8.
- Alexander, R. McNeill (2003). "Muscle, the motor". Principles of Animal Locomotion (2nd ed.). Princeton, NJ: Princeton University Press. pp. 15–37. ISBN 0-691-12634-8.

Permissions

All chapters in this book are published with permission under the Creative Commons Attribution Share Alike License or equivalent. Every chapter published in this book has been scrutinized by our experts. Their significance has been extensively debated. The topics covered herein carry significant information for a comprehensive understanding. They may even be implemented as practical applications or may be referred to as a beginning point for further studies.

We would like to thank the editorial team for lending their expertise to make the book truly unique. They have played a crucial role in the development of this book. Without their invaluable contributions this book wouldn't have been possible. They have made vital efforts to compile up to date information on the varied aspects of this subject to make this book a valuable addition to the collection of many professionals and students.

This book was conceptualized with the vision of imparting up-to-date and integrated information in this field. To ensure the same, a matchless editorial board was set up. Every individual on the board went through rigorous rounds of assessment to prove their worth. After which they invested a large part of their time researching and compiling the most relevant data for our readers.

The editorial board has been involved in producing this book since its inception. They have spent rigorous hours researching and exploring the diverse topics which have resulted in the successful publishing of this book. They have passed on their knowledge of decades through this book. To expedite this challenging task, the publisher supported the team at every step. A small team of assistant editors was also appointed to further simplify the editing procedure and attain best results for the readers.

Apart from the editorial board, the designing team has also invested a significant amount of their time in understanding the subject and creating the most relevant covers. They scrutinized every image to scout for the most suitable representation of the subject and create an appropriate cover for the book.

The publishing team has been an ardent support to the editorial, designing and production team. Their endless efforts to recruit the best for this project, has resulted in the accomplishment of this book. They are a veteran in the field of academics and their pool of knowledge is as vast as their experience in printing. Their expertise and guidance has proved useful at every step. Their uncompromising quality standards have made this book an exceptional effort. Their encouragement from time to time has been an inspiration for everyone.

The publisher and the editorial board hope that this book will prove to be a valuable piece of knowledge for students, practitioners and scholars across the globe.

Index